Is This
Your Child?

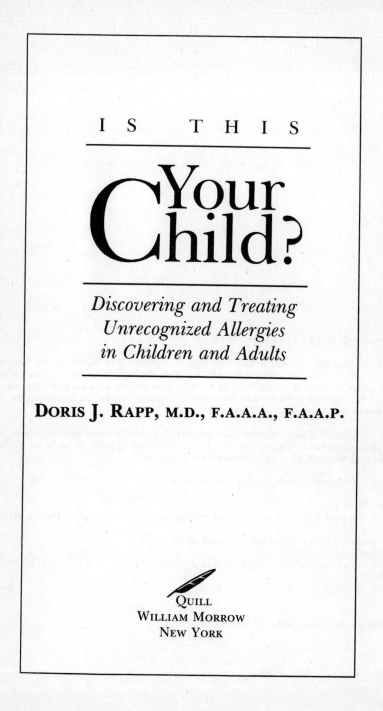

IS THIS

Your Child?

Discovering and Treating Unrecognized Allergies in Children and Adults

DORIS J. RAPP, M.D., F.A.A.A., F.A.A.P.

QUILL
WILLIAM MORROW
NEW YORK

It is the policy of William Morrow and Company, Inc., and its imprints and affiliates, recog-nizing the importance of preserving what has been written, to print the books we publish on acid-free paper, and we exert our best efforts to that end.

Library of Congress Cataloging-in-Publication Data

Rapp, Doris J.
    Is this your child? : discovering and treating unrecognized allergies / Doris J. Rapp.
      p. cm.
    Includes bibliographical references and index.
    ISBN 0-688-11907-7
    1. Allergy in children—Popular works. I. Title.
RJ386.R373   1992
618.92'97—dc20   92-8944
                                                       CIP

Printed in the United States of America

19 20

DEDICATED
TO
PHIL DONAHUE

With thanks and appreciation to Phil and his staff for the opportunity to share so much information, which changed the lives of so many children and their families.

BLESS YOU FOR HELPING SO MANY!

How Can You Use This
Book to Help Your Child?

It is my sincere hope that this book will not only enable you to determine whether your child has an unusual form of allergy but that it will help you to detect exactly what causes your child to feel unwell or to act inappropriately. In many instances you should be able to eliminate the cause and significantly help your child. However, if your child's problems are more complex, you may need to secure additional knowledgeable medical help.

Of course allergies are not a problem with every child. Only some children have physical illness and/or emotional, behavioral, and learning problems that are partly or mainly related to allergies or environmental exposures. Other children's problems are entirely unrelated to these factors and are totally due to other medical problems. For that reason after reading this book you must be certain to discuss *everything* you decide to do with your child's physician.

This book does not need to be read from cover to cover. Read only the chapters or areas that pertain to your child's or family's complaints.

Chapters 1 through 3 will help you recognize whether typical or unusual forms of allergy could be the cause of your child's illness or behavior, activity, or learning problems. If your child has allergic relatives or classical allergy, it is possible that his or her physical, personality, or educational problems might also be due to a less frequently recognized form of allergy. Your child's appearance, as well as the way she or he acts, writes, or draws, may provide important clues.

Chapters 4 through 7 discuss many of the different characteristic ways that allergy can affect children of various ages (infants, toddlers, children, and adolescents).

Once you believe that your child might have a typical or unusual form of allergy, you will probably want to find out how you can detect what could be causing the problem. Sometimes it can be amazingly simple to find the cause of an allergy. Some parents will determine that foods appear to be the major concern. The short, simple diet in chapter 8 might provide easy, rapid answers in four to seven days.

Chapters 9 and 10 give practical, at times subtle, pointers to help you find out if your child is having an allergic reaction and will help you detect the exact cause. These chapters also tell you what *you* can do to possibly help your child feel, behave, or learn better by keeping detailed health records, learning to take a pulse, and/or monitoring an asthmatic child's ability to breathe.

Chapter 11 explains how you can sometimes merely change something inside your home, such as a child's pillow, and thereby resolve a chronic medical illness.

If a child's problems are due to chemicals, outside pollen, or pollution, suggestions in chapters 12 through 13 might quickly provide beneficial answers.

If your child has a specific major health or personality problem, read the individual pertinent chapters from 14 to 23. If fatigue is your child's major problem, for example, you may want to read only chapter 20. Various chapters discuss other common, unrecognized forms of allergy or environmental illness—hyperactivity, depression, aggression, learning problems, delinquency, recurrent infection, intestinal symptoms, and so on. As you read the detailed histories, you'll realize that not only do these children have symptoms often dating back to infancy but they often have one medical complaint after another until the allergy problem is recognized.

Chapter 24 helps you learn to construct a diet that will enable many children to eat most of the foods to which they are sensitive.

Chapter 25 compares typical allergy testing and treatment with the newer methods.

Chapter 26 discusses the drugs commonly used to treat allergy.

Everyone should read chapter 27. This chapter tells how you might be able to strengthen your child's immune system. When that is stronger, allergies and chemical sensitivities may no longer be a problem.

Chapter 28 discusses the need for counseling. When children have not felt well or acted properly for years, both the child and the parents can, at times justifiably, develop secondary psychological and emotional difficulties.

Additional typical histories of children who had specific types of unrecognized environmental illness or allergies are discussed in Appendix E. You might be able to relate some of the detailed information discussed in this section to your child's specific problems. It helps to realize that other parents have been faced with similar challenges and to know what they did to help their children.

An extensive, detailed bibliography is provided for parents, educators, psychologists, counselors, physicians, and paramedical personnel who want to expand their knowledge and read more about certain aspects of environmental illness. This section should also provide scientific information for skeptics who doubt the efficacy of the newer treatment methods.

The index is purposely detailed so that you can quickly find information about the kinds of complaints that bother your child.

The Donahue *Show*

Some readers may wonder why this book is dedicated to a talk-show host. Throughout the book, in fact, I frequently discuss many of the patients who came to see us as a result of our *Donahue* shows in 1987 and 1988. It was truly an accident that I was asked to be on that initial program. Dr. George Shambaugh, a past professor of otolaryngology, was originally asked to be on the show because of his observations and publications indicating that ear problems, allergy, and hyperactivity occurred together in certain children. He suggested that I be invited instead because he had seen and been impressed by some of the films taken in our office that showed hyperactivity in children due to foods.

A vast number of mothers who subsequently came to our office said they were amazed to see the videotape of the hyperactive boy on that initial show. During that program many said that they realized for the first time that their child's behavior problem might be allergy-related.

In 1988 I was called, late on a Tuesday afternoon, to ask if I could find three mothers and their children to appear on an upcoming *Donahue* show. The families were all to be in New York City by the next day. You can imagine all the preparations that would be necessary for parents to be ready in less than twenty-four hours. I called five mothers, rather than three because I was certain some would not be able to get baby-sitters, clothing, beauty parlor appointments, and so forth on such brief notice. All the parents said they would come, and that videotapes of their children could be viewed nation-wide. Most of the parents on the 1988 show had previously seen the 1987 program, and the information on that original presentation had changed their children's lives. Now they were eager for the opportunity to share with other parents who didn't know where to turn for help. Most of the children discussed in this book were subsequently helped because of the knowledge parents gained from the 1988 show.

That *Donahue* program definitely hit a vital chord. The response from truly desperate parents was overwhelming. Phones rang throughout the country, and that show generated over 140,000 letters. Our staff cried on more than one occasion as we read the letters about the unbelievable anguish and grief in some families. Many mothers wrote us that tears of joy and relief streamed down their cheeks as they listened to Phil Donahue talk about the unusual types of allergy that could affect some youngsters. They recognized their child.

May the increased awareness you gain from this book give you not tears, but immense joy and genuine encouragement so that you can not only help your child and yourself but you can in turn help other family members, friends, and acquaintances.

It's all thanks to Phil Donahue!

Doris J. Rapp, M.D.

Acknowledgments

Special Gratitude

To the many parents who shared so many personal details about their children so that other parents and children might be healthier and happier.

To the nurses whose skillful testing enabled the children to *enjoy* coming to our office: Janet Telban, R.N.; Sandy Brzezinski, R.N.; Helen Goeltzenleuchter, L.P.N.

To the nurses who verified and clarified many details in the children's histories, thus ensuring the utmost accuracy: Barbara Rellinger, R.N.; Helen Goeltzenleuchter, L.P.N.

To the physicians and nurses who so kindly read and critiqued parts of the manuscript. Their suggestions were greatly appreciated: Kalapana Patel, M.D.; Ellen Gail Harkness, R.N., Ph.D., Lynn Miller, M.D.; Ben Park, M.D.; Joanne Brown, R.N.

To the patient, careful typists who repeatedly corrected and retyped the manuscript: Patricia Bruce, Norah Liszewski, Arlene Mazikowski.

To the editor, Pamela Altschul and copy editor Daia Gerson, whose suggestions and expertise together made this book more readable and practical.

To my office manager, Nancy Dlugokinski, who has always been there when we needed more help with this manuscript.

To Marlaine Selip, who cared so much she suggested that this book be written.

Without each and every one of you, this book would never have been possible.

My sincerest thanks and wholehearted gratitude. To all of you and to my family, Lou, Teddy, and Katie, who were alone too much and too often so there was time to write this book.

Contents

Tables and Charts

AUTHOR'S NOTE

My Change From a Traditional to an Expanded Concept of Allergy

When I initially began to study allergy in 1958, I was frequently perplexed by some young patients who appeared to have symptoms of classical hay fever or asthma but they had had little or no response to traditional allergy skin tests, nor did their blood reveal evidence of allergy. Yet these children looked and acted allergic and they had allergic relatives. We treated these patients with the typical drugs used to relieve allergies but assured the parents that their children did *not* have an allergy.

Thirty-five years later I wonder how often we missed the diagnosis. Were we unable to detect the cause of certain elusive forms of allergy at that time because of our limited knowledge, myopic viewpoint, and restricted methods of diagnosis? Newer, more precise methods of detecting allergy, for example *provocation/neutralization testing*, might readily have revealed the cause of some of these children's problems.

There are many facets to the problem of allergy. I recognized mostly the typical allergies, such as asthma, hay fever, and eczema, for the first eighteen years of my practice. Then I attended a conference on food allergies in 1975 in an attempt to learn about better ways of detecting food sensitivities. There, I learned that almost any area of the body could be affected by almost any item known to cause allergies, including foods. I also learned about the role of chemicals and pollution in environmental illness.

During the last fifteen years, while practicing allergy and environmental medicine, I found out how much I was *not* taught during my training as a pediatrician and as a children's allergist. Most well-trained board-certified allergists for children have *never been directly exposed* to these newer methods of diagnosis and treatment. If I had not been so fortunate in 1975, I, too, would surely have found much that is written in this book totally unbelievable. This expanded view of allergy is analogous to allowing a mouse into a cheese factory. Never has a physician had such an opportunity to pinpoint the specific causes of so many illnesses.

There is one general theme that is dominant throughout this book: Most patients clearly illustrate that *regardless of how old they were when they initially sought medical care, they usually had obvious clues strongly suggesting allergy beginning in infancy.* Some even showed evidence of hyperactivity when they were in the uterus. The challenge is to help parents, physicians, and educators become more aware of these problems *at the earliest possible stage* of each child's life. If we can do this, an immense amount of needless heartache, illness, and hardship will not have to be endured by so many children and their parents. Hopefully the increased awareness that this book provides will help some youngsters feel truly well for the first time in their lives.

Unfortunately when I was trained in pediatric allergy and immunology in the late 1950s, I was also told that the types of environmentally induced brain and body allergy described so well by physicians during the period of the twenties to the fifties did not exist. It is, however, clearly evident that many children and adults suffer enormously, and at times unnecessarily. In time, it is hoped, much that is detailed in this book will be accepted by the academic allergists who dictate policy. Until then it is anticipated that the information in this book will enable you to:

- recognize whether your children or family members have this problem by the way they look or behave;
- increase your awareness so that you can possibly detect the most probable causes of some of your children's physical or emotional illnesses or learning difficulties;
- decide which forms of therapy you personally believe would be most helpful.

Glossary

Acidophilus—A type of lactobacillus, which is a beneficial microorganism usually found in the intestines.

Addiction—A craving for a drug, food, odor, etc.

ADD (Attention Deficit Disorder)—A term applied to children who are easily distracted, impulsive, and unable to concentrate. If it is associated with hyperactivity, it is called attention deficit hyperactivity disorder (ADHD).

Adhere—To stick to something, in contrast to the word *absorb*, which refers to soaking up or being soaked up into something.

ATFS (Allergic Tension Fatigue Syndrome)—A medical problem that can cause tension, irritability, hyperactivity, and/or fatigue, depression, and apathy.

Alka-Aid—An alkaline tablet, that contains sodium bicarbonate (baking soda) and potassium bicarbonate. It is sold in health food stores. It frequently relieves allergic reactions, particularly those caused by foods.

Alkali—A basic substance, such as baking soda, that has a high pH, in contrast to something that is acidic, which is a substance with a low pH, such as vinegar.

Alka-Seltzer Antacid Formula—An alkali that is a combination of sodium bicarbonate (baking soda), potassium bicarbonate, and a citric acid flavoring. It is sold in drugstores and does *not* contain aspirin.

Allergen—Something that causes an allergic reaction. Common allergens are dust, molds, pollen, pets, and foods.

Amino Acid—Very simply speaking, it is a combination of an alkali or an amino group, such as ammonia, with an acid group, such as acetic acid or vinegar. Some amino acids stimulate the mind and help control depression or sleep patterns. When the amino portions of amino acids are removed, the basic amine that remains becomes a messenger in the nervous system.

Antibody—This substance combines with an antigen like a lock and key. When this happens, chemical mediators, such as histamine, are released that cause allergic reactions.

Antigen—The same as *allergen*.

Aphasia—Impairment in the ability to pronounce words or name common objects.

Apraxia—The inability to perform coordinated movements.

Aspartame—A form of synthetic sugar found in NutraSweet.

Baseline—How a child acts, behaves, and feels **before** allergy skin testing.

Behavior Modification—A method taught by psychologists and counselors to help parents and their children cope more effectively with inappropriate behavior.

Candida—The same as *yeast* or *monilia*. It is a normal organism found on the skin and in certain areas of the body (intestines, vagina, etc.).

Carcinogen—A substance that causes cancer.

Chemical Mediators—Substances that are released when an allergenic substance, for example dust or food, reacts with its corresponding antibody. These mediators—histamine is one example—circulate throughout the body and cause allergic illness, such as hay fever, asthma, and so on.

Conner's Hyperactivity Score—A measure of a child's level of hyperactivity. The score can range from 0 to 30. A score of 0 to 15 is normal. A score above 18 indicates hyperactivity, and the closer the score is to 30, the more hyperactive a child is. This score does not measure changes in behavior.

Cubic centimeter—A cc. or cubic centimeter = a ml. or milliliter. 5 cc or 5 ml = approximately one teaspoon.

Culture—A gelatinlike substance on which molds and bacteria are grown so that they can be identified.

Dermatologists—Physicians who are experts in diagnosing and treating skin problems.

Diuretic—A substance that makes you urinate more than normal so that your body fluids decrease.

Digestive Enzymes—Substances to help digest or break down foods so that they are absorbed more easily from the stomach and intestines into the blood. If foods are well digested, they are less apt to cause allergy.

Double-Blind Study—A way of helping to eliminate bias from a scientific study. Neither the doctor nor the patient (double) knows if the patient was given or exposed to the test item or something that looks, smells, and tastes like the test item. The latter is called a placebo and should have no effect on the patient. The object is to see whether the patient can tell the difference between the real test item, which may cause some symptom, and the mock test item, or placebo, which should not.

Dr. Jekyll/Mr. Hyde—A dramatic change in personality that can occur in some individuals. A child who drinks red sweet beverages, for example, often changes from being a nice, pleasant Dr. Jekyll-type youngster to an impossible or uncontrollable Mr. Hyde. The actions or behavior of a Mr. Hyde type are unacceptable and inappropriate.

Ecologists—Physicians who are particularly interested in environmental medicine. They have special expertise concerning how allergenic items or the chemicals or pollution in our air, water, food, clothing, and homes can affect our physical health and emotional well-being.

Electroencephalogram (EEG)—A type of brain-wave analysis that shows certain characteristic patterns if an individual has seizures or some abnormality in the brain. More precise interpretation of brain function can be obtained from a computerized-line form of EEG called neurometrics.

End-Point Titration—This is also called Intradermal Serial Dilution Titration or the Rinkle Method, another newer, more helpful variation of allergy testing. It uses five-fold dilutions of allergy skin-extract tests to identify substances to which someone is sensitive and to determine the dilution of antigen with which to begin treatment.

Endorphin—A natural painkiller or tranquilizing hormone produced in the brain. It provides a sense of well-being.

Eosinophil—A type of white blood cell that often indicates an allergy when the level is increased in the blood or mucous secretions of the body.

Esophagus—The food tube, which extends from the back of the mouth to the stomach.

Ethynol—A hydrocarbon derived from decayed wood such as coal or oil.

Expiration—The action of breathing the air out of the lungs.

Gastroenterologist—A specialist in stomach, intestinal, or bowel diseases.

Grimace—A twitch, jerk, or tic located on various parts of the face.

Groin Area—The area near the crease of the skin at the junction of the thigh and lower abdomen.

GTT (Glucose Tolerance Test)—A test to detect hypoglycemia. The patient drinks a solution of flavored glucose or sugar. The blood is then examined every thirty to sixty minutes for three to five hours to determine if the blood sugar level follows a normal pattern or falls into a hypoglycemic range (below 60 mg%).

Histamine—One chemical mediator that is released when an antigen, such as a food, pollen, dust, or mold, combines with the corresponding antibody.

Hydrocarbons—Numerous organic compounds that contain only hydrogen and carbon, for example benzene and methane.

Hypoglycemia—A blood sugar below 60 mg%. This can cause hunger, irritability, temper tantrums, fatigue, unclear thinking, and aggression.

IgE (Immunoglobulin E)—One type of antibody. If it is elevated, it suggests that a person is allergic.

Immune System—The part of the body that defends or protects us.

Intradermal Allergy Skin Test—An allergy test in which a solution is injected into the outermost layers of the skin.

Lactobacillus—A type of "good" intestinal bacteria that aids digestion.

Lactose Intolerance—An inability to digest or break down lactose or milk sugar because of a lack of the digestive enzyme called lactase.

Larynx—The voice box located near the Adam's apple of the throat.

Leach—To lose or release soluble matter into a liquid. For example, the chemicals in the plastic of a container can leach into the liquid held inside and alter the taste and contents of that liquid.

Metabolism—A complex series of physical and chemical processes that break foods down into forms or particles that can be utilized in the body. Protein substances, for example, are broken down into simpler peptides and amino acids, which eventually release energy needed by the body.

Mite—A pinpoint-sized colorless organism that lives in stuffed furniture, carpets, and mattresses. It is the major component in house dust that causes allergy.

Monilia—A type of yeast that is also called candida.

Organic—Anything derived from something alive, such as plants and animals, in contrast to *inorganic,* such as stone.

Peak Flow Meter (PFM)—An inexpensive plastic tube with a gauge that measures how well an asthmatic child can breathe out. If used properly, it helps parents pinpoint the cause of their child's asthma.

Placebo—A substance that looks, tastes, smells, and appears identical to a test item. For example, if you want to determine if a certain white pill stops pain, you would give someone in pain two sets of identical-appearing and tasting white pills to be taken on separate occasions. The one set might be a placebo, such as sugar pills, the other a form of aspirin, for example. The object is to see which of the two pills makes a difference, if any, in the patient's symptoms. Placebo tablets help eliminate preconceived bias.

Plethora—An excess of something.

PMS (Premenstrual Syndrome)—Symptoms of fatigue, irritability, depression, or anxiety, sometimes noted a day or two before some women develop their menses.

Practical Rotary Diet—A diet that consists of four lists of foods. Each day's diet is selected in a repeating four-day pattern from one of four different lists. This diet enables people to identify specific food allergies quickly because symptoms repeatedly occur in a patterned sequence. For example, if milk is always ingested on Day 2 of the four-day pattern, and if milk causes asthma and hyperactivity, then the child will wheeze or become hyperactive, but only on Days 2, 6, 10, and so forth, when some form of dairy is eaten.

Prick Allergy Test—A way of conducting an allergy skin test. The skin is pricked with a needle through a drop of allergy extract, which has been placed on the skin. If the test site becomes sufficiently red or swollen, it indicates a probable allergy to the test item.

Prophylactic—A preventative.

Provocation/Neutralization (P/N)—A newer, more precise way of doing allergy testing, that consists of two steps. *Provocation* refers to a skin test that provokes a change in the skin-test site and/or causes symptoms after a drop of an allergy extract is placed under the tongue or into the outer layers of the skin. This dilution helps confirm that a patient is allergic to a test item. *Neutralization* refers to a weaker dilution of the same allergy extract that eliminates, or neutralizes, the reaction caused by the provocation. This dilution can be used to prevent or relieve allergy symptoms, so drugs may not be needed.

RAST (Radioallergosorbent Test)—A blood test. If this test is positive, it indicates that a person is allergic to the particular substance tested, such as a specific food, mold, dust, or pollen.

Rotation Diet—*see* Practical Rotary Diet.

Scratch Allergy Test—A type of allergy testing that is performed by putting a drop of an allergy extract in a premade indentation in the skin. The site is scratched with a toothpick, and if it becomes sufficiently red and swollen, an allergy is indicated.

Single-Blind Study—A scientific study in which the doctor, for example, but not the patient, is aware of what is being given or done to a patient. It is a method aimed at helping to eliminate preconceived opinions or bias, but only on the part of the patient.

Subcutaneous Treatment—A form of allergy treatment in which an allergy extract is injected into the upper arm or leg. The injection is given beneath (*sub*) the surface of the skin (*cutaneous*).

Sublingual—Allergy testing or treatment that is administered by dropping the allergy extract under (*sub*) the tongue (*lingual*) instead of by means of injections.

Terpines—Crude botanical extracts prepared from the growing parts of plants. Terpines are responsible for the odor and taste of plants, which in turn determine whether insects will be attracted or repelled by them.

Traditional Allergy Testing—The type of allergy testing used by most allergists. A tiny droplet of allergy extract is carefully inserted into the outer layers of the skin. The skin-test area is examined ten minutes later. If there is significant localized redness or swelling, the test indicates a probable allergy. If the skin-test site remains essentially the same, this suggests there is no allergy.

Volatile—Something that forms a gas.

Yeast—An egg-shaped organism, also called monilia or candida, that normally grows on and in certain parts of our bodies, as well as on plants and in foods.

Yeast Connection Syndrome or Yeast-Related Complex—A yeast imbalance that appears to be associated with a certain characteristic pattern of medical illness.

Xenobiotics—Any type of foreign chemical.

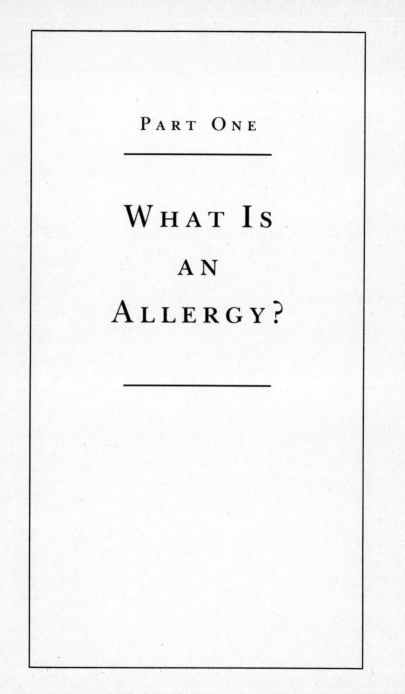

PART ONE

WHAT IS AN ALLERGY?

CHAPTER 1

How Many People
Have Allergies?

In 1950, it was thought, about 14 percent of the U.S. population had allergies. The 1985 estimates say that this number may have risen to about 33 percent, or 75 million Americans. All of these figures may be low estimates. For example, physicians interested in environmental medicine estimate that the number of children and adults who have food allergies or sensitivities exceeds 75 percent. They detect and confirm food allergies using short, informative diets and newer variations of traditional allergy skin testing.

If one parent has allergies, one out of every four of his or her offspring will have some form of this problem. If both parents have typical allergies, about 60 percent, or two out of three, of their children will tend to develop allergies. It is most unusual, however, to have more than one exquisitely sensitive child in the same family.

Does Your Child Have Allergies?

Many parents already know that someone in their family is unwell because of hay fever, asthma, hives, or eczema. These are the typical, major accepted forms of allergy.

There are other areas of the body that can be affected by allergies, however. Unfortunately these are not always recognized, suspected, or even agreed upon. Parents may be told repeatedly by their physicians that their children's complaints could not possibly be an allergy. Yet the parents' observations are often entirely valid.

Many adults are totally unaware that some of their children's or their own medical or emotional complaints could be solely due to an allergy. They often attribute chronic congestion, stuffiness, or throat clearing to a chronic sinus problem, but they don't go one step farther to ask *why* the sinuses are always infected. They attribute their persistent cough to a postnasal drip but never ask *why* they always have a postnasal drip. Sudden irritability and mood changes, as well as fatigue, are sometimes erroneously attributed solely to the stresses of daily family life or to challenging situations at school or work, when they are in reality unusual manifestations of allergy.

Adopted Children

An inordinate number of allergic children appear to have been adopted. This seems to be particularly true for environmentally ill children. Maybe this is related to the prenatal attitude and health care of the mother. Maybe sometimes the infant cried so much because of an undetected milk allergy that the mother was overwhelmed and placed the infant for adoption. We simply don't know.

What Is an Allergy?

Surprisingly there is much confusion at the present time about the definition because the word *allergy* does not represent the same thing to all physicians. There are two distinctly divergent differences of opinion.

The original definition referred simply to any adverse reaction to a substance that does not bother most other individuals. The majority of people, for example, do not develop illness after they are exposed to dust, molds, pets, freshly cut grass, or after eating certain foods. In contrast allergic individuals commonly develop hay fever, asthma, hives, eczema, or intestinal symptoms from these types of exposures. The tentative diagnosis of allergy was originally based mainly upon the patient's history and physical examination, which suggested allergy. For example, if someone's nose repeatedly and suddenly became watery and itchy while cutting the grass, it was diagnosed as hay fever due to grass pollen.

In 1925, however, allergy was redefined, and the scope of what could be called an allergy became strictly limited. The majority of traditional allergists currently accept three basic concepts in relation to what is or is not an allergy:

- An allergy must affect only specified areas of the body.
- The source of an allergy must be due to established and acceptable causes.
- An allergy must be scientifically confirmed by certain accepted immunological tests.

This restricted definition may have to be updated and liberalized, however. There simply are too many children and adults who do not fit into the current restricted traditional definition of allergy. When too many individuals are the exception, the rules may need to be changed.

Let us examine each concept in a bit of detail.

Areas of the Body That Can Be Affected by Allergy

Many traditional allergy specialists believe that allergies can only affect limited and specific parts of the body. The nose, eyes, lungs, skin, and intestines are accepted areas. They strongly doubt, however, that a slice of bread, for example, could cause a toddler suddenly to be unable to walk or that a peanut butter sandwich could cause a child to fall asleep in school. They would not believe that the brain functions of children could be influenced by a food or other environmental factors, for example dust or mold, in such a way that the children would develop hyperactivity or behavior or learning problems. Articles published over forty years ago, however, as well as recent publications, indicate that a wide variety of medical complaints, including overactivity, fatigue, bed-wetting, inappropriate behavior, and even epilepsy, in *some* children, may be due to allergies.[1] Specialists in environmental medicine believe it is possible that *any* area of the body can be affected by an allergy or a food or chemical sensitivity. Substances called chemical mediators are released during allergic reactions and travel all over the body, not just to "accepted" areas such as the lungs or nose.

Substances or Exposures That Can Cause Allergy

Traditional allergists believe that only certain specific substances or exposures can cause an allergy. They recognize that dust (mites),

1. See Bibliography.

molds, pollen, pets, feathers, and a few foods cause hay fever or asthma, but they would strongly doubt that these same items could cause behavior, personality, activity, or learning problems. Most allergists would scoff at the idea that the latter problems or a wide range of typical medical illnesses could be caused by a wide range of foods or by chemical odors. There is no doubt, however, that *some* children's unacceptable behavior or inability to learn can be eliminated by certain diets or avoidance of specific chemical exposures. These symptoms can be repeatedly reproduced after certain suspected foods are eaten or during newer methods of allergy testing. Classical toxic reactions to chemicals are accepted, but a claim that either hay fever or a behavior problem could be caused by a smell of a chemical or an allergy skin test with a weak nontoxic solution of allergy extract made from an offending chemical would be doubted. Specialists in environmental medicine, however, believe that almost *any* exposure or food can cause an allergy or sensitivity response in some individuals.

Immunological Tests to Confirm an Allergy

Current immunological tests provide many valid answers, but *not for all allergic patients*. Some people do not manifest the typical immunologic abnormalities required by traditional allergists to diagnose an allergy. In spite of apparent cause-and-effect relationships, some individuals show no evidence of typical allergy in their blood or by *routine* allergy skin testing. These same patients, however, not only show evidence of typical or unusual forms of allergy using newer, more precise methods of allergy testing but they often respond favorably to allergy extract therapy. The bottom line is the patient's response to treatment, not the immunological evidence of allergy in the blood.

Which Allergy Skin Tests Help Confirm an Allergy?

The most common tests to help confirm or diagnose a traditional allergy are allergy skin tests by either the scratch or intradermal method. Most traditional allergists agree that although scratch (or prick) tests are not entirely reliable, they do provide clues *if* a child is very allergic to a test item. Many, but certainly not all, allergists believe that intradermal allergy skin tests using stronger concentrations of allergy extract are helpful in detecting some weaker but definite allergies routinely missed by scratch allergy tests. Many allergists either scratch or inject a number of allergenic items, all at one time, on or into the skin. They look at the skin-test areas after ten minutes, and if these test areas have not become red or swollen, they assume the child is not allergic to those items.

Some different variations of traditional allergy testing and treatment have been used since the 1940s. One method is referred to as Intradermal Serial Dilution Titration, End-Point Titration, or the Rinkel Technique and is used by over two thousand ear, nose, and throat specialists. Another is called provocation/neutralization treatment, or the Miller method. Both appear to pinpoint quickly specific substances to which a person is sensitive and the recommended allergy extract treatment seems able to relieve symptoms in some to many patients in a relatively short period of time. This book will only discuss patients treated by the P/N method.

This method is presently being used by a growing number of physicians both in America and abroad. Although enormously time-consuming, P/N appears to be both more informative and more precise. P/N testing is basically performed in the same manner and with exactly the same allergy extract solutions as the ones used by the traditional allergists. One key difference, however, is that each item is tested separately so a physician can often see whether that item causes a specific symptom or not.

In P/N testing, tiny droplets of different dilutions of a potentially allergenic item are injected into the upper layers of a child's skin. If the test causes a significant local reaction or if it provokes or reproduces a miniature form of a child's exact medical symptoms, the test is considered positive. It is not essential, however, to replicate a child's symptoms during provocation allergy testing. When it does, however, this manner of testing can convincingly confirm a parent's or physician's suspicions that an allergy exists.

After provocation testing it is routinely possible to stop the provoked symptoms, or neutralize them, with a weaker or more dilute solution of the same test item. If a mother sees that a drop of an allergy extract suddenly reproduces her young child's hay fever, headache, or hyperactivity within a few minutes, it can be most reassuring that one cause of the problem may have been found. Parents are then often relieved, reassured, and impressed to see their child's stuffy nose, headache, or hyperactivity subside within a few minutes after neutralization treatment with a weaker solution of allergy extract. The ultimate aim is to help a child so that there are no symptoms *and* no need for drugs. Although drugs can be gratifyingly effective, we must strive to eliminate the cause of an illness, not simply provide temporary relief with drug therapy.

A Detailed Example of How P/N Testing Is Done

A child's major complaint might be a recurrent headache, which a parent thinks is due to eggs. This type of conclusion is often reached after a child has been placed on either the Single or Multiple Food Elimination Diet (see Chapter 8). Before any allergy testing is begun, the nurse, as well as the parent, should note exactly how the child looks, acts, and behaves. One must, for example, determine if the child has a headache and how severe it is *before* testing is begun. The nurse also records the child's pulse and asks the child to write her or his name. This is called the baseline. The aim is to compare what happens during the egg allergy test procedure with how the child was before testing began.

A placebo or nonallergenic item is customarily tested first. This test should be negative. The patient is then often tested with histamine, which should cause a positive skin test reaction in allergic or normal individuals. These tests help the doctor determine if the parent's and/or child's interpretations of changes related to testing are reliable or not. Ideally, to help diminish any preconceived bias, neither the child nor the parent should know what is being tested at any time.

After the doctor has taken a detailed history and completed a thorough physical examination, testing of suspect allergenic substances can begin. One tiny droplet of an egg allergy extract would be placed intradermally into the skin of the upper arm. Both the parent and the nurse must observe the child carefully at all times during the entire testing procedure. Every seven minutes the skin test site, symptoms, appearance, pulse, and writing are again evaluated and recorded. An allergy to egg in a child may be present if any of the following occurs:

- The skin test site enlarges significantly. Sometimes it looks like a large mosquito bite.
- The child holds his head or complains of a headache.
- The child suddenly develops some other medical or emotional complaint.
- The pulse suddenly increases by over 20 points.
- The child can no longer write his name as well as before.

If a child had a slight headache before the test was started, and seven minutes after the first egg test, the headache is extremely severe, this would strongly suggest that egg was the cause of the headache. If the child develops head pain, when none existed before the test, it means that the egg allergy extract probably provoked the headache. The nurse then injects a tiny droplet of progressively weaker 1:5 dilutions of allergy extract every seven minutes, i.e., $\frac{1}{5}$, $\frac{1}{25}$, $\frac{1}{125}$, and so forth. When the correct neutralization dosage is found, the child should say that his headache is gone. The skin test site, pulse, writing, and the child's appearance at that time should all have returned to normal. This neutralization dose of allergy extract should be effective to either prevent or relieve that child's headache whenever it is caused by eating eggs or foods that contain eggs.

Each child needs to be watched in a slightly different way. If a child has asthma, the lung function would also need to be checked every seven minutes to detect if the testing decreased the child's ability to breathe (see Chapter 10). If someone had an irregular heartbeat or high blood pressure, these could similarly be monitored to note the effect of each allergy test item on the heart or blood vessels. When the correct dilution of extract is given, the lung or heart changes should return toward normal. Of course these changes will be noted only if an allergy to a test item is related to these particular medical problems. Dust might cause asthma, whereas egg might cause a headache.

If there is any reason for concern because of a patient's history of a frightening reaction to some item, a blood test called an IgE RAST can be performed prior to the first allergy skin test for that item. The doctor must be very careful so that the patient does not have an alarming reaction to any test. In general if a food is repeatedly eaten, even if it makes a child somewhat ill, it can be safely tested without a RAST. If there is a doubt, ask your doctor for a RAST *before* a skin test for that item is done.

After testing, the patient who reacts to an egg test, for example, is given bottles of allergy extract that contain the neutralization dose for egg, and any other items that were positive during testing. Three drops of extract initially are taken sublingually (under the tongue) three times a day, or 0.1 cc can be injected subcutaneously, or just under the skin, once or twice a week. Either form of treatment should enable many patients to eat most foods for which they are treated without difficulty. The choice often depends upon the child's and the parents' personal preference.

If the drops or injection of the neutralization dose for egg, for example, are given *before* an egg is eaten, this treatment should prevent a headache. If the drops or injection are given *after* eggs have already caused a headache, the treatment should relieve the headache. If there is any doubt about the effectiveness of the treatment, parents are encouraged to feed their child eggs at a four-day interval or in such a way that the extract will prevent and/or eliminate the symptoms.

Most Allergists Do Not Believe in P/N Testing

Most traditional allergists do not believe that provocation/neutralization (P/N) tests are reliable. This is perplexing because this method appears to be a more sensitive, accurate, and exact method of detecting allergies. Those who disagree often lack personal experience or are not properly knowledgeable about this technique. The P/N method basically tests one item at a time, in contrast to many, and uses 1:5 rather than 1:10 dilutions of the same allergy extract used for traditional allergy testing. It is a much more meticulous and precise method of detecting an allergy.

Are Allergies Psychological?

Maybe you've heard of people who are allergic to roses. Every time they smell a rose, they develop asthma or hay fever. Some people say that the "proof" that this type of response is purely psychological is that these same individuals sometimes react similarly to "the smell of plastic roses." This argument has been used repeatedly to indicate that allergies are a purely psychological problem in some individuals. More and more evidence, however, indicates that the mind and the body are one. The recognition of this interconnection has led to a new science called psychoneuroimmunology.

A controlled scientific study by Michael Russell, et al. in *Science* (1984) showed, for example, that it is possible to design a study in such a way that guinea pigs can be made allergic to a protein at the same time that they are exposed to a fishy odor.[2] In time these guinea pigs will have an allergic-type of histamine release merely from an exposure to a fishy odor, without any contact with the protein. If a guinea pig can do it, why can't people? It is hard to believe that the guinea pig developed a psychological problem related to the odor of fish.

Of course some allergic individuals do have psychological problems. It would be difficult for a child or adult not to ask "why me?"

2. Michael Russell et al., "Learned Histamine Release," *Science* 23 (1984): pp. 733–734.

after a lifetime of illness, restrictions, reprimands, and various forms of denial and rejection. But in many youngsters it is not the psychological problems causing the allergies but the allergies causing the psychological problems.

Examples That Create Confusion in Present-Day Allergy Practice

Every allergist has seen and been perplexed by the occasional patient who has yearly flare-ups of classical hay fever during the grass-pollen season but surprisingly has entirely normal skin and blood allergy tests for grass. When such an individual is treated for a grass allergy, however, she or he often shows significant improvement. We must therefore conclude that although allergy skin tests are usually accurate, they unfortunately do not always provide definitive correct answers.

Allergists often see children and adults who claim to feel well when they stop eating specific foods and develop symptoms whenever some problem food is accidentally or purposely ingested. Sometimes the cause is an allergy, even though traditional allergy skin or blood tests for that food indicate no allergy.

Another confusing occurrence is the more typical individual whose traditional food-allergy tests appear to be positive for almost every food tested, even though these foods do not *appear* to cause any symptoms when they are eaten. Most allergists are perplexed by this common finding and say that these positive allergy skin tests represent "a past, present, or future allergy." What parents want to know, however, is whether a food causes their child to be ill or not right now. Diet challenges that consist of eating individual suspected foods at five- to twelve-day intervals sometimes provide fast, easy, inexpensive, and valid answers. Each of the many foods that test positive by traditional allergy tests needs also to be confirmed using this type of diet.

In contrast, if a problem food is not eaten for a month or longer, it is possible to find that it no longer *appears* to cause symptoms when it is *initially* added back into the diet. The symptoms can recur so gradually that the cause-and-effect relationship between the food and a symptom is not recognized.

A lack of appreciation of the significance of this latter observation prevented me from recognizing the scope of food allergy during my first eighteen years in pediatric allergy. To detect a food allergy, the food must be eaten no more often than every five days and no less often than every twelve days.

Many well-trained allergists continue to believe that food allergy cannot be treated with an allergy extract. This is what I was told when I studied allergy in the late fifties and this belief continues to be taught today in many training centers. Fortunately, there are newer and better methods to detect and treat food allergies which undoubtedly appear to be effective in some patients. These methods include a combination of the Practical Rotary Diet and/or food extract therapy. When these are effective, the need for daily medication to control food-related allergies is often diminished or eliminated. Even more important, after treatment, most patients can eat the majority of the foods which previously caused symptoms.

Some children have a clearly elevated RAST blood test indicating a food allergy. During P/N testing for that food, that child will develop hay fever, for example, or a distinct personality change. Another food will produce identical hay fever or personality changes during P/N testing, but that RAST blood test will be entirely normal. This suggests that although it can be very helpful, the RAST blood test does not always provide a reliable, accurate answer to help diagnose the cause of an allergic problem. When the test is positive, it probably indicates an allergy, but when it is negative, it does not indicate an absence of allergy, but rather a "maybe."

Some children are wheezing from some obvious exposure, such as grass, when they come for allergy testing. When their lungs are examined using a stethoscope and their lung function is properly measured on a machine, there is evidence suggesting asthmatic spasm. When some, but not all, of these children are P/N tested and treated for the suspected item, it is not unusual for their lungs to clear and their breathing tests to improve remarkably, without the need for any drugs. Regardless of what the RAST tests showed, it is possible to produce and eliminate asthma in some children merely by using droplets of different dilutions of an allergy extract.

Some children are depressed to the point of suicide each year during the pollen season. If such a child comes into the office at that time in a withdrawn, negative, depressed state, it is often possible to see an obvious dramatic personality change within a few minutes after the "correct" neutralization dose of allergy extract. Allergists would not doubt that hay fever or asthma can be caused by pollen. Depression, however, is certainly not the type of illness that many traditional allergists, psychiatrists, or psychologists would consider as a possible manifestation of allergy. Most physicians strongly doubt that common allergenic substances can cause allergic reactions in certain "off limit" areas of the body.

In spite of what is taught in allergy training programs, some infants have characteristic allergy problems due to foods, sometimes even seasonal flare-ups due to pollen, before the age of one year. They urgently need allergy treatment but this is often denied because they are "too young." With P/N testing and treatment they often respond quickly and well.

After Testing, Then What?

Regardless of whether scratch, standard intradermal, or the newer P/N variation of allergy testing is used to confirm a suspected allergy, the next step is usually recommendations to make the home more allergy-free and/or some form of diet. In addition, allergy extract treatment is often begun. Such treatment is thought by most but not all allergists to help prevent, diminish, or eliminate symptoms of allergy. Parents can judge the effectiveness of traditional versus P/N therapy by comparing how well their child feels and how many drugs a child uses, both before and after each form of treatment. For eighteen years I practiced traditional allergy medicine and many patients were significantly helped. Treatment consisted of allergy-extract injections three times a week for about thirty weeks, then once a month for several to many years. Many patients needed drugs to control their symptoms. Some needed cortisone or steroids.

In the past fifteen years, although it certainly does not always provide the perfect answer or help all children, the newer P/N allergy testing method appears to be unquestionably superior. Many children can be treated with three drops of allergy extract either under their tongue three times a day or via an injection once or twice a week. The injections can safely be given by the parents. The treatment is often needed less and less frequently and in time can be discontinued completely. Drugs are still required by some patients but their need is often diminished, and at times, abolished. Many physicians specializing in environmental medicine have had similar gratifying experiences.

No, Everything Is Not an Allergy

All hyperactivity, fatigue, depression, physical complaints, and behavior or learning problems, of course, are not due to an allergy. In some children, however, one possible unsuspected cause of these problems can be an allergy. This is particularly true when no one knows why certain children are "always" ill or can't behave. If these children have many allergic relatives, suffer from hay fever or asthma, and/or look allergic, it is possible that allergies also make them unable to behave or learn appropriately. This statement is true even if the usual blood or traditional scratch or intradermal allergy skin tests show no evidence of allergy.

I prefer to think of allergy as a large pie. Allergists are routinely taught to investigate one or two pieces. If the tests do not reveal an allergy, it is thought that this is not the patient's problem. Environmentally oriented physicians, who adopt a more expansive viewpoint, however, believe that there are many pieces of the pie that still elude the understanding of our best academic medical scientists. It certainly appears that in spite of impressive recent medical advances, human beings are much more perplexing and complicated than present-day medicine seems to appreciate. These newer approaches of allergy testing and treatment represent a small but impressive step in the right direction. These methods enable us to relieve symptoms quickly in some patients, even though we do not presently fully understand the fundamental physiological reasons why these methods are so helpful. Having tried it, I could not with a clear conscience ever practice allergy again in the manner that I was originally taught.

CHAPTER 2

Typical Allergies

Allergies are prevalent in today's society. About 22 million people have hay fever, about 10 million have asthma, and about 11 million have some form of skin allergy. At least 20 percent of all visits to pediatricians are due to a major allergy-related illness. Let's see if this is a problem in your family and then discuss some simple measures that might help to decrease or eliminate this tendency to develop allergies.

How Classical Allergies Affect Children

Hay Fever

Hay fever is rarely due to hay and does not cause a fever. Hay fever usually means that the nose or the eyes are congested. Sometimes the roof of the mouth or the ear canals become itchy, and children try to scratch these areas.

If hay fever symptoms occur for only a few weeks in the spring, summer, or fall, they are probably due to pollen and/or molds. Not uncommonly, however, these complaints are noticed all year long, either every day or intermittently. Year-round hay fever is more apt to be due to foods or allergenic items such as dust, molds, or pets. It is not unusual for young children who initially have year-round symptoms to develop definite seasonal flare-ups when pollen and molds are in the air as they grow older.

Eye Allergies

When your child's eyes are affected by allergies, one or both eyes will tend to itch, tear, and become red. Surprisingly, some children who have hay fever have more trouble with their eyes than with their nose. If the symptoms are very severe, the eyes can swell shut or appear as slits. On rare occasions eye allergies cause the white part of the eye to become extremely swollen and look like jelly.

Many people with eye allergies have "bags" directly below their eyes or a swelling in the area of the upper cheekbones (see Figure 2.1). Dark eye circles can make children look as if they have "black eyes." Sometimes, however, the eye circles look pink or blue rather than black (see Figure 2.2). They can have wrinkles under their eyes

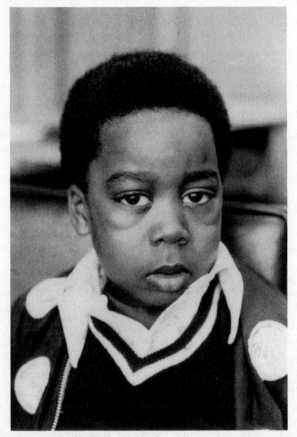

Figure 2.1. Puffiness under the eyes

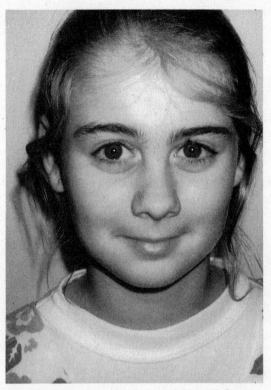

Figure 2.2. Dark black, blue, or pink eye circles are a prevalent signal for allergies.

just below the lower eyelids (see Figure 2.3). Some allergists and dermatologists believe these are characteristic of allergy. The upper lids in particular sometimes appear swollen because of allergy.

Allergic eyes are often rubbed by the child because they are intensely itchy. If a child's hands aren't clean, germs can infect the eyes when they are rubbed. This can cause the characteristic colorless allergic eye secretions to become gray, yellow, or green. These secretions can cause the lids to stick together, especially in the morning. (See David, Appendix E.)

Nose Allergies

Nasal allergies cause either varying degrees of stuffiness or a runny, drippy nose. Nose mucus caused by allergy is usually colorless. If

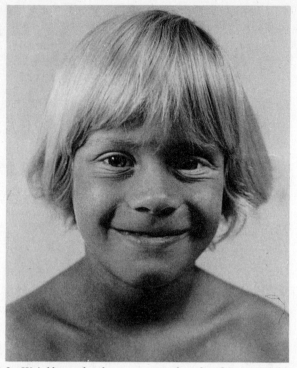

Figure 2.3. Wrinkles under the eyes are another clue that your child may have allergies. (Photograph by Bob Sacha)

mucus constantly drips from the nose, the area between the nose and upper lip can become red and sore. The nose can be so itchy that many children or adults rub their nose upward with the palm of their hand (see Figure 2.4). This causes a permanent horizontal crease across the middle of the nose (see Figure 2.5). Others wiggle their nose like a bunny rabbit or pick their nose. Hay fever is also characterized by bouts of sneezing, repeated throat clearing, or clucking throat sounds. The latter is a characteristic clue suggestive of a milk allergy.

Children who have nose allergy often sound nasal and breathe with their mouths open. This can cause dried, cracked lips. If it is a chronic problem, nose allergies can alter the development of the roof of the mouth so that orthodontia may be subsequently required.

Nose allergies can begin anytime from early infancy to late maturity. If the cause is not eliminated, antihistamines are often needed for years. Many antihistamine drugs make children and adults tired. This can also hinder a child or adult's ability to learn, think clearly, excel in sports, or engage in activities that require coordination.

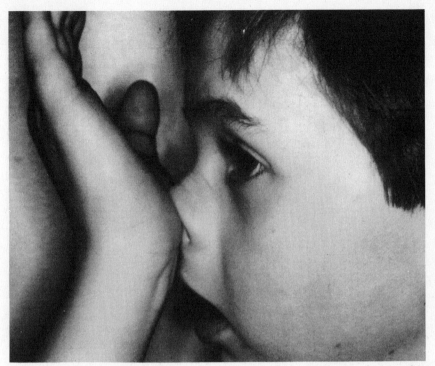

Figure 2.4. This method of stopping a runny nose is called an "allergic salute," and is a sure bet that your child has allergies.

Newer preparations such as Tavist, Seldane, or Hismanal are believed to cause less fatigue than the antihistamines used in the past. (See David and Bryan, Appendix E.)

Untreated Nose Allergies Can Lead to Chronic Throat, Ear, Sinus, and Lung Infections

Allergies cause the tissues inside the nose to swell. There is a tendency for hay fever sufferers to develop recurrent nosebleeds and infections. We all have germs inside our noses, but normal tissue with an adequate blood supply tends to resist infection. Allergies sometimes indirectly cause the adenoids, located in the back of the nose, to become infected and enlarged. This can cause snoring and a nasal voice. Large adenoids or swollen nasal tissues often block the connecting doorways that lead from the inside of the nose to the area behind the eardrums or to the sinuses. If this swelling is not eliminated, it can cause repeated ear and/or sinus infections. (See Eve and Jimmy, Chapter 13.)

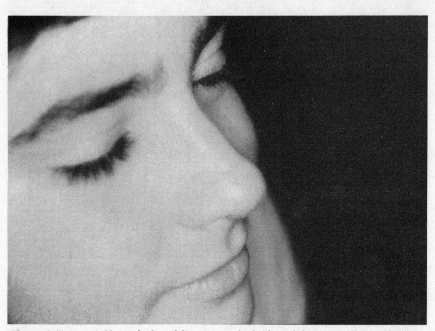

Figure 2.5. A wrinkle or darkened line across the bridge of the nose will form from repeated rubbing upward—one permanent result of the allergic salute.

Sometimes unsuspected and untreated allergy leads to nose, throat, ear, or sinus surgery. In some allergic children the tonsils tend to become chronically enlarged and infected. If the tonsils become so big that they interfere with a child's ability to swallow, they often need to be removed. Unfortunately the tonsils and adenoids tend to grow back, because they serve a necessary function; they help provide a barrier to confine infection to the throat area in an effort to help protect the rest of the body. In some allergic children the adenoids or tonsils need to be removed before a child is three or four years old, and then again later on.

You should develop the habit of looking into your child's throat with a flashlight. In time you'll be able to notice if the throat looks red or swollen in certain spots. If you see that there is only a little opening in the back of the throat because the right and left tonsil press against each other, check with your doctor. It is not unusual for the tonsils to swell temporarily during an infection, but with an allergy these tissues can stay swollen for years. When the tonsils and adenoids shrink to normal size and are not infected, surgery is not necessary. Sometimes this problem subsides completely after allergy treatment or if surgery can be delayed until the tonsillar tissue normally shrinks at the age of nine or ten years. (See Laurie, Appendix E.)

I saw two children in the same family who had recurrent fluid behind their eardrums for years. One child had had tubes placed in his eardrums nine times, the other six times. Their ear problems subsided for the first time shortly after their home was made more allergy-free and they followed a simple allergy diet. It is possible for early allergy treatment to eliminate the need for this type of repeated surgery in some youngsters.

Nose Allergies and Coughing

Nose allergies commonly cause a cough. This cough is due to a post-nasal drip. It is usually worse during the night and is thought to be due to mucus dripping from the nose and accumulating in the back of the throat during sleep. This type of cough often disappears with exercise or running because activity tends to clear an allergically stuffed nose.

Asthma and Allergic Coughing

This problem can begin at any age, from infancy to advanced maturity. Asthma appears to be on the increase. Between 1982 and 1986 the number of asthmatic children rose by 25 percent. Hospitalization for asthma increased 33 percent between 1982 and 1987. Asthma tends to occur more often in families who have asthmatic relatives in contrast to those who do not, but this is certainly not a hard-and-fast rule. Allergic coughing may be the first clue that an asthmatic tendency is present. Asthma can make a child prone to infection, so that an allergic cough can progress rapidly to asthmatic bronchitis. An allergic cough frequently precedes the first asthma attack by a few months to a year or two. This type of cough is often worse when a child exercises, laughs hard, drinks cold liquids, eats cold foods, breathes cold air, or becomes excited. Allergic coughs, which are worse on rainy days or in damp places, suggest a probable mold sensitivity.

Bronchial asthma means that the air tubes in the lungs are inflamed, swollen, and have gone into spasm. If they are a little tight, there will be a squeak, whistle, or wheeze when your child breathes out. If the asthma is severe, there is difficulty both breathing in and

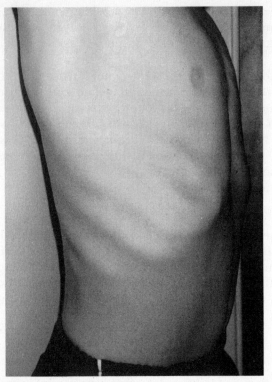

*Figure 2.6. Typical appearance
of chest during severe asthma*

breathing out. If the attack is very severe, the skin on the lower neck
and between the ribs will be sucked in and out with each breath (see
Figure 2.6). At that time, the respiratory squeaks and whistles can be
easily heard in the next room.[1]

Asthma is different from pneumonia or a cough due to an infection, such as bronchitis. These illnesses characteristically cause
more difficulty breathing *in* than breathing *out*. They are often but
not always associated with a fever and yellow or green mucus. If a
child has bronchitis, parents tend to complain about the child's persistent cough. If the problem is asthma, the complaint is more apt to
be that their child can't breathe.

Flaring nostrils tend to be somewhat more common during infections, such as pneumonia, than with asthma, unless the latter is

1. J.F. Soothill and J.O. Warner, "Control Trial of Hyposensitization to Dermatophagoides
Pteronyssinus in Children With Asthma." *Lancet* 9 (1978): 912–915.

very severe. When nostrils flare, the lower edge of the nostrils open wider than normal. They seem to grab a gulp of air each time a person takes a breath.

First asthma attacks can occur at any age, often before the age of five years. The initial asthma attack in children usually occurs during a viral infection, but in time wheezing commonly occurs, especially at night, for no apparent reason. Asthma also tends to occur after a stress such as an accident, the loss of a loved one, a move to a new home, or a change of schools. (see Jean, Chapter 6; Megan, Chapter 25.)

Similar to the nose, if there is swelling inside the air tubes of the lungs and too much mucus in that area, there is an increased tendency to infection. (See Laurie, Appendix E.) The first clue in infancy is often an illness called bronchiolitis. These infants have up to a 55 percent chance of developing asthma during early childhood, and respiratory illness later in life. This tendency is much greater if an infant has allergic relatives, obvious personal allergy, and positive blood or skin test evidence of allergy. In these infants it is thought that the RSV virus that is associated with bronchiolitis can damage the airways so that they would be more prone to asthma later on. For this reason parents of such infants should be more cautious than most in making sure that the children are not exposed to tobacco smoke or chemical pollution, which could further irritate their lung tissues. Asthma medications and extremely expensive antiviral drugs are of limited value in treating infants who have bronchiolitis.

Some children (and adults) have one episode of asthmatic bronchitis after another. (See Jean, Chapter 6.) This means the doctor hears asthma or wheezing sounds and there is also evidence of infection, such as green or yellow mucus, or a fever. The cough with bronchitis due to infection tends to be hoarse, deep, or barky, rather than the throat-clearing type of cough due to a postnasal drip.

One type of asthma noted in some children (or adults) is called exercise-induced asthma. After a few minutes of moderate to heavy exercise, affected children begin to wheeze, and the attacks can last from twenty minutes to several hours. These types of asthmatic episodes can sometimes be prevented if they are treated with a drug called Intal, or cromolyn sodium, before exertion. Sometimes this problem improves after a comprehensive allergy treatment program.

When the chest is affected by allergies, it is not unusual for the lungs to be quite sensitive or twitchy. Cold air or irritating odors such as tobacco, fire smoke, or pollution can cause sudden spasm in the airways of the lungs. This is often called irritable or reactive airway disease. Sometimes touchy airways become stable if the basic cause of the problem can be eliminated with comprehensive allergy care.

Many parents know their allergic child wheezes but do not realize that a wheeze can be the same as asthma. Parents are afraid to hear that their child has "asthma"; the term wheezing is less frightening. Many medical problems can cause wheezing, but in allergic children the cause is usually bronchial asthma. Be assured, children rarely die from asthma. Only one child in 100,000 expires from asthma, but this illness certainly disables many children so that they cannot run and play normally. If the cause of asthma can be found, it is often possible to help some asthmatics to have fewer attacks so that they need much less or no drug treatment.

If your child wheezes, always think back to the first time it happened. Can you recall if your child had an alarming choking episode a few weeks or months earlier? Sometimes a wheeze is due to some food particle that is stuck in one of the air tubes. This type of problem differs from asthma in that a wheeze due to a foreign substance is usually repeatedly located in one confined or discrete area of one lung, rather than in scattered areas throughout both lungs, which is so typical of asthma. Special X rays will often detect certain types of foreign bodies in the air tubes and help your doctor to diagnose this type of problem. X rays will not, however, detect such nonopaque substances as a piece of grass or food. If a foreign particle is found and removed, this type of wheeze usually stops entirely.

Buy an inexpensive stethoscope at a physician's supply store for about ten dollars. Learn to listen to your child's lungs when she or he is mouth breathing. The child must breath deeply and force all the air from the lungs. You may be able to detect when you need your doctor earlier. The only normal sound you should hear should be the sound of the whish of air that you normally make when you breathe deeply in and out with your mouth open.

In allergic families this tendency for children to develop asthma or asthmatic bronchitis might be prevented if parents were more aware about what causes asthma. They should take prophylactic measures to avoid excessive exposure to common allergens such as dust, pollen, mold, and pets. Also, do not forget to think about foods and chemicals. New chemicals are being used in innumerable products, and most have not been evaluated by our government for either safety or health factors. Many parents may not realize that chemical sensitivities can cause wheezing.

Of course it is certainly not always possible to find and eliminate the cause of asthma in allergic children, but it is gratifying that with a bit of thought and effort some asthmatic children can be signifi-

cantly helped. The paramount challenge should be to find and eliminate the cause of asthma, not to try another newer and better drug.
(See Bryan and Jay, Appendix E.)

Hives or Urticaria

Hives are similar in appearance to a mosquito bite. They typically
cause a central raised, slightly firm, white circular area surrounded
by a halo of red skin. Sometimes hives appear as itchy pink spots or
patches. They can vary from the size of a pea to larger than a grapefruit in diameter. They tend to appear and disappear over a period
of several days.

Hives can be caused by an immense variety of things. Commonly
they are due to drugs such as aspirin or antibiotics such as penicillin.
Also suspect foods such as milk or peanuts, infections, parasites,
insects, or unusual contacts with items such as a new fabric softener,
body or laundry soap, the chemicals in new clothing, or some new
preparation that is used on your body. Contacts with animals, pollen,
molds, and dust can also cause hives. Some people develop hives in
sunlight, others when they are exposed to cold. Some even develop
hives from pressure on their skin such as under a tight waistband.

If detailed records are kept of what was eaten and touched for
the eight-hour period before the first hive, the cause is often clearly
evident. If hives are caused by an antibiotic or drug, they tend to
appear within a few hours or days after the medicine is begun and
to disappear within a few days after the drug is discontinued.

If the cause can be found and eliminated, hives are much less apt
to reappear suddenly when children wear tight clothing or become
overheated after a hot shower, exercise, excitement, or a fever. The
latter factors do not really cause the hives; They merely enable the
body to tell you to recognize that some allergenic substance is present
in the body and ready to reveal itself. Eliminate the cause of the hives,
and a hot bath or exercise will no longer cause this problem.

If hives recur for a period over three or four weeks, it is called
chronic urticaria. Prolonged hives often come and go over a period
of years, and the cause can remain elusive. The answer can sometimes
be found if parents will keep detailed records of everything eaten or
touched during the few hours prior to the onset of the first hive or
any new severe flare-up of hives.

Routinely parents will insist that nothing unusual was eaten or
touched—until they sit down with a pencil and pad. Then parents

quickly recall some rarely eaten item, a food binge, a new fabric softener, or some other unusual contact. Good records often reveal elusive answers that relieve hives on a permanent basis.

Angioneurotic Edema

Hives are located on the outer surface of the skin. If they are deeper under the skin, they tend to cause less itching but much more swelling. This form of hives is called angioneurotic edema. If large areas of the body such as the face swell, you might not even recognize your child. Do not be fearful. When the swelling subsides, the appearance will return to normal. Fortunately this type of edema or swelling is usually not dangerous unless the back of the throat or tongue swells. If the area of the voice box swells, it can interfere with your child's ability to speak clearly and cause a hoarse voice or difficulty breathing. Contact your physician immediately if the tongue or throat are not right. An antihistamine and/or an injection of long-acting adrenaline may be most helpful. The latter can be obtained from your physician or at the nearest emergency room. If this is a recurrent problem, ask your physician to teach you how to give your child long-acting adrenaline. It is not difficult to do, and this knowledge will give you confidence and peace of mind. Keep adrenaline and syringes at home and in your car and purse at all times for emergencies.

Sometimes special blood studies indicate that angioneurotic edema is not an allergic reaction but is due instead to an inherited deficiency of a specific enzyme called C_1 esterase inhibitor. A problem of that sort requires the diagnostic expertise of a well-trained allergist.

Eczema or Atopic Dermatitis

Eczema is a general term that refers to many types of red, scaly, or itchy skin patches (see Figure 2.7). Atopic dermatitis is a specific type of allergic eczema that is intensely itchy. Many but certainly not all dermatologists and allergists doubt that allergy skin tests, special diets, or allergy extract therapy are helpful. Dermatologists have great expertise in the use of various creams and ointments to heal the skin. These certainly enhance healing, but unfortunately the relief may be only temporary. If the major cause of atopic dermatitis can be found and treated, affected children can sometimes be helped on a more permanent basis. The cause of eczema is often due to certain foods, dust, molds, yeast, chemicals, or contacts. (See Katie, Chapter 4.)

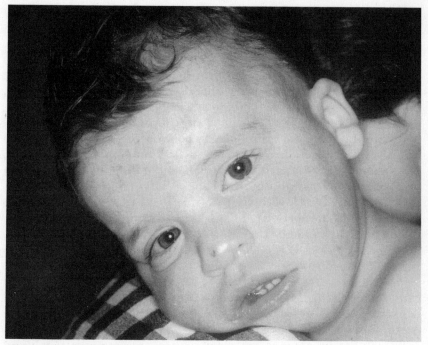

Figure 2.7. Typical rash of atopic dermatitis or eczema

Eczema often begins at about six months of age or near the time when breast feeding is tapered or discontinued. Mothers also frequently start giving their infants solid food, such as cereal, at that time. The rash appears first on the cheeks, wrists, ankles, and near the creases of the arms and legs. In some children the rash appears in small to large coin-shaped patches, which can be located on any area of the body. Many children scratch so much that their skin bleeds and their fingernails have a smooth, polished, shiny appearance. Although it is claimed that the palms of eczematous children are extremely wrinkled, this is infrequently noticed in my practice.

Atopic dermatitis is frequently associated with asthma and hay fever. If a child is fortunate, the skin rash may disappear at about the age of two years and new forms of allergies will not develop. Commonly, however, eczema is simply replaced with another type of allergy. If a child is extremely allergic, the eczema not only persists but other manifestations of allergies, such as hay fever or asthma, also become evident.

If your infant or young children have soft skin, eczema is much less apt to persist as they grow older. Children who have dry, scaly skin, however, tend to have atopic dermatitis, which continues through adolescence and well into adulthood. As children age, eczema tends to localize mainly in the arm and leg creases, on the back of the neck, and as cracks on the finger and toe tips. Some eczema patients improve after allergy extract treatment for dust, mites, molds, yeasts, and foods such as eggs and oranges, in particular. Contact with wool, mohair, or certain fabrics or personal-body-care products may also have to be avoided. Sometimes eczema improves if children take nutrients such as vitamins A, E, B$_6$, biotin, pantothenic acid, bioflavinoids, and essential fatty acids. Care must be taken not to take too much of these nutrients. More is not necessarily better. Check with your doctor if you want to try these.

If a child's atopic dermatitis is worse during the warm months, pollen or molds could be the cause of these seasonal flare-ups. Again, appropriate newer P/N allergy extract treatment can often help to resolve this problem.

Detailed records often reveal the cause of skin flare-ups. If a food causes eczema, the affected skin areas can typically become red and itchy while or shortly after the problem food is eaten. Immediately make a list of the foods and beverages eaten. Although the typical rash may not be obvious for a day or two, the immediate itch and redness provide excellent clues to help you pinpoint the specific cause of eczema. (See Linda, Appendix E.)

Intestinal Allergy

When allergies affect the digestive system, this is called intestinal allergies. Many parents recognize that certain foods repeatedly appear to cause abdominal complaints in their children. There is no question that the slightest contact with fish, eggs, buckwheat, or certain nuts can cause some very allergic individuals to become alarmingly ill. Some vomit, swell up with an itchy rash, can't breathe, or even collapse. These symptoms, however, are not the common, typical, frequently seen forms of intestinal allergy.

The intestines often send subtle reports to allergic individuals indicating that a food is causing an early, mild form of allergy. They transmit personalized messages, but someone must be listening. Some people only have bad breath; others merely have sudden bloating, a noisy abdomen, or excessive gas. The stomach wisely tends to hold back a problem food. This can cause belching and the problem food surprisingly can be tasted in the mouth. The stomach, however, will allow the "good" foods to pass along into the intestines without any telltale backup. Other common intestinal messages that could indicate allergy include abdominal discomfort, pain or cramps, diarrhea, constipation, nausea, vomiting, and at times blood or mucus in the bowel movement. (Constipation is sometimes a clue that strongly suggests a milk and dairy allergy.)

If your child continues to eat a food that offends the digestive system or if the only treatment to quiet the stomach is an antacid-type drug, the intestines may have to send stronger and stronger signals. In other words digestive problems can become progressively more serious in time if a person continues to eat the wrong foods, year after year.

In some patients irritable bowel, Crohn's disease, ulcers, mucous colitis, and even ulcerative colitis can be due to undetected allergies, especially to foods such as milk, wheat, eggs, chocolate, corn, and sugar. In others we do not know the answer. Stress can certainly make these and many other medical illnesses worse, but anxiety and emotional upset may only be aggravating factors, not the cause of a disease. (See Linda's mother's history, Appendix E.)

You should not ignore the early warning signs of an abdominal complaint in your child or in yourself. You should find out why the digestion is not normal. What did your child eat that could have caused the problem? Detailed records, again, often provide valuable answers. Suspect foods if all the intestinal symptoms stop when you don't eat or when you're fed only intravenous fluids.

Nonintestinal Symptoms Caused by Foods

Although not routinely recognized, food-related allergies can cause a wide variety of complaints that are unrelated to the intestines. For example, headaches, nose or chest complaints, fatigue, hyperactivity, depression, agitation, muscle aches, skin rashes, joint tightness, heart irregularities, and problems remembering or thinking are sometimes caused by food allergies.

If You Eat the Wrong Food, When Do You Become Ill?

Symptoms of classical food allergies are usually noted within fifteen minutes to an hour after a problem food is eaten. The relationship between a food and an illness is often obvious to parents and even to some children. Reactions to foods can last from ten minutes to six days, but most subside within twenty minutes to two hours.

Some foods typically cause delayed health problems that routinely occur several hours to a day or two after a problem food is eaten. Children or adults who awaken at 3:00 A.M. feeling alert, restless, or ill may be having a delayed reaction to their dinner. Some allergic adolescents or adults find that they feel best if they eat late at night, so that their reactions are over by morning and then they can work more effectively in the daytime.

Many affected individuals are totally unaware of the relation between the offending food and their recurrent medical problem. Delayed food reactions, for example, can cause otitis (ear fluid), bed-wetting, eczema, canker sores, colitis, irritable bowel, ulcers, Crohn's disease, and arthritis.

Special IgE RAST blood tests for immunoglobulin-type IgE allergy often confirm food sensitivities that cause obvious and sometimes severe reactions shortly after a small amount of a food is eaten. Other food reactions, however, which require larger amounts of food, can repeatedly cause either immediate or delayed symptoms. These foods do not routinely cause an elevated IgE RAST blood test, suggesting that there is no allergy when one may in fact be present. At times these negative IgE RAST foods can cause a strongly positive IgG type of RAST, suggesting that another form of food allergy is present. There must still be some missing pieces, however, because sometimes both the IgE and IgG RAST tests can be negative, even though some of these patients develop symptoms during provocation/ neutralization (P/N) allergy testing. These same patients can also respond favorably to allergy extract therapy.

I must add a strong word of caution here to emphasize that there are *many* other medical reasons that can cause each of the medical complaints mentioned earlier. Although allergy certainly should be considered, it is only one possible answer. It is not necessarily an allergy when young, spirited boys belch, but maybe this is why some boys can do it so readily. Sometimes they do it purposely to annoy, perplex, or attract attention.

The challenge is not so much to seriously consider other common diagnoses for chronic digestive complaints but to think of food allergy as one possible cause of the problem. Many food-allergic patients have had extensive medical evaluations by intestinal specialists that have not detected any reason for a persistent digestive problem. Some "take these pills and learn to live with it"–type medical problems, however, can simply be an unrecognized allergy.

Why Do Food Allergies Develop?

The tendency to develop food sensitivities is increased if the intestinal lining has been damaged for any reason. For example, if someone has diarrhea, the intestinal wall becomes more porous, and in addition it loses some of its normal protective lining or its immune barrier. It is therefore most unwise, for example, to drink an eggnog if you have diarrhea because large unbroken food particles of both highly allergenic egg and milk protein can enter the bloodstream more easily and possibly cause a subsequent allergy to these foods. In addition, if the linings of the stomach and intestines are damaged, digestive enzymes may not be optimally efficient, leading to improper breakdown and absorption of foods.

How Can You Find the Answer to a Food-Related Illness?

Parents and older children must learn to pay attention when their intestines complain. They should keep records of what was eaten when the gut warns in "belly" language that the wrong food has entered the intestinal system. By studying diet diaries it is often easy to detect an offending food item, even if the basic problem is not a food allergy. A milk problem due to a lactose intolerance is one example. This approach can also be helpful at times for some adults who have had intestinal problems for years.

In today's world of working parents it is not always easy to keep records. It fortunately takes only a little while to help figure out why some children are not well. If parents simply haven't the time, their child's problem may persist and worsen. Remember, no one knows a young child as well as his or her parents do. The answers may be a pencil and pad away. You should also give grandparents and baby-sitters the opportunity to help find answers by keeping diet records. If they resolve your child's medical problem, they will feel immense personal satisfaction and you will have an opportunity to be exceedingly grateful.

Two Basic Concepts to Understand Allergies Better

To properly analyze your records relating any medical complaint to an allergy, there are two necessary basic concepts that might help: The first is the barrel effect; the second is adaptation.

The Barrel Effect

Specialists in environmental medicine explain why something causes an illness one time but not the next time by what is called the barrel effect. In essence this means that each potentially allergic person has a barrel. If the barrel is empty or partially filled, there are no allergic symptoms. This is seen all the time: The pollen count is low and the pollen-sensitive patient feels great; when the pollen count rises above a level that is critical and specific for that individual, hay fever or asthma are suddenly evident. The barrel has overflowed.

In most allergic individuals it is not that simple. Usually the barrel is filled with a combination of allergenic dust, pollen, molds, foods, pet hair, and chemicals. If it is overflowing, the patient has the typical and/or less commonly recognized symptoms of allergy.

You can empty your barrel by

- making your home more allergy-free and ecologically sound;
- modifying your diet;
- avoiding chemicals and pollution.

If enough of any of these allergenic substances is removed, the barrel is not overflowing and there may be no evidence of illness. This is true even though you continue to be exposed to all the other allergenic items that are left in the partially empty barrel.

You can make your barrel larger by

- taking allergy injection therapy;
- improving your nutrition;
- decreasing stresses in your life.

With a larger barrel, you can be exposed to more allergenic items before becoming ill.

You make your barrel smaller when you develop an infection, eat junk food, or have too many stresses in your life. A move, a separation, a divorce, the death of a relative or pet, the loss of a job, or simply becoming emotionally upset over anything can make your barrel smaller. This means that a previously half-filled barrel is suddenly overflowing. This is one factor that contributes to asthma attacks, for example, which are associated with infection or major life stresses.

The barrel effect logically explains why something causes allergy symptoms one time and not on other occasions. Merely try to empty your barrel. You can make your home allergy-free and then you may be able to eat certain foods that previously bothered you. Or, conversely, you may be able to keep your pet dog if you adhere to an allergy diet, clean up the moldy basement, dust the house more often, use an air purifier, and receive allergy extract treatment for dog hair and dandruff.

It must be admitted, however, that it is not always possible to empty an overflowing barrel. It is possible for someone to be so extremely sensitive to something that in spite of doing everything possible, there is no improvement. If you live in a very damp home in a moldy city, you can try everything, but if your barrel is tiny and your mold exposure too great, you may not feel well until you move to a dry home and/or area.

In summary, not everyone can be helped, but many surely improve with the comprehensive program outlined in this book and used by specialists in environmental medicine. You can lower your total allergenic load by changing your house and diet and avoiding known allergenic substances and chemicals as much as possible. You can take measures to eliminate harmful chemicals from your body. You can enhance your immunity with proper nutrition and healthier living. This combination appears to help many individuals. If these measures don't help, find a doctor who can test and treat the twentieth-century type of allergy. Drugs are the answer only while these measures are being implemented and if they are not sufficiently helpful.

Adaptation

Normal human adaptation responses make up one major built-in defense response to help protect our bodies. Alarm reactions from food or chemical sensitivities occur if allergic reactions are obvious or unmasked. These supersensitive individuals recognize their alarm symptoms very quickly after eating the wrong food or after the slightest exposure to an offending chemical. They immediately develop symptoms, such as asthma, hay fever, a headache, increased activity, irritability, fuzzy thinking, and so on.

The second stage is the addiction phase, or one of adaptation or masking. Cause-and-effect relationships are no longer obvious; they are masked. The person's body adjusts to some food or odor in such a way that illness is not noted. The body is saying, "Gee, I can handle this." Some handle it so well that they get a pick-me-up or actually feel better after certain exposures. Most of these people are totally unaware of their sensitivity. They think they are well, as do their family and friends. To unmask someone in this stage, the offending food or odor must be avoided for about four days. If this is not done, it is easy to be deluded into thinking that no sensitivity exists, when in reality it does.

If this masked stage is prolonged, the "fixes" last less long and more and more of the addicting substance is needed at more frequent intervals to remain well. At this stage the body is saying, "Gee, I thought I could handle it, but the load is too great." Symptoms of illness can change from infrequent to often after an illness has been unmasked. It is no longer possible to prevent illness by taking one more bite of a food or one more smell of a chemical. The defenses have broken down. Both family and friends notice something is wrong, and at that point a doctor often enters the picture. Some children and adults feel sick in some way and tend to become withdrawn, tired, irritable, depressed, or complain about having difficulty thinking.

In this third stage the body is exhausted. The body is saying, "Sorry, I did my best, I've given my all. I can't protect you any longer." Each exposure causes immediate symptoms. Patients realize they are ill. The illness can be constant and incapacitating if the exposure is daily and unavoidable. These patients will require intensive evaluations and individualized care to reverse their illness. At a cellular level they have literally "run out of gas." Most children are not that ill, and it is hoped that the information in this book will help prevent the progression of illness from obvious to adapted to exhausted.

CHAPTER 3

How to Recognize
Unsuspected Allergies

It is often easy to recognize typical allergies, such as hay fever, asthma, or eczema, merely by looking at a child. These children are sneezing, wheezing, or scratching. The clues in this chapter provide different and at times more subtle but equally important evidence of allergy. Once they are pointed out, they will be clearly obvious to many parents. They will vividly recall seeing these physical clues in their child, but they simply were not aware of their significance. The changes in appearance or behavior that are discussed may be present on a daily or on an intermittent basis. If you suddenly see any of these changes, notice how your child looks at that time and see if "that look" is associated with other symptoms or changes in personality. For example, are dark eye circles noticed in relation to your child's temper outbursts and inability to speak clearly? Do the red ears, headaches, and inability to write or draw all occur at the same time? In this way you may be able to recognize that certain physical changes in your child's appearance provide warning signals that predict that a medical complaint or problem with learning, activity, or behavior is about to become evident. Dramatic changes in appearance, health, and personality can all be due to unsuspected allergies, and if you can spot the early clues, you may be able to prevent many problems and make your family life much less stressful.

Physical Clues Suggesting Possible Allergy

Skin

Ticklishness

Dr. Lendon Smith has said for many years that allergic children are extremely ticklish, and this has certainly been true in my practice. He is also correct in his observation that blond, blue-eyed boys are predominant in the practice of physicians who see children who have behavior and learning problems related to allergy.

Excessive Perspiration

Some infants and children always perspire much more than normal, even when it is not too hot. This may be evident anytime, but especially at night. Infants and very young children who have recurrent ear infections, in particular, tend to perspire more than normal on their forehead, or at times over their entire head. Some allergic infants or young children need their entire clothing changed several times a day. Aware parents can sometimes pinpoint exactly what is causing this intermittent problem.

Perspiration, which normally has no odor in young children, can at times be particularly offensive in some extremely allergic children. The odor can become very pungent and can permeate an entire room when some adolescents ingest or have been exposed to some highly allergenic item. These adolescents complain that the odor is difficult to eliminate with bathing. Aware adolescents or parents can relate the sudden appearance of a specific body odor directly to foods or factors known to cause certain changes in their affect, behavior, or physical well-being.

A YOUNGSTER WITH UNPLEASANT FOOT ODOR

Paul

One pleasant adolescent young man, Paul, complained that the odor of his feet was simply horrible. He was embarrassed because the smell was similar to "rotten cheese." His father had complained about the same problem for years. Both of them perspired profusely. We tested and treated Paul for two weeks for molds, and at the same time he also stopped eating all grains and milk products. He was amazed to find that although his feet continued to perspire, there was absolutely no odor. In time we found that wheat was the cause of this problem. If he binged on wheat, the odor quickly returned.

His father then decided to stop eating wheat. Two days later his feet smelled so nice that his wife kissed them! We assume that Paul's wheat allergy extract therapy has helped relieve his wheat-related foot odor because he can presently eat wheat, in moderation, without developing smelly feet.

Pale Face

The face of an occasional allergic child can appear so abnormally pale that many people comment that the child looks anemic. In older children or severely allergic chemically sensitive adults, the face may be a characteristic ashen or a peculiar gray-yellow color, associated with pale cheek areas and a slight yellowish swelling of the outer lip edges.

Expressionless Face

Many youngsters develop a spaced-out look when they are having an allergic reaction. They lack their usual animation and their face looks expressionless. At that time they often are not thinking well or correctly. They look as if they do not hear what you are saying. If this look is associated with red earlobes, wiggly legs, and dark eye circles, it helps parents recognize that the child's brain may be affected by an allergy.

A Nine-Year-Old Boy Who Reacted to Corn

Mike

His teachers complained because Mike simply could not concentrate and inexplicably seemed to be unable to learn in spite of the fact that he was usually an honor student. He lived in a somewhat rural area where they were harvesting the corn at that time. We decided to test him for corn, and ten minutes after we found his treatment dosage for corn, he appeared to be more alert and animated immediately. (See Figures 3.1a and 3.1b.) After treatment with his allergy extract for corn he was much more alert in school and his school performance returned to its original superior level.

Nose

An unusual clue is the red nose tip. This happens in both children and adults. The cause and effect happen so quickly that it is often easy to pinpoint which food, beverage, or exposure is at fault. This is frequently noted after the ingestion of grape juice or wine in allergic adults. It is usually attributed to the dilatation of blood vessels normally caused by alcohol, but at times it may provide a vivid clue to an unsuspected allergy.

Eyes

Typically allergy can cause red, itchy, watery eyes. The following specific eye symptoms are often noted in many allergic children, but particularly in children who have activity or behavior problems: They frequently have bags under their eyes or dark eye circles (see Figures 2.1 and 2.2). Many have wrinkles under their eyes (see Figures 2.3 and 3.2), which are particularly, but not exclusively, evident in children who have eczema (see Figure 2.7). Some children develop glazed

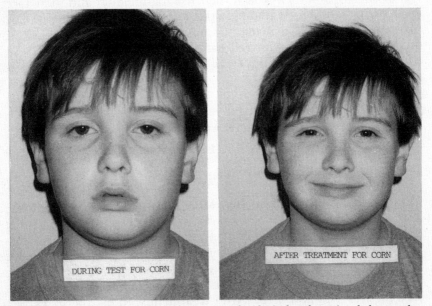

DURING TEST FOR CORN

AFTER TREATMENT FOR CORN

Figures 3.1A, 3.1B. These photos demonstrate the physical and emotional changes that occur during allergy testing.

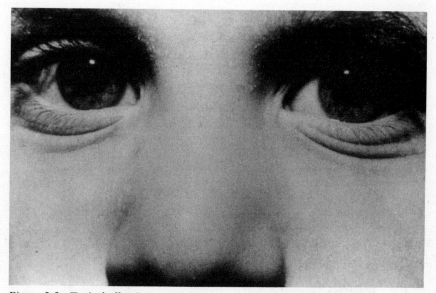

Figure 3.2. Typical allergic eye wrinkles

eyes and appear spaced out during allergy-related temper tantrums. You scream, "How many times do I have to tell you," but you see that your words do not even register. This can be due to allergies affecting the brain. Sometimes these children really don't hear until they look, act, and feel normal again. At times they truly don't remember what they did that was wrong.

Eye allergies sometimes cause such an extreme sensitivity to sunlight that dark glasses are needed whenever a child is outside, at times even when a child is indoors.

One adult clearly illustrates how vision can be affected by odors. She had extreme chemical sensitivities, and her eye physician had just built a beautiful new office building that had an overwhelming odor of the many chemicals found in new construction materials. After her eye examination she found she could not see with her new glasses. She returned to the same office with a portable oxygen tank. During this eye exam she breathed oxygen from the tank constantly. This eye examination revealed that the previous lens prescription had not been correct; when the new glasses were prepared, she could

see well. Scientific studies by Dr. Satoshi Ishikawa's group have documented that aerial chemical sprays with malathion certainly can
adversely and measurably affect eye function.[1]

Ears

Red Ears

Children often suddenly develop one or two brilliant red earlobes
after specific allergenic exposures (see Figure 3.3). These children
(or adults) may comment that their earlobes feel very hot. This often
precedes or accompanies the so-called Dr. Jekyll/Mr. Hyde personality changes. These children suddenly switch from being adorable
to being impossible. This typically occurs within an hour after some
children ingest certain foods, beverages, or medicines that contain,
for example, sugar, dyes, or corn. Molds, pollen, dust, and mites can

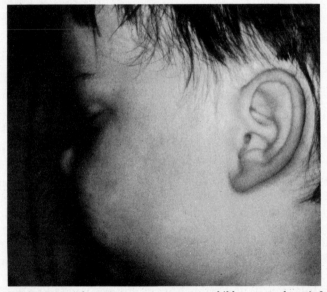

*Figure 3.3. Outward symptoms can appear on children as early as infancy.
Notice the discoloration of the ear on this toddler.*

1. S. Shirakawa, Satoshi Ishikawa, M.D. et al., "Evaluation of the Autonomic Nervous
System Response by Pupillographical Study in the Chemically Sensitive Patient," *Clinical
Ecology* 7 (2) (1990).

cause similar changes during P/N allergy testing or after direct exposure to these items.

One word of caution in relation to this and the other clues mentioned in this chapter: There are often innumerable causes for the same physical change or complaint. Fair-skinned children can develop red ears just from being in a hot room, so please don't interpret every red ear as an allergic reaction.

Some children develop an acute sensitivity to normal sounds when they are having an allergic reaction. If someone speaks in ordinary tones, they cover their ears, scream that the voice is too loud, and run to some silent sanctuary. This same response can occur at home after exposure to allergenic substances, as well as during routine P/N allergy testing.

Recurrent Ear Infections

Beginning in early infancy and through early childhood it is not unusual for some allergic children to develop fluid behind their eardrums and to have one ear infection after another.[2] This can cause some infants of normal intelligence to speak late and learn more slowly, because they cannot hear well. In addition, these children often have associated nose, sinus, or lung infections. They receive antibiotic after antibiotic, and this in turn can cause an overgrowth of candida or yeast, which upsets the delicate balance of microorganisms normally present in the intestines. (See Chapter 23 and Eve and Jimmy, Chapter 13.)

Cheeks

Bright, red, circular, rougelike cheek patches are seen in many allergic children, particularly if they eat a food to which they are sensitive. These patches look like round circles of rouge and are particularly evident in children ages one to four years (see Figure 3.4).

Lips

Certain foods or substances that touch the lips, such as toothpaste or bubble gum, can cause a rash below the lower lip or around the entire mouth. Occasionally children or adults who have food allergy ner-

2. R.J. Hagerman and A.R. Falkenstein, "An Association Between Recurrent Otitis Media in Infancy and Later Hyperactivity," *Clinical Pediatrics* (1987) 26, pp. 253–257.

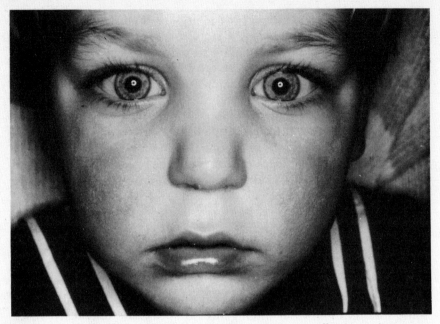

Figure 3.4. Red patches on the cheeks often appear during an allergic reaction.

vously lick some area around their lips. Sometimes the lips are dried and cracked, especially if a child has to mouth-breathe because of nose allergies. Rarely, the lips swell until the child's appearance is distorted. During some allergic reactions the swollen lips can feel like hard rubber.

Many older children and adults have a distinct yellowish discoloration and slight puffiness along the entire outer border of their lips. This is especially evident in severely food-allergic adults.

Excessive Drooling

At any age, from infancy on, excessive drooling can be directly related to exposure to certain offending beverages, foods, or odors. All normal infants drool when their teeth develop, but allergic infants can drool so excessively that their socks are wet. Some need constant bib changes all day long. Some normal and many retarded children also can drool an extreme amount of saliva. After an allergic exposure this problem can suddenly become so severe that a stream of thick, frothy saliva can extend from a youngster's mouth all the way to the floor. (See Laurie, Bill, and Roger, Appendix E.)

If your dentist comments about the extreme amount of saliva in your child's mouth, think about allergy. Excessive saliva can cause unintentional spitting during ordinary conversation. In some children and adults it can cause a rash or irritation in the corners of the mouth. A vitamin B_2 deficiency can also cause the corners of the mouth to be excessively moist.

Gums and Cheeks

Some children tend to develop ulcers or open sores on their gums and inner cheeks called canker sores. These can be caused by eating too much of certain foods. One frequent cause is an excessive amount of orange juice or vitamin C. Certain flavors of toothpaste, salty foods such as potato chips or pretzels, or acid foods such as pickles, tomatoes, or vinegar salad dressings are also common causes. Detailed diet records may provide answers.

Remember, however, there can be a delay of a few to twenty or so hours between eating a food and the appearance of a canker sore in the mouth. Once a sore has developed, it takes several days for that area to heal.

Tongue

Patchy Tongue

Normally your tongue should be evenly coated so that it seems to have a generalized pink color. If you see bare islands of naked, reddish tongue surrounded by the normal pink color, it often indicates a food allergy (see Figure 3.5). This is called a geographic tongue because the bald, naked patches make the tongue look like a map. These changes can occur within a few hours after certain offending foods are eaten. The tongue may appear abnormal for several days.

Teeth Marks on the Tongue

Teeth indentations on the edges of the tongue can indicate a digestive disturbance. Check with a nutritionist or gastroenterologist.

White Tongue

If someone's tongue has a very thick white or grayish-white coating most of the time, this suggests a possible chronic overgrowth of yeast. At times the tongue can also appear geographic and this is unrelated

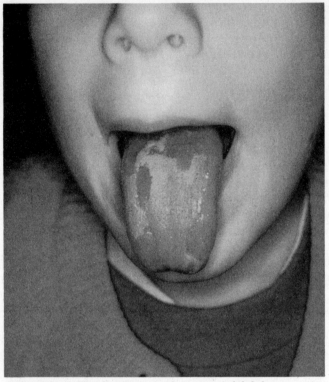

Figure 3.5. A discolored and patchy tongue is labeled a "geographic" tongue, another symptom of previously unrecognized allergies.

to an allergy. This is commonly noted in children who have needed frequent and prolonged courses of antibiotics (see Chapter 23) and the tongue improves after treatment with mycostatin or nystatin.

Excessive Thirst

Excessive thirst is not always associated with a hot day or exercise. Sometimes it can indicate infection, a kidney problem, diabetes, an essential fatty acid deficiency, or an allergy. Some children who have ecologic illness have an insatiable desire to drink and/or eat. If these symptoms are due to allergy, they often subside after the children respond to a comprehensive allergy treatment program or after the Multiple Food Elimination Diet (see Chapter 8).

Speech

Motor Mouth

The speech of children who have allergies can change dramatically. Parents commonly complain that their child has a "motor mouth," along with hyperactivity. These children ramble on and on endlessly, yet the content of their speech is limited. Such children may never be at a loss for words, but after allergy therapy their speech tends to contain more substance.

Whining Repetition

Young toddlers or children tend to whine and repeat the same sentence over and over again. Even if you give them what they want, they continue to ask for it or something else. If they repeatedly ask for a specific food in this manner, they are often telling you exactly what causes their allergies.

Stuttering or Unclear Speech

Allergies can make some children speak very quickly, others to stutter, and others to talk unclearly or slur their words. These are usually intermittent problems, but be suspicious of a food if your child's speech changes occur shortly after some food is eaten or after an exposure to some odor.

High-Pitched Voice

Adolescent girls and women who have unrecognized allergies tend to intermittently develop a high-pitched rapid manner of speaking. At those times their shoulders may be raised, and they frequently complain about sore upper-back and neck muscles.

Unusual Sounds

Some young children bark, grunt, moan, mimic a crow, dog, or rooster, or make other strange sounds. Surprisingly these sounds, at times, can be related to eating certain foods or exposures to specific allergenic substances. Teachers will often complain that their noises interfere with classroom teaching and learning. Yes, some children do it only for attention, but at times it can indicate an allergy. Look for associated facial or ear changes.

Hoarse Voice

The most common causes of a deep, hoarse voice are yelling, screaming, or an infection. Sometimes, however, it indicates a potentially serious allergic reaction in the larynx or voice box. Chemical odors and foods, in particular, can sometimes cause sudden hoarseness or a total inability to speak. This indicates a need for immediate medical attention to prevent suffocation. Sudden swelling of the laryngeal area in the back of the throat is a medical emergency. Although an antihistamine or an asthma pill may be helpful, a spray-type asthma medicine or an injection of adrenaline would be more effective. (See Chapter 26.) A physician's expertise should be secured as soon as possible to prevent or treat such episodes. If it is a recurrent problem, the older child himself or a parent should be taught how to give an injection of adrenaline.

Hands and Feet

Most children and adults who have ecologic illness complain about cold hands and feet. We really do not know why, but it may reflect a problem with their histamine blood levels. This is a particularly common complaint in allergic females. Correct treatment for allergies will at times relieve this problem.

Some children with yeast problems have an odor to their hands and feet that lingers, even after bathing. Occasionally mold-sensitive allergic individuals complain about smelly, moist feet. Food allergies also sometimes cause this problem.

Legs

Leg aches at night, either in the calves, ankles, or thighs are extremely common in children aged two to five years. Mothers are familiar with this complaint because they have to rub their child's legs at night or carry their child in malls or home from school because of leg pain. Older children are less frequently bothered. They sometimes wrap their legs in warm towels to obtain temporary relief. These aches are unrelated to exercise or tight shoes or socks. Again, milk or dairy products are common but not the sole cause of this problem. (See Linda and David, Appendix E.)

A few infants, but many children and adult males, in particular, tend to have wiggly legs. Others don't just wiggle their legs, they have to move frequently when they sit in order to reposition their lower extremities or they feel uncomfortable. Some children and adults wiggle their legs rapidly back and forth shortly after they have eaten allergenic foods. Restless legs that do not ache or hurt are a common complaint of some schoolchildren who simply can't sit still. This can be caused by many factors, but it is commonly due to a sensitivity to dairy products in particular.

Some very chemically sensitive older children and adults complain that their calves and feet burn if they wear plastic shoes, vinyl shoe inserts, or stand and walk for long periods of time on synthetic carpets. Muscle aches; strange, localized tender skin spots; and weak extremities are not uncommon in some allergic children or adults. These complaints occur, in particular, when a chemically sensitive person walks through a typically highly air-polluted shopping mall or hospital.

Less obvious causes include chemicals, for example contact with a synthetic carpet or sitting on plastic chairs or furniture. Even electromagnetic emanations from fluorescent overhead lights, television sets, or computers can cause some children to wiggle and act agitated, especially in school. Coffee, tea, or chocolate can also cause non–allergy-related wiggling due to the excessive stimulation of caffeine, but not all wiggling due to chocolate or beverages is due to caffeine. It can be due to an allergy to the cocoa bean or coffee bean.

FATHER AND SON WITH INCREASED ACTIVITY DUE TO CHOCOLATE

Bart and His Dad

We saw Bart initially because he became hyperactive after eating chocolate. He and his dad both had wiggly legs from chocolate. His mother determined that cocoa was one of Bart's problem foods. She gave him some chocolate after he had not eaten it for two months, and within a half hour he was screaming and kicking.

His father was a classic confirmed chocoholic. He had craved chocolate for years and admitted that all his baby teeth had cavities because he was always drinking or eating chocolate. As a young child he routinely received chocolate bunnies that were almost as large as he was from his loving aunts. He said he often ate so much he would have morning nausea and almost vomit or pass out.

As an adult his addiction persisted. He would start his day with a cup of hot chocolate. In the car he would have another cup and then eat a couple of chocolate bars. He drank cola for lunch. (Cola is in the same botanical family as chocolate and can cause an interchangeable type of addiction.) He ate more chocolate intermittently throughout the day. In the middle of the night he often awoke in need of another fix. M&M's were always close by. He said he was truly apprehensive, anxious, and ready to panic if there was no chocolate within arm's reach. His history sounds similar to that of an alcoholic or heroin addict because he needed a steady supply of chocolate to feel well.

When he ate chocolate, he noticed that his ears would tingle and become hot and red. He and his wife noted that his perspiration seemed to have a strong odor after he binged on chocolate. He was oblivious to the noise that his restless legs made banging away against the side of his metal desk at work. He tended to combine the disturbing repetitive sounds of his vibrating desk with pencil tapping as he fidgeted. His co-workers were often upset by his aggravating "nervous" habits. Chocolate also tended to make him irritable, which at times led to some serious interpersonal problems at work and at home. His wife said that chocolate caused his voice to become high-pitched, and he would speak so rapidly he sometimes stuttered.

We reproduced the typical wiggly legs in both Bart and his dad with a few weak drops of cocoa allergy extract during P/N testing. Bart also became hyperactive, whereas his father developed his characteristic rapid speech, red ears, increased perspiration, cough, and throat clearing. After each one received a drop of his appropriate dilution of a cocoa extract, all symptoms subsided in both Bart and his father.

A Boy With Weak Legs

Don

This youngster had a slightly different problem with his legs. His complaint was weakness. He simply could not stand up.

Don (age three) told his mother his legs "would not hold him up," and he would fall down repeatedly. We eventually determined that wheat was the major recurrent cause of this problem. We could produce and eliminate this weakness at will either by feeding him wheat or by using the newer methods of P/N allergy testing.

On one occasion, when he was five, his kindergarten teacher called to state that he could not get up from the floor. His mother immediately asked, "What did you feed him?" Cookies was the answer. She reminded the teacher that wheat caused this type of problem and rushed to his school. After being given his neutralization allergy treatment for wheat and a dose of an alkali he was up and walking within a few minutes. (See Chapters 8 and 25.)

He responded favorably to his extract treatment and his comprehensive allergy treatment program and in time he was able to eat wheat without any further episodes of leg weakness.

Joint Stiffness

Joints that are painful on damp days suggest a possible mold sensitivity. Stiff fingers in the middle of the night often indicate that some food eaten during the previous evening was not well tolerated. Ask which of the following foods was craved? Red meats (such as beef or pork), grains, tomato, potato, peppers, or tobacco are a few common causes of this type of discomfort. Sometimes the cause is a beverage such as coffee, tea, or cola. Think of an individual's favorite foods or beverages first. Again, do not forget chemicals, especially exposure to natural gas stoves or furnaces. Handling chemically treated school papers or meat-wrapping paper also can cause this type of complaint in some sensitive persons.

Sometimes arthritic adults find their joint pains disappear shortly after they go on a vacation but recur as soon as they return home. They should carefully evaluate their home environments. The answer is probably something inside their houses or in the air in their hometowns.

A tall, handsome fifteen-year-old noted that he could not sit on his legs. His mother discontinued all grains and milk for two weeks while he received allergy treatment for grains and molds. He was amazed to find that for the first time in about six years he was able to sit on his knees without any difficulty. He was more limber and could change from a sitting to a standing position much more easily. His mother added these foods back one at a time and noticed that when he ate an excess of wheat products, this problem recurred.

Every May a forty-three-year-old woman was seen in my office. She repeatedly complained of fatigue and pain in her knee, elbow, and hand joints when the grass pollinated. When her sublingual grass allergy extract dosage was correct, these symptoms subsided quickly. Another woman found that orange, in any form, repeatedly caused severe back spasm. This observation prevented her need for back surgery. Some nutritionists claim that niacinamide in conjunction

with a comprehensive nutritional program relieves some osteoar-
thritis.[3]

Bladder Problems[4]

Some allergic children seem to have spasm of their bladder rather
than their lungs. Their allergies cause them to wet their pants, not
to wheeze. They can wet their clothing in the daytime, but it is more
frequently only a nighttime problem. Most children do not wet the
bed beyond the age of five years. If bed-wetting persists, a pediatric
urologist is sometimes needed. (Se Eve, Chapter 13, and Julius, Chapter 20.)

At times when the bladder is affected by allergies, these children
will have to race wildly to the toilet, or else they wet or "have an
accident." Mothers often believe the children are so busy playing,
they don't want to take the time to urinate. In reality the cause may
be an inability to delay the need to void for a normal period of time.
Others tend to need to urinate much more often than normal. Of
course there are many physical and emotional reasons for these types
of complaints, but if your child has other evidence of allergy, think
about foods, dust, molds, and chemicals. The major beverages that
cause urination problems of this type are milk and apple, orange,
grape, or pineapple juice. This is particularly true if any of these are
a favorite beverage.

You can readily determine whether these drinks are a factor by
not giving your child any fruit and then for the next five days giving
only water as a beverage. Then add back milk on one day, apple juice
the next, and so on. Some mothers notice that their children are
totally dry for the first time in ages during the two-week Multiple
Food Elimination Diet. In a few days it may be obvious that the bed-
wetting has stopped, and during the second part of the diet it is easy
to see which foods cause a wet bed. If the cause is molds or dust, a
child may wet only on humid days or after exposure to a dusty place.
Some tend to wet their pants shortly after a meal that contains an
offending item. This can cause embarrassing school problems, which
can be made less evident if a child wears dark-colored trousers.

Your suspicions can sometimes be confirmed easily during P/N
allergy testing. I vividly recall one little boy who was being skin-tested
for pineapple. He immediately pulled down his pants and created a

3. Jonathan Wright, M.D., *Dr. Wright's Guide to Healing with Nutrition*, Emmaus, Pa.: Rodale
Press, Inc., 1984.

4. Patrick Kingsley, *Conquering Cystitis* (London: Ebury Press, n.d.).

wavy pattern of urine on the floor and carpet as he ru
the bathroom. Other children merely go to the bathro
quently when an item is being tested that causes their bladder
suddenly feel full.

Sometimes a child's bed-wetting improves on a particular diet but
some accidents still persist. A youngster might wet only twice rather
than seven times a week. If your regular doctor can't find the answer
and your child's urine examination is entirely normal, your child may
need to be seen by a pediatric urologist. There may be some ana-
tomical defect that is contributing to the urination problems, and
once that is corrected, there may be no further difficulty. In other
words, if bed-wetting improves but persists, it may respond to a combination of allergy treatment plus therapy for some physical or emotional problem that can easily be remedied.

Sleep Problems

Some allergic children cannot get to sleep, stay asleep, or get up very
early in the morning. At times they are inordinately restless and the
bedding is a jumbled mess when they awaken. Other children have
frightening nightmares. Merely keep records of what was eaten at
bedtime or during the evening meal. The answer many be obvious.
In other children the sleep problems are related to some change in
the bedroom, such as sheets dried with a fabric softener or a new
furniture polish. (See Chapters 6 and 27.)

Pimples on the Buttocks

Food-sensitive children often have little pimples scattered about the
rounded portion of their buttocks. This can be noted from early in
infancy to adolescence.

Scalded Buttocks

Mothers often notice that their infant's buttocks look lovely, yet by
the time of the next diaper change the buttocks are suddenly red
and appear scalded. This commonly occurs when an offending food
has been passed in a baby's most recent bowel movement. The cause
in a totally breast-fed infant can be a food the mother ate that passed
from the breast milk into the infant. (See Chapter 4.)

Of course sometimes diarrhea can also cause red, irritated buttocks. Yeasty diaper rashes also cause redness, but the buttocks do
not appear scalded. A yeast rash is usually quite red. It has a distinct

border with little spots scattered along the outer edge. The rash is often worse in the groin area between the legs and abdomen or in the folds of the skin.

Some babies are sensitive to some ingredient in disposable diapers or the soap or fabric softeners used to wash cotton diapers. A change to another type of diaper or soap often resolves this type of problem. (See Linda, Appendix E.)

Soiled Underwear

Some children's bowels leak so there is a spot of feces on their underwear. This can be caused by foods such as raisins, grapes, apples, or even by pollen.[5] One little boy routinely soiled his underwear whenever his grass allergy extract treatment dosage was not correct. This same youngster stuttered and blinked excessively during the fall months when ragweed and molds were prevalent and had an increased pulse rate in the early spring months when tree pollen was a problem. These symptoms were evident only when his extract treatment for these items were not exactly right. As soon as his neutralization allergy extract treatments were adjusted, these varied seasonal symptoms subsided.

Red Ring About Anus

Children who have had repeated prolonged courses of antibiotics for infections often develop a red ring around the anus (see Figure 3.6). This can indicate a yeast (candida or monilia) problem. (See Chapter 23.) This responds well to appropriate treatment.

Genitals

Infants often begin to touch or "dig at" their genitals as soon as their diaper is removed and sometimes even while it is being worn. Young children cause disturbances in the classroom and at home because they can't stop touching their genitals. This is often attributed to tight underwear or clothing, or to pinworms. In my experience this is very commonly due to an unsuspected overgrowth of yeast after the repeated need for antibiotics. After proper therapy this complaint dis-

5. Doris J. Rapp, M.D., *The Impossible Child*. 1989. Practical Allergy Research Foundation (PARF), P.O. Box 60, Buffalo, NY 14223-0060.

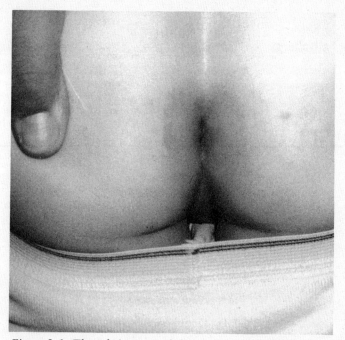

Figure 3.6. The red ring around the rectal area often indicates a candida or yeast infection in a child.

appears, along with the red rectal area, white-coated tongue, and smelly hair and feet.

Of course, the various medical conditions of many of the children just described are not scientifically documented observations. They do, however, represent cause-and-effect relationships helped by the recognition and treatment of the source of their illness. Surprisingly, many parents can find answers in a similar manner merely by watching their children more carefully.

Changes in Writing and Drawing Can Also Reveal an Allergy

When some allergic children react to foods or exposures, their writing can change quite dramatically within a few minutes. The child who abruptly becomes moody, depressed, or withdrawn will write very tiny (see Figures 3.7–3.9) or refuse to write anything (see Figures

Writing before school-air allergy test	Writing during allergy test	Writing after school-air allergy extract therapy

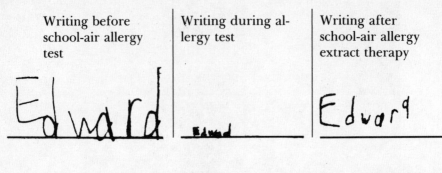

Feels well, acts normal	Withdrawn, throwing toys, headache, red ears, earache	Ears less red, headache and earache gone, behavior appropriate

Figures 3.7–3.9. Writing size changes during allergy extract testing.

Before disinfectant exposure	During disinfectant exposure	Peak of disinfectant reaction	After oxygen treatment for disinfectant exposure

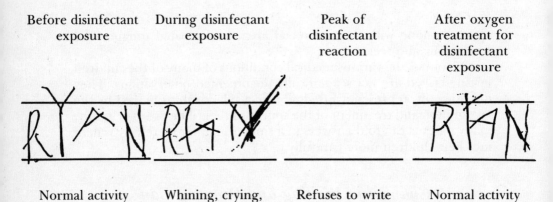

Normal activity	Whining, crying, tired	Refuses to write	Normal activity

Figures 3.10–3.13. Child refuses to write during allergy extract testing for disinfectant aerosol.

Before test	During test	After mite (dust) treatment
	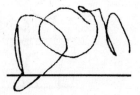	
Quiet and calm	Rocking in seat, kicking on floor, earlobes red	Quiet and calm

Figures 3.14–3.16. During a test with mite (house dust) allergy extract, this eight-year-old boy's handwriting becomes very large.

3.10–3.13). The hyperactive child will write very large (Figures 3.14–3.16) and often sloppily (Figures 3.17–3.20). The angry, aggressive child will stab or crumple the paper and then break the pencil and throw it at you. The child who becomes vulgar will write an explicit, embarrassing note (Figures 16.1–16.3, page 348). The learning disabled or very young child will suddenly write backward (see Figures 3.21–3.23), upside down, in mirror images (Figures 3.24–3.26) or be unable to write clearly or correctly. They will be unable to write the alphabet (see Figures 3.27, 3.28) or a sequence of numbers.

Similarly, the ability to draw can be altered during allergic reactions. Young children will suddenly be unable to color within the outlines in coloring books. Hostile children will draw bloody knives, skulls (see Figures 21.1, 21.2, page 414) and cemetery headstones in dark colors (see Figures 18.1, 18.2). Within a few minutes after appropriate allergy extract treatment, such drawings can change to brightly colored hearts and flowers. Figures 3.29, 3.30, and 3.31 show how an eight-year-old will draw a happy picture before a test for molds, become angry and draw himself unhappy during the test, and then after the neutralizing dose, his picture is again happy, showing a smile and butterflies. These changes provide dramatic evidence that the brain can be altered quickly and reversibly by an allergenic exposure followed by appropriate allergy extract treatment.

Baseline
P. 68

During Test
P. 72
Hungry, can't concentrate

During Test
P. 72
Hungry, can't concentrate

After Test
P. 64
Not hungry,
can concentrate

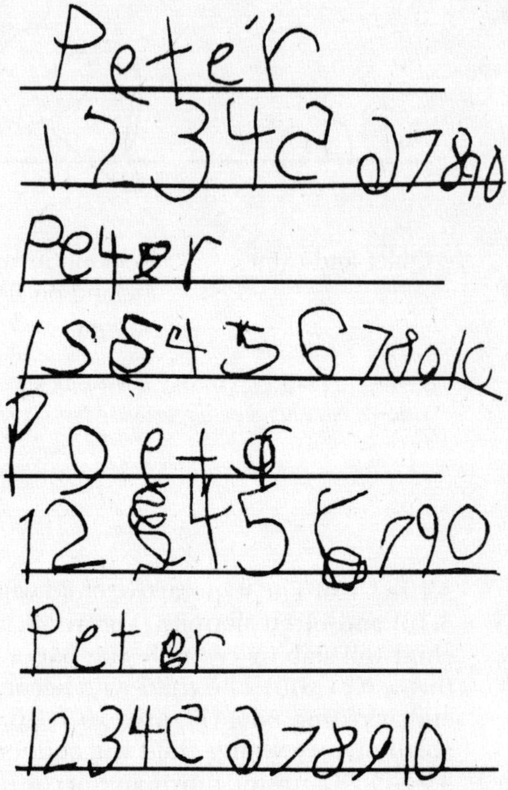

Figures 3.17–3.20. During a test with peanut allergy extract in a six-and-a-half-year-old boy, his handwriting becomes sloppy.

Other Common Problems That Might Be Related to Allergy

Although not frequently recognized, it appears that hypoglycemia, obesity, and alcoholism can sometimes be related to an undetected allergy.

Hypoglycemia

One major area of confusion for children, parents, educators, and physicians is hypoglycemia. You can sometimes tell if this is a problem

Before test	During test	After egg treatment

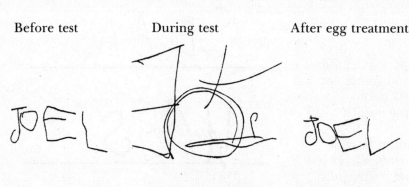

Normal activity	Very red earlobes, hyperactive	Normal activity

Figures 3.21–3.23. During a test with egg allergy extract in a four-year-old, his handwriting changes to backward and upside-down.

by noticing if your child asks for food or demands it immediately (see Table 3.1). Does your child kick the refrigerator when he's hungry? Does your child tend to become irritable, tense, argumentative, tired, impossible to please, show a change in personality, or seem unable to concentrate at about 11:00 A.M. and again sometime between 3:30 P.M. and 5:00 P.M.? We find that an inordinate number of allergic children appear to have hypoglycemia. Fortunately the hypoglycemic and allergic symptoms both tend to subside when certain children respond favorably to comprehensive allergy care. (See Sidney, Chapter 28.)

Drs. William Philpott and Dwight Kalita discuss their observation in their book.[6] They note that the blood sugar of some children changes dramatically due to exposure to allergenic substances. They suggest that in these cases the pancreas can be the area of the body affected by allergies. In other words, instead of developing asthma after eating a problematic food, some people develop an alteration in the insulin production of their pancreas, causing a temporary abnormal lowering of their blood sugar. If the pancreas is affected instead of the lung, a child can develop low blood sugar instead of

6. William Philpott, M.D. and Dwight Kalita, M.D., *Brain Allergies: The Psychonutrient Connection* and *Victory Over Diabetes* (see bibliography).

SEAN

Before mold test:
Handwriting normal
PFM normal
Pulse normal

ИАƎS

During reaction
to mold allergy test:
PFM decreased
Pulse increased
Handwriting backward
and written right to left

SEAN

After correct
mold allergy treatment:
Handwriting normal
PFM elevated
Pulse normal

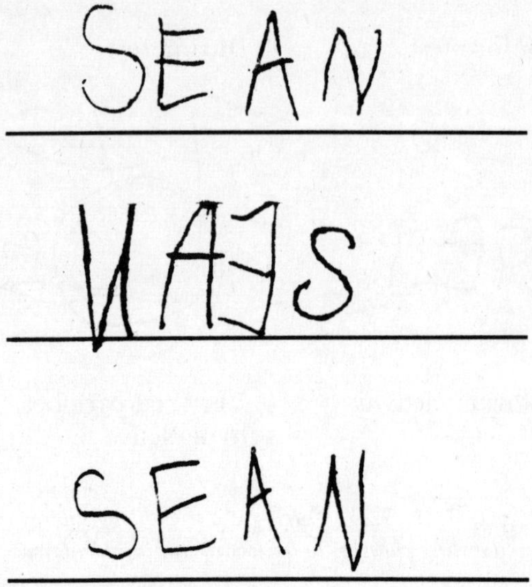

Figures 3.24–3.26. A learning-disabled child demonstrates writing in mirror-images during allergy extract treatment.

Baseline 1234 26 78 9 0

After exposure 1 3 4 [6 9 0 1 1 3] [8 0 0

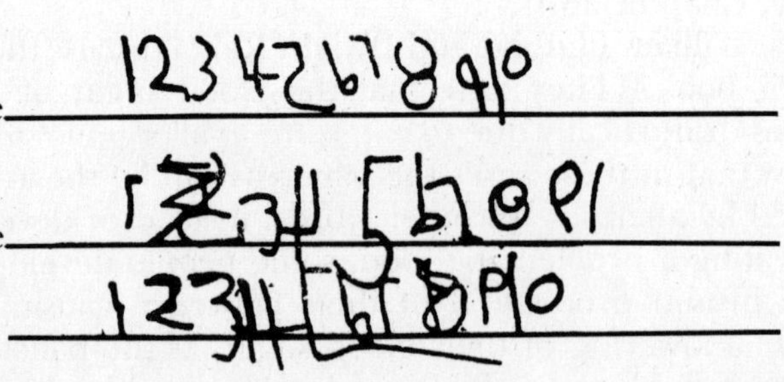

Figures 3.27–3.28. Notice this child's inability to write numbers correctly minutes after exposure to cleaning fluid.

Before mold test   During mold test   After mold test

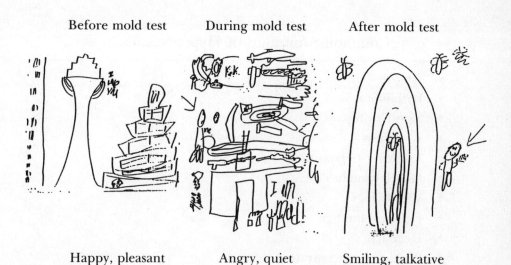

Happy, pleasant   Angry, quiet   Smiling, talkative

Figures 3.29–3.31. Personality changes during allergy extract treatment are noticeable through drawing samples.

asthma. If an allergy can affect different areas of the body in each individual, why not the pancreas?

Dr. Philpott has studied many children who have hypoglycemia. He found that some children develop a sudden drop in their blood sugar when they are skin-tested for an allergy. These children often respond, as do patients who have classical asthma or hay fever, to appropriate comprehensive allergy and environmental therapy.

Hypoglycemia is one example that clearly illustrates how the beautiful balancing that automatically takes place in healthy bodies can sometimes fail. When our innate system of checks and balances works improperly, hypoglycemia can develop.

Most substances in our blood must be present within a specific range, which is called normal. When anything is either too low or too high, some marvelous biological factors come into play to bring everything into balance again. When hypoglycemia occurs, however, it indicates that these biological changes need a bit of fine-tuning. The blood sugar should ideally range between 80 and 120 mg/cc. If it is below 80 or above 120, there can be a problem. In very simple terms, if your fasting blood sugar is too high, or above 120 mg/cc, you might have diabetes. If that blood sugar is too low, or below 60 mg/cc, you probably have hypoglycemia.

TABLE 3.1
Common Symptoms of Hypoglycemia

- Fatigue
- Irritability
- Mood swings
- Weakness
- Excessive perspiration
- Muscle twitches
- Wiggly legs
- Extreme hunger
- Headaches
- Problems concentrating
- Dizziness
- Anxiety
- Heart palpitation

To illustrate what happens, let's imagine you ate a hot fudge sundae. This quickly causes a surge in your blood sugar level. A silent alarm goes to your pancreas saying, "We must immediately correct this deluge of glucose." The message indicates a need for more insulin to lower the blood sugar level back to the normal range. Usually just the right amount of insulin is released and everything is fine. But in hypoglycemics the pancreas can be too exuberant and too much insulin is released. If the mark is overshot, the blood sugar can dip too low, causing symptoms of hypoglycemia. Then another silent signal goes to the sugar storehouse in the liver saying, "Please release more sugar into the blood as soon as possible." In this way the blood sugar level is again brought into the normal range and a proper glucose balance is restored.

A low blood sugar level is not always due to an enthusiastic pancreas. The liver may be nonresponsive. The release of sugar may be delayed or the liver may not have enough sugar in storage. The result is the same: The body's blood sugar falls below the normal range.

If the blood sugar level in humans falls below 60 mg/cc, it can cause the brain to act sluggish or confused so that it becomes difficult to think, learn, remember, or act appropriately. Some children have this problem and learn poorly every day. They can't remember, get tired, become irritable, or misbehave, usually late in the morning and again late in the afternoon. Sometimes a small snack, maybe a tablespoon of some type of nut or a few carrot sticks, midmorning and midafternoon, will prevent the unnatural dip in blood sugar and improve a child's scholastic performance, as well as provide a sense of well-being.

One must be cautious about eating candy or sweet fruit as a snack, because an enthusiastic pancreas might produce too much insulin too quickly, thus allowing the blood sugar to dip too quickly and too much. For this reason it is better to snack on a vegetable, nut, rice cake, seeds, a hard-boiled egg, cheese, or a protein such as meat. Be certain to select a food item that does not cause a known allergic reaction.

As in much of medicine, what you've just read is not unanimously agreed upon among doctors. Some believe that a single fruit as a snack will not cause any problem. The bottom line is which snack seems best to prevent or relieve your child's symptoms.

When we obtain a five-hour Glucose Tolerance Test (GTT), certain children appear to have obvious hypoglycemia. They often develop typical symptoms at the same time that their blood sugar drops. The reactions usually occur about three to four hours after they drink a glucose test solution made of corn sugar or dextrose and flavored with lemon.

Surprisingly we also see a rather large number of children who appear to act hypoglycemic every day at the same time, but their blood sugar is perfectly normal. We also give them a snack and in a few minutes they, too, act normal. It appears there is still much we do not know about hypoglycemia. Maybe they have hypoglycemia that is unrelated to the sugar, corn, and citric flavor in the beverage commonly used when a GTT is performed. Others may have hypoglycemialike symptoms because they are addicted to a certain food. If that food has not been eaten, or they need their "fix," they may have withdrawal symptoms.

There are other factors, however, that might explain why some children appear to have hypoglycemic symptoms in spite of a normal GTT. It can be due to the time when their blood samples are taken. For example, suppose a child becomes tired and irritable at 11:15 A.M. but the next blood is not drawn until 11:30. In that fifteen minutes a compliant liver may have released enough sugar so that by 11:30 the blood sugar is again in the normal range. For this reason when a GTT is performed, you must insist that a blood sample be quickly taken at the very time your child is complaining or acting hypoglycemic. This greatly increases the chance of documenting a low blood sugar problem.

One other common cause of confusion is the traditional three-hour GTT. If the blood sugar does not fall until four hours after a child eats sugar, a three-hour test will miss the diagnosis. A five-hour test, however, would possibly provide proof.

Some physicians justifiably disagree about the value of the GTT, because it is not a natural challenge that mimics real life. Children rarely drink a large amount of a very sugary solution on an empty stomach and then stop eating for the next five hours. This in no way simulates a normal eating pattern, but this is how a typical GTT is conducted. In addition a GTT indicates that about 25 percent of normal, healthy people are hypoglycemic, when they supposedly are not. As with most medical tests, a GTT does not always provide the final correct answer.

Because this test is not natural, some physicians suggest that it is more sensible to eat a typical meal and then check the blood sugar at various intervals to see how the pancreas responds. Even better, try to obtain a blood sugar level at the very time when symptoms are evident. This would help detect hypoglycemia related to foods other than sugar and simulate what happens in real life.

If eating frequent small snacks quickly reverses the moodiness, irritability, or fatigue noted when no food has been eaten for several hours, this suggests that hypoglycemia might be a problem. If this relieves your child's symptoms, it provides a sensible solution, even if the GTT or blood sugar indicates that there is no hypoglycemia. Until we know more, if snacks help, use them.

Your doctor can write a note for school so that your child can eat every two hours or more often if necessary. This is truly a common problem and one frequently unrecognized reason for daily poor school performance late in the morning or afternoon. If a child eats no breakfast, however, the symptoms might be evident earlier in the morning.

A Young Adult With Hypoglycemia

Paul

At fifteen years of age, Paul came to see us because he was bright but doing poorly in school. He was always tired and he had trouble concentrating. He had no allergic relatives, but his mother said he could also sleep anyplace, anytime.

Before Paul's office visit he had tried our Multiple Food Elimination Diet and after the first week he was more even-tempered. During the second week, after he ate chocolate, his ears became red and he became irritable. When he added milk back into his diet, he seemed grumpy and his knees hurt. None of the foods, however, seemed to cause him to become sleepy.

His mother said he had mild nose allergies and tended to have wiggly legs and red earlobes. When he was younger, he cried easily and had nightmares. He often complained about knee aches and headaches. The key clue, however, finally came when one teacher commented that late in the afternoon his mood often changed and he tended to become impatient and even angry. This portion of his history suggested that he possibly had hypoglycemia, in addition to some other less commonly recognized forms of allergy.

During P/N allergy testing he developed red ears, a headache, and seemed more tired than usual during the oat, dust, and mite test. He was extremely tired when we tested for histamine and corn. Corn also caused wiggly legs. When we tested him for milk at 11:50 A.M., he was exceedingly tired. His blood sugar dropped to 67 mg/cc. At 3:40 P.M. he developed a headache, and at that time his blood sugar was 69 mg/cc. In spite of the fact that his blood sugar was not below 60 mg/cc., on both occasions shortly after he ate a snack, he immediately perked up and was more alert. This suggested that his fatigue might not be related to the item being allergy tested, but possibly due to hypoglycemia.

We therefore ordered a GTT. During this test he became tired and slow by 10:45 A.M. He commented that he felt the way he did at school. Unfortunately no blood sample was taken at that time. His blood sugars fifteen minutes before and after that time were normal. At 11:30 A.M., however, his blood sugar dropped to only 58 mg/cc.

We believe that at least part of Paul's poor school performance was related to a combination of hypoglycemia and allergy. He began to eat small snacks every two hours while he was in school and he also received allergy extract therapy. He no longer had problems staying awake and alert in school.

Do You Spend Your Whole Day Feeding Your Child?

Some children are always famished. They eat one snack and meal after another. It is not a craving for a particular food, but for any food.

Sometimes this type of problem is hypoglycemia. But it also could be, for example, a thyroid or pancreatic problem, parasites, an emotional or nutritional problem, or even an allergy. Sometimes children are so hungry we can barely find time to skin-test them because they must eat every hour or so. At times this intense food craving is due to a food sensitivity. Surprisingly it can even be due to a mold allergy. We often find that after children receive allergy extract treatment for the foods they eat and for molds, in particular, they stop begging for more food and eat more normally.

Alcoholism and Obesity

Many children discussed in this book have relatives who are alcoholic or obese. Ecologically oriented physicians often care for environmentally ill adults who are, at times, thought to be alcoholic because they are addicted, in particular, to the type of grains used in the preparation of their favorite alcoholic beverage. For example, some men find they feel unwell whenever they drink beer. Most beer is made from corn, but if these same individuals drink Michelob or Budweiser, which are derived from rice, they may notice no adverse effects. It is possible that the corn in beer, not the alcohol, causes symptoms, such as headaches, in some individuals. The grain can also cause the craving, leading to the alcoholism.[7]

Three unusual but scientifically unconfirmed observations have been noted in relation to alcoholism:

- Individuals at AA meetings often have a positive allergy history.
- Some very allergic adolescents appear to become addicted to alcohol after their first drink.
- Some alcoholics have found that they feel and act drunk, even though they did not drink any alcohol. They literally act drunk after they eat the grain that was used as the source grain in their favorite alcoholic drink.

Some individuals are obese because they tend to have inordinate cravings for common fattening foods, such as wheat, dairy, corn, or sugar. Sometimes very overweight women find they have repeatedly

7. Theron Randolph, M.D., *An Alternative Approach To Allergies* (New York: Harper & Row, 1989).

and diligently dieted without success. Once they detect, for example, that they have a wheat sensitivity, some find that they can lose weight easily for the first time. They merely stop eating the one problem food to which they were sensitive and their weight not only goes down but it stays down. Again, sometimes nutritive deficits are the cause of inordinate appetites. There are many reasons for obesity, and emotional problems are often only part of the problem.[8]

Drs. Theron Randolph, Marshall Mandell, and Joseph Beaseley have all written informative practical books that provide invaluable insight to help individuals who have alcoholism or obesity problems.[9]

8. Jonathan Wright, M.D., *Dr. Wright's Guide to Healing With Nutrition* (see bibliography).
9. Marshall Mandell, M.D., *Dr. Mandell's 5-Day Allergy Relief System* (New York: Pocket Books, 1981) and *It's Not Your Fault You're Fat* (New York: Harper & Row, 1983); Joseph Beasley, M.D., *How to Defeat Alcoholism* (New York: Times Books, 1989); Randolph, *An Alternative Approach to Allergies*.

PART TWO

GENERAL CLUES TO ALLERGY IN VARIOUS AGE GROUPS

CHAPTER 4

Infant Allergies

In essence the approach to an infant allergy is the same as it is for children or adults. One merely has to ask, Is the infant worse after eating, when indoors or outdoors, or if near chemicals or certain odors? With a little observation and increased awareness the answers sometimes become obvious. Infant allergies often date back to before birth.

AN UNHAPPY ALLERGIC INFANT

Aaron

Aaron was an attractive eight-month-old little blue-eyed blond baby, but he appeared to be extremely unhappy and irritable. His mother looked worried, distraught, and exhausted.

His mother noted he was overactive (as are many allergic infants), even before he was born. His mother tried to do everything right when she was pregnant. She drank three to four glasses of milk every day so that she would have a very healthy baby. Her unborn baby, however, seemed to hiccup much more than she thought was normal and he wiggled and moved constantly in the uterus.

After he was born, she was surprised, as was his pediatrician, because he walked before eight months of age. Most infants don't walk until about twelve to fifteen months. As an infant Aaron simply did not sleep. He was up three or four times every night. His mother said he never sat still and that he wiggled constantly. He would not tolerate quiet cuddling. The only way she could keep him quiet was to repeatedly bounce him up and down. He tended to whine and fuss. He had one temper tantrum after another. He drooled so much his bib was constantly soaked. His nose was always stuffy. He had dark eye circles and his eyes were often glassy or glazed, especially during his emotional outbursts. He coughed, wheezed, and had too much mucus. He made clucking throat sounds and funny chest noises whenever he tried to swallow his formula. He was a gassy baby with a bloated belly and constipation.

His history strongly indicated a simple cow's milk allergy. We diagnosed a milk allergy using P/N allergy tests during this initial office visit and quickly found the "right" milk dilution for his allergy extract neutralization treatment. His mother was surprised because during that initial office visit, *for the first time in his life,* he was not restless and seemed calm and content. He even drank his next bottle without the need to be bounced constantly. In addition, the funny chest sounds he always made during his feedings suddenly stopped. His mother was amazed because he began to smile a few minutes after he was tested for milk. That night he slept all night. Within a week, and in the following months, his mother was astonished and delighted because he continued to be quiet, happy, and content. He has remained remarkably improved for over two years.

The next patient illustrates the type of infant we commonly see. Not all have such severe symptoms and not all respond as dramatically, but Bruce certainly exemplifies many of the typical characteristics that we associate with infant allergies.

A DISTRAUGHT INFANT AND FAMILY

Bruce

Bruce was seen by us at the age of six months. His mother looked almost as exhausted, ill, sad, and upset as the baby. The baby had the most distressing frown we have ever seen on any infant. His history was typical of allergic infants. He had not responded either to the conservative management of a pediatrician or to the care of a specialist in environmental medicine.

Bruce had a multitude of allergic relatives. As a fetus he kicked and hiccupped *much more* than normal. His mother was very uncomfortable during the latter part of her pregnancy. She was drinking a half gallon of milk a day at that time.

His mother described Bruce's infancy as "terrible." He screamed at times for twelve hours straight. He never slept more than a total of five hours in a twenty-four-hour period. He would nap for thirty minutes and then frantically sob for the next two hours. Even when he was sleeping, he moaned as he rolled and tossed about.

He spit up his formula, always had diarrhea, passed gas, burped repeatedly, and had puffy eyes. His parents tried several different infant formulas, but none seemed to be well tolerated.

His parents said he was extremely restless. If they placed him on the mattress, they had to pound it so that he would be thrust vigorously up and down. If they carried him, they not only had to bounce him for hours but he seemed more content if they also walked up and down a flight of stairs. His mother traversed them so often she thought she had worn holes in the steps. His parents took turns all through the night attempting to quiet him with never-ending up-and-down movements.

His mother wondered why his feet smelled and why he disliked loud sounds. By five months of age he already had typical nose allergies.

During the first office visit we tested him for a possible allergy to several infant formulas, using the newer provocation/neutralization method. As soon as his correct allergy treatment doses were found, he *immediately* stopped frowning and was happier. He slept for the entire two hours it took to drive home and, amazingly, he did not need his usual bouncing. When he was put to bed that night, he slept for a surprising additional six hours without screaming. The next morning he awoke happy for the first time! In two days, after treatment for seven items, his parents said he was 50 percent better. He was less active, and his bowel movements were less loose. In eight days he was 70 percent improved, and his foot odor was gone. By two weeks he was over 80 percent better and no longer appeared to have abdominal pain. He was sleeping fourteen hours per day. His bowel movements were formed. For the first time he could play by himself. He was calm and content and routinely awoke with delight, rather than dismay.

To accomplish this, however, his mother returned to our office frequently during the first few weeks, and we had to treat him for four different infant formulas so that he could drink a different one each day. He simply could not drink the same formula every day. When his mother began to feed him foods, each one had to be tested, treated, and, similar to his formula, fed to him no more often than every four days.

He is presently twenty-one months old and is doing very well. He rarely needs to see us. His parents have made their home more allergy-free, are feeding him a four-day rotation diet, and avoid chemicals as much as possible. In addition he is receiving his allergy extract under his tongue. Our treatment appears not only to have relieved his present allergies but we also hope we have prevented some future medical and emotional problems.

Before-Birth Symptoms of Food Allergy

Aaron's and Bruce's histories illustrate many characteristics that are typical of infant allergy (See Tables 4.1 and 4.2). Allergic infants frequently hiccup or kick excessively in the uterus. Some mothers describe their allergic unborn infants as a football player inside their abdomen. Other mothers complained that their ribs were bruised black and blue and sore because the fetus was so restless and kicked so vigorously. Some state that neither they nor their husbands could sleep because the baby kicked so hard and so often. Some mothers watched their abdomens go up and down as their infants kicked away. One mother said the unborn baby's kicking caused waves in her bath water. Another mother put an ashtray on her abdomen and showed friends that her unborn baby could kick it across the room.

Knowledgeable mothers often notice after they eat a particular food or are exposed to a certain odor that their unborn infant will suddenly start to kick or hiccup. Different foods, such as milk and dairy products, chocolate, bananas, cabbage, corn, and spicy foods, have been noted to do this. It can be any food or beverage, however.

TABLE 4.1
Common Symptoms of Allergy Before Birth

- Extreme overactivity
- Prolonged hiccupping
- Vigorous kicking
- Mother's ribs bruised

TABLE 4.2
Common Symptoms of Possible Infant Allergy

- Prolonged colic
- Excessive spitting
- Repeated vomiting
- Diarrhea and/or constipation
- Congestion of nose or chest
- Eczema or itchy rashes
- Restlessness
- Screaming or prolonged crying
- Dislike of cuddling
- Need to be walked and bounced
- Excessive drooling
- Extreme perspiration
- Excessive crib rocking
- Head banging
- Walking by seven to ten months
- Repeated ear infections
- Genital touching
- Reluctance to stay dressed
- Rapid pulse
- Demand for constant attention

By observing when an unborn infant suddenly seems extremely uncomfortable, it is often easy to think back and detect a possible offending food or odor.

One mother, for example, noted that when she picked up her husband's check in a chemically polluted office on Friday afternoons, her unborn infant kicked wildly for the next half hour. After he was born, he routinely became very active, but only when he accompanied his mother to that same polluted office.

After-Birth Symptoms of Food Allergy

After babies are born, the allergic infants often respond unfavorably to foods that their mothers loved and ate in large quantities during the pregnancy. Excess milk or dairy products are by far the most common offenders. The pattern is thought to be as follows: Before the infant is born the mother eats a food, and broken-down or partially digested particles from that food pass from her intestines into her blood and then into the blood of the baby in her uterus. This causes the baby to react. After birth the mother eats this same food and again certain food particles pass from her intestines into her blood and then these particles pass into her breast milk. The baby drinks that breast milk and again reacts. When the baby is older and he directly eats that same offending food, again these same food particles are absorbed directly from the infant's own intestines into the blood. Again reactions occur, each time from the same digested food particles. Once mothers are aware, they often repeatedly note such relationships.

A BREAST-FED INFANT WITH MILK AND OTHER ALLERGIES

Emily

Emily was only eight months old when she came to our office. Her mother had learned much from Emily's older allergic sister. If Emily's mother ate turkey, egg, chicken, soy, or nuts for lunch, she could expect Emily to have a reaction during and after the 5:00 P.M. nursing. Emily would develop a skin rash and become very discontent and refuse to sit or play. She would whine, pass gas, and want to be nursed every five minutes. This response was noticed *only* after her mother had eaten the above foods, not on other occasions. A trace of these foods in the mother's breast milk appeared to be sufficient to cause these complaints in Emily. Her mother has continued to watch Emily very carefully now because Emily is beginning to eat these foods. Emily's response to these problem foods is presently similar to, but not exactly like, the type of reaction she had in the past when she was being breast-fed. At the present time she develops a rash only if she eats these foods.

Allergic infants are frequently a challenge to feed. When allergies affect a baby who is totally breast-fed, the cause is usually the cow's milk or dairy products that the mother is ingesting. Many mothers believe or are told to drink milk and eat dairy products so that their infant will have strong bones. Of course other foods that a mother eats also can cause symptoms, but milk seems to be the prime offender. To find answers, all a mother has to do is keep some records of what she has eaten (or smelled) prior to the time when her breast-fed infant acted upset in some way. If dairy products are a problem, a calcium supplement can be prescribed by the obstetrician for the mother and the infant.

If a breast-feeding mother suspects a food such as bananas or potatoes, for example, all she has to do is eat each questionable food only every fourth day. If the suspected item is ingested on Monday and not again until Friday, a mother may notice that her infant is distraught only on Monday and Friday. These were the days when the suspected food was eaten.

Symptoms in breast-fed infants usually occur two to four hours after a mother eats a problem food. Often both the breast-feeding mother and the infant have numerous allergies to the same food. When the infant begins to eat solid food and is still continuing to breast-feed, both the mother and the infant may feel better if they both adhere to a similar four-day rotation diet. In other words if the baby and mother both eat oats only on Monday and again on Friday, for example, it is easier to see if a food is causing illness in either of them at a four-day interval.

Milk-Allergic Mothers Fall Into Several Categories

Some pregnant mothers know that milk makes them ill in some way, but they force themselves to drink it anyway so that they can have a healthy baby. These mothers can be sensitive to milk or have a lactose intolerance that causes gas and diarrhea. If they develop other medical complaints, their problems are more apt to be a milk allergy. These mothers tend to be ill in some area of their body whenever they ingest an excessive amount of dairy products.

Others do not recognize their own milk sensitivity. They just know they hate milk and love cheese, yogurt, or ice cream. These mothers eat the dairy products that they enjoy and often continue with their own "learn to live with it"–type medical problems. For example, many mothers also have recurrent headaches or intestinal complaints, but they do not realize that the cause could be milk products. In addition to making themselves ill in some way when they are pregnant, they may unknowingly contribute to their infant's discontent by consuming cheese and yogurt, even though they totally avoid milk.

The last group of milk-sensitive mothers includes those whose favorite foods include *every* dairy item. A craving for milk and dairy products, in every form, strongly suggests a milk sensitivity in any individual. These mothers again often have some unrecognized form of milk allergy, causing, for example, nasal stuffiness, coughing, irritability, depression, fatigue, muscle aches, tight joints, or difficulty in thinking clearly.

To investigate this type of allergy, a mother who routinely eats some dairy should stop *all* milk products *in every form* for four days. When no dairy product has been ingested during the previous four days, on an empty stomach binge solely on milk and plain cottage cheese or "the" favorite dairy product. For the first time the effect of milk or dairy may be clearly evident to that mother. Most milk or dairy-product reactions occur within an hour, but they can cause some delayed medical problems up to twenty-four hours later in some sensitive individuals. These late reactions can include eczema, earaches, acne, colitis, joint pain, canker sores, or the need to urinate too frequently in the daytime or at night.

Which Type of Milk Is Best for Infants?

For many reasons the best milk for infants is breast milk. There is an immense amount of individuality in babies, and some do well on typical milk formulas, others on soy-milk preparations, and some on either powered or liquid goat's milk. Your doctor will have to help you decide which to try if your baby seems to have a feeding problem.

If untreated or raw cow's milk is allowed to sit, it separates into two layers. The top, which is clear and slightly yellow, is called whey. The bottom becomes clumped white curds and is called casein. It is used to make cottage cheese.

Various infant milk formulas are prepared from these different parts of milk, so the response of each baby may be dependent upon exactly what is contained in each formula. A very allergic infant can be challenging. Some seem to be unable to tolerate any form of either the usual milk or soy formulas.

If an infant also can't tolerate sugar or glucose in dextrose water sold in drugstores in the form of Pedialyte, the problem could be a corn sensitivity. Corn, in the form of dextrose, is frequently used to sweeten commercial milk or soy formulas. If only cow's milk and/or corn are a problem, the answer is easy. Ask your doctor if the baby can be placed on a formula that contains no milk or corn, such as Nursoy liquid or I-Soyalac formula. Nursoy powder contains corn, so it can't be used in corn-sensitive infants (see Appendix A).

A new preparation called Ricelyte contains a natural fruit flavor and rice-syrup solids instead of dextrose or corn. If a baby tolerates this well, but not Pedialyte, this suggests a corn sensitivity. If an infant takes Pedialyte well, but does poorly on Ricelyte, this suggests a rice sensitivity. Both are available without a prescription to help relieve diarrhea.

Alimentum and Nutramigen are similar in that they both contain casein that has been altered by hydrolysis, so they are both better tolerated by some unusually allergic infants. This new corn-free formula, Alimentum, appears to be well tolerated by some allergic infants. Alimentum contains some soy oil but no corn, whereas Nutramigen contains corn oil and corn syrup. These differences might make some infants tolerate one better than the other. Good Start contains both whey protein and soy lecithin, so it may or may not be tolerated by some milk- or soy-sensitive infants. These special formulations can be quite expensive.

Formula or Feeding Problems in Infants

Some allergic infants push away their formula but eat food vigorously. This often indicates a sensitivity to some ingredient in the formula. Some spit up too much and too often. Other allergic babies vomit so vigorously that the diagnosis of pyloric stenosis may be considered. Some have colic, not for the first three or four months but for the entire first year. Sometimes these infants never have a normal bowel movement. They have either diarrhea or constipation. Although diarrhea could indicate a milk sensitivity, many other digestive problems can also cause this. In contrast some infants or older children have chronic constipation, which is more apt to be an unrecognized cow's milk or dairy allergy. When all dairy is stopped, they often improve.

Remember, infants must have calcium, so if no dairy or soy milk are ingested, check with your doctor. For calcium supplementation Neocalglucon liquid is recommended. The mint flavor of this can cause symptoms in some infants and children. One tablespoon provides 345 milligrams of calcium. An infant dose is usually one teaspoon, five times a day. The dose varies according to the weight of the infant.

Excessive Perspiration and Drooling

It is not unusual for allergic infants to perspire so much that their clothing must be entirely changed several times a day. Some also tend to drool so excessively that they require a body-length bib. Some allergic infants use one bib after another, all day long. More than one mother has had to place a towel under her infant's head because the saliva was so copious. One must wonder if these copious secretions are efforts on the part of the body to excrete an excess of unwanted substances.

Early Hyperactivity

Allergic infants can be so hyperactive that they begin to walk earlier than normal. A few infants even walk at seven months. Many over-active infants walk before ten months of age. They can sometimes barely be held because they arch their head back and walk up their parent's chest. They sometimes rock their cribs about the room or bounce them off the walls until the crib is broken or the wall is dented. Some bang their heads against the floors, crib, or walls at times until they are bloody. Some parents have to turn the crib upside down to make a cage to keep the baby from falling out. These infants may be sending an early message. Maybe they will be the problem school-children of tomorrow. They sometimes become the children who cannot sit still in school, cannot concentrate, and cannot learn. If their food problems are recognized during infancy, some hyperac-tivity and behavior and learning problems in later life could possibly be prevented.

Sleep Problems

Allergic infants tend to sleep very poorly, and sometimes this lasts for years. Some sleep for less than an hour, then scream, not cry, for the next four hours. The result is a baby who frowns or does not smile and parents who are desperate and exhausted. Allergic infants are typically not content just to lie still or be quietly held or rocked in their parent's arms. They often need to be walked and bounced, hour after hour, day after day, week after week, and month after month.

Nose Allergies

An inordinate number of allergic infants have stuffy noses. This can not only interfere with their ability to breathe and suck from the breast or bottle, but nose allergies predispose infants to one infection after another. Allergic swelling makes the tissues of the nose, ear, chest, and sinus passageways more prone to infection.

Ear Problems

Allergic infants, in particular, often tend to accumulate fluid between their eardrums and their nose. This fluid can interfere with hearing and subsequent speech. When this fluid becomes infected, they require constant antibiotics. The ear problems often start at less than six months, and some have one ear infection every three or four weeks. These infants often have tubes surgically placed through their eardrums before the age of two. It is possible that the early recognition of the cause of nose allergies can completely resolve some chronic ear problems in infants, toddlers, and children, eliminating the need for surgery.

Bright Red Buttocks

Many allergic infants have scalded red buttocks; the condition appears suddenly when a highly allergenic food is passed in their bowel movements. If parents will keep a few records of what was eaten in the few hours before the buttocks look scarlet, the culprit food may be obvious. If an infant is totally breast-fed, think about the foods eaten by the mother.

It is not easy to find either baby powders or disposable diapers that do not smell of perfume. The odor can cause some infants to have allergic symptoms. Use plain cornstarch, providing your baby is not sensitive to corn.

Some allergic infants are not able to tolerate the newer, supremely absorbent-type diapers. Some allergic babies even have difficulty with cotton diapers from a laundry service. Unfortunately, mothers of such extremely chemically sensitive infants may have to use 100 percent cotton diapers, which they must personally launder because their infants can't tolerate the usual laundry soaps. Dimple diapers are new fitted reusable diapers that are 100 percent cotton.

Eczema

Eczematous itchy rashes often appear on an allergic infant's cheeks, around the wrists, and in roundish patches about the body. Eventually, classical infant skin allergies tend to localize in the creases of the arms or legs. These are often caused by dust, molds, or certain foods. Laundry soaps and fabric softeners, as well as wool, polyester, or acrylic clothing also contribute to some infant skin irritation. These little babies can be immensely unhappy because of the constant itch. (See Figure 2.7, page 57.)

AN INFANT WITH SEVERE ECZEMA

Katie

Little Katie was seven months old when her parents brought her to see us because she had developed severe eczema when she was only one month old. Clues of a possible milk allergy dated back to when she was in the uterus. Her mother was very perceptive and on her own recognized that whenever she ate ice cream while she was pregnant with Katie, the baby kicked and hiccupped much more than usual.

After Katie was born, she tended to be extremely overactive, wiggly, and restless. She always slept poorly. She was totally breast-fed, and in time Katie's mother again noted that if she ate oats, carrots, or celery, the baby's skin rash worsened. If she ate a strict diet, avoiding these foods, Katie's skin cleared.

When Katie was six months of age, therefore, her mother sought the help of a traditional allergist to determine if other foods were related to her baby's skin rash. Although he confirmed the diagnosis of severe eczema, he felt that the mother's observations about foods were completely irrelevant and were unrelated in any way to the infant's skin allergy. He said, however, that Katie's blood and prick allergy tests indicated definite reactions to many foods, dust, molds, and pets.

Two weeks before Katie came to our office, her mother stopped breast-feeding and found that Katie could not tolerate several different formulas because they caused excessive spitting up and hives.

During the first visit Katie was tested for Alimentum, rice, yeast, and dust. By the next morning her skin looked less red, but she was still itchy and continued to be restless in her sleep. The second day we tested Katie for mites, a mold, squash, apple, and oats. That night she slept well for eleven hours, not her usual eight. She awoke without itching and her skin was definitely much better. Her mother said she was 95 percent better. Four months later she remained 75 percent better.

Coughing, Bronchiolitis, and Asthma

Allergic chest problems in infants cause noisy breathing. Some develop wheezing sounds, with or without infection. Bronchiolitis is common in allergic infants and sometimes precedes asthma by a few years. Excess coughing, with or without infection, can be allergic in nature, even during the infant period. If proper allergy and environmental precautions are taken early in life, it should be possible to prevent, lessen, or possibly delay the onset of asthma.

Pulse Changes

We have found that many allergic infants appear to have an increased pulse if they eat or smell some item to which they are sensitive. Normally an infant's pulse is about 110 beats per minute until about the age of six months and about 100 at the age of one year. After infants eat a problem food, their pulse can suddenly increase to 140 beats per minute or more. By taking a quiet infant's pulse over the heart or the left chest for a full minute, both before and again fifteen minutes after eating, it is sometimes easy to detect some problem foods. An inexpensive stethoscope from a medical supply store can make it easy to count the heartbeat when the baby is quiet. (See Chapter 10.)

A SENSITIVITY DISCOVERED BY PULSE CHANGES

Donny

I recall one infant who was responding very well to allergy treatment and then suddenly developed asthma and a rapid pulse. This was evident mainly when he was in his own home and not in my office. A leak was discovered in the gas furnace at home, and when it was repaired, his pulse returned to normal and his asthma was relieved. The normal pulse in our office and elevation at home, even when he was sleeping, helped us to pinpoint that some change in his house had created this new medical problem.

Another infant had an elevated pulse whenever he was in a moldy place. After appropriate mold therapy, his pulse decreased to a normal level.

Common Causes of Typical Infant Allergy

Some babies develop rashes or other medical problems because of the chemicals or perfumes in certain diapers or body powders. Others have difficulty when they crawl on new chemically laden synthetic carpets or old dusty, moldy woolen rugs. Some scream if they nap on a bedspread that was dried with a fabric softener. Some become ill from the odor of cleaning solutions, waxes, furniture polish, aerosols, or disinfectants. Some can't be held without screaming, simply because their parent is wearing an acrylic sweater.

Personality changes or physical illness have also been noted shortly after the use of fumigants, pesticides, or termiticides in or around homes. The scope of contacts that can cause infants to feel unwell and unhappy appears to be endless.

Some infants seem well until their family moves into a trailer. Trailers are commonly contaminated with an extreme amount of formaldehyde and other chemicals. In a few weeks or months a previously happy active baby can become tired, irritable, withdrawn, overactive, and prone to temper tantrums. Other family members may also feel ill or behave in a different manner because of the chemicals used in trailer construction. (See Chapter 13.)

It is possible to make changes in a home and in an infant's diet, as discussed in detail in Parts Three and Five of this book. These measures should help to decrease your infant's present symptoms and perhaps prevent some future ones. Be sure to discuss any planned changes, however, with your infant's doctor.

Serious Severe Infant Allergies

Very rarely an infant will collapse after being fed a food or drinking milk. Some babies can suddenly become weak, pale, and perspire. This can indicate anaphylactic shock and needs *immediate* medical attention. These types of extreme food allergies can be caused by such foods as peanuts, eggs, buckwheat, or fish. It is extremely difficult or impossible at this time to treat these sensitivities. Most allergists would not attempt to treat an infant or child for foods that cause anaphylaxis, although on rare occasion such therapy has been shown to be both safe and successful. The blood of these infants would usually indicate a very elevated IgE-type RAST result for such an offending food.

Common Misconceptions About Infant Allergy

Are Infants Too Young to Be Treated for Allergies?

It is thought that it is difficult to determine the cause of an infant allergy because these patients are so small. Sometimes it is embarrassingly easy. Just stop cow's milk and try soy, or stop all formulas that contain corn (dextrose). Be sure you discuss any change, however, with your infant's doctor. Babies must have adequate nutrition or they won't grow and develop normally.

Can Infants Be Treated With Allergy Extract?

If simple dietary changes do not relieve an infant's symptoms, it is possible for physicians who are knowledgeable about environmental medicine to skin-test and treat infants for food or other allergenic substances. Parents are often told to wait until their infant is three years or older before they can be treated. It is possible, however, to test and treat infant allergies at any age. Some babies simply can't wait several months or years before receiving appropriate help. Fortunately they tend to improve much more quickly than adults. The key is to find an allergist or specialist in pediatric allergy or environmental medicine who is experienced in testing and treating infant food allergies (see Appendix D).

Are Infants Too Young to Develop Pollen Allergies?

Some allergists are taught that young infants are not supposed to be allergic to dust, molds, or pollen. Unfortunately infants don't know that, and some develop hay fever, asthma, or personality changes when they are near freshly cut grass, in a moldy basement, or in a dusty home. They can develop classical symptoms at less than one year of age. Alert parents can readily detect whether outside pollen or pollution have a bad effect on their infant. These are the babies who develop symptoms or appear unwell as soon as they are taken outside during the pollen season or whenever the air is polluted with

chemicals. We cared for a precocious one-year-old boy who immediately screamed and said his arms hurt when he stepped off the
plane into polluted Los Angeles. He was all right indoors, but whenever he was taken outside, he said, "Hurt," as he pulled on his skin.

Most babies remain fine if they stay indoors, unless they are sensitive to house dust or molds inside their home. Some seem to have
seasonal difficulty

- in the early spring when the trees pollinate;
- in the middle of the summer when the grass needs cutting;
- on damp, wet days or in the early fall when molds are in the
  air;
- in the late summer or early fall when weeds are evident.

Can Infants Have Brain Allergies?

Many physicians do not believe that a child's or adult's nervous system
could be affected by an allergy. They would consider the idea that
an infant could have brain allergies to be ridiculous. Unfortunately
some babies in allergic families appear to become irritable, hyperactive, agitated, aggressive, angry, and even depressed from foods
or common allergenic items. Although foods are the most common
cause of typical and unusual forms of allergy in infancy, dust, molds,
pollen, pets, and chemical odors must also be considered.

Are Infant Nose Allergies Due to Dust, to Pollen, or to Foods?

Many doctors believe that an itchy nose indicates mainly an allergy
to something in the air such as pollen, molds, or dust. Foods certainly
are a commonly missed cause of classical nose allergies and should
be suspected in any infant or youngster who continues to have nose
symptoms in spite of appropriate allergy care. This is particularly
true if antihistamines are needed on a daily basis.

Is Bottle Feeding as Good as Breast-Feeding?

For many reasons breast-feeding is certainly the very best way to feed
an infant. It does not, however, assure that an infant will not develop
an allergy. Although breast-feeding has been shown to decrease nose
and chest allergies, eczema is as prevalent in breast-fed infants as it

is in those who are bottle-fed. Other forms of allergy can also develop, especially if a mother craves and binges on certain highly allergenic foods, such as milk or chocolate.

Can Baby Vaccines Be a Problem?

It is possible for babies or children who are allergic to eggs to react to the MMR (mumps, measles, and rubella) or influenza vaccines. Although extremely rare, any vaccine grown on the skin cells of chicks can conceivably place an extremely egg- or chicken-sensitive child at risk during immunization.

If Infants Stop Milk for a Few Months, Is Their Allergy Outgrown?

If an infant avoids a food for several months or a year or two, it does not guarantee that a food sensitivity will be outgrown. The majority of children (about 75 percent) will continue to be allergic. Sometimes, because the allergy appears in another part of the body, it can be difficult to recognize that the previous problem food is still causing symptoms. For example, if milk causes eczema in an infant, it is typically discontinued in all forms for several months. When it is added back, it may not appear to be a problem at first. Then the milk might cause a stuffy or runny nose, asthma, or intestinal problems. No one realizes that the milk is again the problem because it no longer causes eczema as it did before.

The following child typifies how often the clues of a persistent milk allergy can be missed. Our bodies give us clear messages, but we need to listen.

A YOUNGSTER WITH OVERACTIVITY SINCE BEFORE BIRTH

Elisha

Elisha had behavior problems when she came to see me at the age of four years. Elisha was so extremely overactive when she was in the uterus that her parents simply did not know what to do. They finally decided to play music using earphones stretched across her mother's abdomen.

After birth Elisha was an irritable, screaming, and unhappy little baby who had dark eye circles and a runny nose. She could not be cuddled. She had to be bounced and walked, always with a diaper because she spit up or vomited so frequently. She would cry when she was hungry. Then for the next thirty minutes after each milk formula she screamed until she either had diarrhea or vomited. Her clothing needed to be changed three to four times a day because she perspired so heavily. When her milk formula was replaced with soy, at the age of four months, the severe colic finally subsided. On one occasion she accidentally ate some cereal that contained milk powder and she immediately developed severe abdominal discomfort.

In the later part of the first year she tended to jump excessively in her crib. By the age of one year the ear problems began. As a toddler she screamed wildly whenever her parents told her no. Her parents thought it was the "terrible twos or threes." She had three temper tantrums and hitting episodes each day, each lasting about thirty minutes. The dark eye circles and the puffiness under her eyes persisted.

Similar to many allergic infants, Elisha stopped soy milk and began to drink whole milk again at about the age of one year. This caused no apparent difficulty, in spite of her previous milk-formula problems.

She spoke very late and very unclearly. She seemed to understand, but she could not express herself. (This is called apraxia.)

When her parents finally discontinued all milk again at the age of three and one-half years during an allergy diet, she improved remarkably. Her behavior became calm and her disposition was suddenly sweet and lovable. However, Elisha's symptoms returned shortly after her mother decided to allow Elisha to have limited amounts of milk each day because she was concerned about a possible calcium deficiency.

At the age of four years some relatives saw our 1988 *Donahue* show about food allergies. The parents again wondered if Elisha might have a milk allergy. The family saw a traditional allergist, but his evaluation indicated that Elisha did not have allergies. A scratch test for milk allergy was negative. In spite of the allergist's conclusion, however, her parents decided, on their own, to discontinue all milk and dairy again for two weeks. When they gave her milk again, she was sick within thirty minutes. They wondered if milk was the reason she continued to have nose, ear, and hearing problems. Was milk the cause of her excess perspiration? Her father said she "sweated like a pig."

When Elisha initially saw us, she could not sit through a meal or a television program. Her speech was unclear. After three days of allergy testing and treatment, she was 50 percent improved. Her milk-allergy skin test indicated a definite sensitivity. Within three weeks she was 65 percent better. Her disposition, excessive perspiration, tantrums, and eye circles were less evident. When she ate excessive amounts of sugar or candy at Halloween, these symptoms recurred briefly. She now tolerates milk and dairy products, in the normal amount, without difficulty, but only if they are ingested no more often then every four days. Several months after treatment her mother states that her behavior and concentration continue to be greatly improved.

For a few days before her initial visit to see us she was given a small amount of both milk and egg. She not only became much more active but she could no longer communicate as well as before. She reverted to baby talk. She spoke more loudly than usual, unclearly, and could not say certain sounds correctly. It appeared that these foods might be affecting her hearing, as well as her ability to speak clearly.

In retrospect there was clear and abundant evidence repeatedly during infancy and later on, that milk in particular caused major health and emotional problems in Elisha. After four months on comprehensive treatment she continues to be 65 percent improved. In time her mother has noticed that Christmas candy again caused her speech to become unclear. Dusty decorations caused bright red ears and cheeks. The odor of marking pencils or the odor of newsprint caused her eyes to water.

One Special Problem in Infants: Gastroesophageal Reflux

Most infants spit up a bit after their bottle. Some babies, however, spit up and vomit excessively. There are many causes for such a medical problem. In some affected infants the vomiting can be so extreme that it interferes with their growth. One such digestive problem is called gastroesophageal reflux. This diagnosis can be confirmed by newer specialized X-ray techniques. *Reflux* simply means that the infant's formula or food can pass easily into the stomach but that the lower end of the esophagus or food tube does not tighten properly after swallowing. The result is that the formula can back up and be vomited vigorously from the mouth. As the formula backs up, a little can accidentally get into the lungs on its way to the mouth. When the formula falls into the lungs by mistake, it can cause an aspiration pneumonia.

When infants begin to have this type of problem, the doctor frequently suggests that the formula be thickened with cereal, that the nipple holes be made smaller, and that the baby be propped upright after feedings. Sometimes antacids are helpful because they neutralize the excess stomach acid. Sedatives are prescribed to relax the stomach so that there is less spasm and less chance of reflux. These methods usually provide relief, and by the time an infant is six months old, most affected infants no longer have this problem.

If the reflux persists, however, some babies may vomit so continuously that they do not grow and develop properly. At that point surgery may be considered. One common form of surgical treatment is called the Nissen procedure. This means that the upper end of the stomach is wrapped around the lower end of the esophagus like a lasso. This prevents the baby from vomiting. So that the infant can eat, the surgeon creates an artificial hole in the stomach and places a tube through that opening. The mother then uses a large syringe that contains milk formula to feed her baby. She empties the syringe full of milk through the artificial tube so that the milk formula passes directly into the infant's stomach.

Some infants, however, vomit as vigorously through the artificial stomach tube as they did through the mouth. This can occur if the infant is sensitive to some component in the previous formula that is now being forced through the stomach tube. We have seen two infants who appeared to improve and no longer needed the Nissen procedure after we detected and treated their corn sensitivity.

The Nissen procedure is not a one-stage surgical procedure. Once the infant improves, the stomach tube must be removed and the hole in the stomach must be closed. Then the infant often needs the lower end of the esophagus stretched so that food can pass normally into the stomach again. If months have passed without normal feeding, an infant may have problems learning to suck and chew normally. In addition, bowel obstructions can occur after the early or later surgery due to adhesions or intestinal scarring.

The cause of reflux is not always known, but if conservative measures are not helpful, the diagnosis of allergy should be considered. An analysis of the formulas or foods that caused vomiting may provide the essential clue. This certainly should be investigated by a physician who knows how to test and treat food allergy before surgical procedures are contemplated.

The following patient illustrates the types of problems that can arise in rare food-sensitive infants because the diagnosis of food allergy was not suspected or recognized in a baby who had reflux.

AN INFANT WITH MANY SURGERIES

Billy

Billy had allergic relatives. Typical of many allergic children, his symptoms appeared to begin while he was still in the uterus. He kicked his mother so much and so hard that it hurt her insides and he hiccupped much more than her other children.

His parents brought him to see me because he was extremely unhappy and he was a feeding problem. They had just seen our 1987 *Donahue* show about food allergies and behavior problems. Although he was fifteen months old, he weighed only eighteen pounds. He should have weighed about that much at ten months of age. He never slept all night. He was always up from two to five times, not crying but screaming. He could never be held or cuddled. Sometimes he screamed as long as twenty hours a day.

By the age of three weeks he had a very large, tender abdomen and was constipated. His bloated abdomen could not be touched without causing him to cry. His parents' most serious concern, however, were his violent episodes of vomiting, which occurred as often as seven times a day. In spite of many formula changes, this problem did not stop. A diagnosis of gastrointestinal reflux was made but unfortunately the usual medical treatment did not help. The Nissen Fundoplication surgical procedure was performed when he was four months old. Unfortunately he continued to vomit as vigorously as before. Now, however, he vomited through the stomach tube rather than through his mouth.

By the age of six months he needed surgery again, this time for his first bowel obstruction, and by the age of seven months he had two more bowel obstructions due to adhesions, requiring more surgery. When his nurse-mother complained that the surgery did not help and made him worse, the hospital doctors refused to talk to her. They told her they would only talk to her husband. At one point they threatened Billy's mother that they would recommend that her son be placed in foster care if she kept complaining. She was made to feel that her baby's persistent problems were her fault, even though her older son's infancy had been totally uneventful. When she asked questions, she was told that she was defensive and hostile. Her husband was told by a pediatrician that his wife might be having a postpartum depression or some mental illness.

Billy's mother kept trying to tell the hospital doctors that if Billy did not eat, he was not stuffy or congested. This was a critical and most important observation. No one listened. She told them that red antibiotics or red antihistamines caused him to "go crazy," but she was assured that that was simply not possible. In retrospect, if they doubted his mother, it is perplexing why they did not simply give Billy a half teaspoon of the red antihistamines or a few drops of red food coloring and see what happened.

By the time he was seven months of age, he began to have one ear infection after another. In the ten months before he was seen in my office he had had a total of eight ear infections. Ventilation tubes were surgically placed through his eardrums when he was fifteen months old.

By the age of ten months he had asthma. By the age of eleven months he had temper tantrums at least twice a day. He was not talking or walking, but he managed to bounce his crib off the walls. If his parents tried to hold him in their arms, he walked up their chest, arched his head back, and pulled away.

After a thorough history and physical examination in our office, we decided to place him on a corn-free soy formula (I-Soyalac). Analysis of all of his previous formulas indicated they all had contained corn. Maybe corn was his problem. That afternoon he did not awaken for four hours. In the past he had never slept more than an hour or two at one time. That night he slept all night for the first time since he was two weeks old. The next morning his parents did not awaken to his usual screams but to a smiling, contented infant. That day he had fewer temper tantrums than usual and seemed much happier

Using provocation/neutralization, we subsequently videotaped his response when we skin-tested him for a corn allergy. He appeared normal until we provoked the agonizing screaming so reminiscent of the past shortly after one droplet of corn allergy extract was placed in his arm. Soon after we found his neutralization dosage for corn, he became happy and cuddly again. His parents were delighted. In time we found he had many more allergies, but it certainly appeared that the corn in his previous infant formulas had probably contributed significantly to his reflux, poor weight gain, and repeated surgeries.

One Last Word

When allergic infants scream endlessly hour after hour, mothers justifiably can become enormously tired, discouraged, and upset. At times these mothers often eat a food to which they are allergic, which makes them feel moody, depressed, irritable, and fatigued. The same food can make their breast-fed infants equally unhappy, fretful, and discontent. This combination can lead to enormous stress because both the infant and the mother can be victims of a similar unsuspected, unrecognized, and untreated allergy. These mothers need the patience of Job to be able to control their emotions and provide constant loving care to their fragile, endlessly screaming infants. They need the continued support and help of family and friends at this time in their lives so that they are not pushed beyond the breaking point. If you know such a mother, try to be there, for both the mother's and the infant's sake.

CHAPTER 5

Toddler Allergies

Allergic children have both the obvious classical and the more elusive symptoms of allergy throughout the infant period. Sometimes the causes of these problems are recognized and eliminated so that the child does well through the toddler period. More frequently, however, we see children who had problems during infancy but seemed somewhat better when they were about a year old. Then new and somewhat different medical and emotional problems become evident. Sometimes mothers who knew their infants could not tolerate milk begin again to feed various forms of dairy products to their child by the age of ten to eighteen months. It is not unusual for this food, in particular, to appear to be well tolerated *initially*. Then the milk-related physical illness, behavior, or activity problem slowly but surely becomes evident.

When a two- or three-year-old child begins to have tantrums, it is usually assumed to be a passing phase and called the terrible twos or the terrible threes. Some strong-willed nonallergic toddlers simply want to express themselves dramatically. This is a natural "no" period, and this word tends to cause rebellion in many normal youngsters. With some reflection, however, some mothers will find that their child's episodes represent not defiance and self-expression but an unnatural response to a food, odor, or something in the air. If your family has a number of allergic relatives, allergy may be the cause. Look at your toddler. Does your child have red ears, dark eye circles, or very wiggly legs just before the tantrum begins? If the answer is yes, ask what did your child just eat, smell, or touch? It requires some detective work to find out why a child's personality or mood suddenly changes.

The Dr. Jekyll/Mr. Hyde tantrums are easy to recognize. Initially the child is a delightful, well-behaved angel, and then for no apparent reason the change is swift and dramatic. There is no way to control this inappropriate, impossible behavior and activity. These sudden episodes can become excessive in number and duration. They can occur once a day for five or ten minutes or three times a week for fifteen to thirty minutes. At times they can continue on and off, all day or night, and can last for as long as two days after a child merely eats one single food to which he is sensitive. These episodes can be mild and manifested by whining sounds or by the tendency to repeat the same sentence over and over. On other occasions they can be explosive and result in tipped-over bookcases or the child's urinating in a wastebasket or hanging out an open window. These youngsters can cry and scream for hours. They often spit, hit, kick, punch, and pinch. Not uncommonly they attack their mothers, the younger children, furniture, plants, the family dog, or even their dishes. When nothing else is nearby, these distraught children even bite themselves. Some champ their jaws as they approach the target for their aggression. I recall one two-year-old who told her mother, "Mommy, I simply have to bite you," and with gusto she made her way across the room to attack her mother one more time.

More than one mother of an allergic toddler has had to use a leash or harness, to make it possible to take her child shopping. Managers of prenursery day care centers do not know what to do when confronted with such children. Unless you have personally dealt with such a child, it is easy to be critical about futile or even foolish, impractical attempts to control these children. Some unknowing parents will totally disbelieve that any toddler could routinely act this way; others who are less fortunate will recognize their child's habit pattern and hopefully be relieved to realize that their child's problems may not be due to poor mothering skills.

Many parents are afraid to take their child to a doctor because they fear they may be accused of battering. The truth is the child is often self-battered. Allergic hyperactive children often race about wildly banging into walls and furniture. As a result they can be badly bruised. They run and move so fast that their poorly developed depth perception cannot prevent accidental bumps and bruises.

The mothers of these children are often distraught, desperate, and depressed. They feel immensely guilty because they have been told by everyone that there is no reason why they should not be able to control their child. The grandparents and relatives routinely not only refuse to care for the child, they commonly insist that the difficult child be left home whenever the rest of the family comes to visit. The mothers are in an emotional turmoil. They are justly afraid to leave these children with a baby-sitter. Even if they chance it, most baby-sitters won't stay; they quickly move on to care for less challenging children.

Fathers often rationalize their desire to be away by citing socially acceptable excuses, such as a need to work late or to travel. Some fathers dread nights and weekends because their home life is so stressful. They do not want to be faced with constant disciplinary decisions as soon as they enter their home. If the unruly child is an exhausted angel at that time, the father is perplexed because of the tales of woe relayed by his anxious, distraught wife.

Most physicians see only the adorable "between-tantrum" child and reassure the mother with such statements as "It will pass," "Be patient," "It's just a phase," "Try to discipline or modify the behavior, but don't hurt the child," and "It can't be that bad." Physicians cannot order the routine activity-modifying narcotic drugs such as Ritalin because this drug is not recommended for children under six years of age. Antihistamines tend to make these young children sleepy or may not curb the activity or behavior. Sometimes they take the edge off the child's reactions, but they surely do not eliminate the cause of the problem. The dyes, corn, and artificial flavors in these drugs can also precipitate sudden uncontrollable episodes in some toddlers.

Counseling is often needed, not only for the child but also the typically guilt-ridden mother. Both parents can be frustrated because they sincerely want to care for their child properly but feel upset and even a little resentful because they earnestly would like to have a bit of peace and quiet after working all day. The toddlers are often so physically ill, disturbed, or demanding, both night and day, that many mothers cannot work, in spite of their desire, capabilities, and a family's financial need.

Typical Allergies

Allergic toddlers can have a wide range of associated physical or behavioral complaints, which characterize the full spectrum of allergy (see Tables 5.1, 5.2, and 5.3). These children typically have classical nose allergies, which makes them prone to recurrent ear infections in particular. Chest infections can cause bronchitis, and this often precedes their initial asthma attack by months or years. After about

Table 5.1
Major Physical Symptoms of Possible Allergy in Toddlers

- Red earlobes
- Red cheeks
- Dark eye circles
- Bags under the eyes
- Wrinkles under the eyes
- Glassy, glazed eyes
- A "spaced-out" look
- Wiggly, restless legs
- Dislike of being touched or cuddled

two years of age, seasonal hay fever or asthma commonly begin because of repeated exposure to various highly allergenic pollens or molds.

Digestion and Behavior Problems

Infant digestive problems gradually reappear, especially after the milk or soy formula is stopped when cow's milk is restarted. In a few weeks or months some children may begin to gag and vomit clear mucus, almost at will. Periods of hyperactivity and aggression become apparent. Some toddlers walk up to strangers and kick them. Others will tear down the curtains, fly off the banister, try to climb out an open bedroom window, or try to ride their tricycle over the neighbor's toddler.

Sleep Problems

Many times these children have never slept well, even as infants. They arise tired and irritable, after thrashing about all night. They tend to have nightmares. They often have difficulty going to sleep and staying asleep. They hate to be awakened in the morning. Mothers often dread beginning each new day and dislike the challenge of

TABLE 5.2
Major Physical Complaints of Allergic Toddlers

Recurrent infections:

- Ear
- Chest
- Sinus

Intestinal complaints:

- Bloating
- Belching
- Gagging and vomiting
- Diarrhea
- Constipation
- Abdominal pain
- Nausea
- Rectal gas
- Halitosis
- Leg aches
- Headaches
- Nose rubbing, wiggling, picking
- Runny or stuffy nose
- Wiggly legs
- Coughing or wheezing

rousing them. These children are apt to greet mom with a scream and an emphatic "I hate you."

Excessive Clinging

Some toddlers cling to their mothers. They almost have to be peeled off their mothers' bodies. Their mothers learn to cherish any few precious moments they can be entirely alone. Some children need to

TABLE 5.3
Major Behavioral Characteristics of Allergic Toddlers

Temper tantrums
Whining
Screaming
Clinging
Hyperactivity
Aggression:

- Biting
- Hitting
- Spitting
- Pinching
- Punching
- Kicking

Repetition of the same phrases

- Desire for a craved food
- Nonstop, senseless talk

Reluctance to smile
Excessive fatigue
Depression
Refusal to stay dressed
Refusal to be touched
Desire to crouch in dark corners or under furniture

---

be touching constantly and insist on invading their mother's space at all times. Although these children are deeply loved, even mothers require a bit of personal time for themselves and at times they feel guilty because they resent the child who is persistently too close and clinging to them.

Dislike of Being Touched or Held, Withdrawal

Sometimes toddlers are too quiet. These children tend to crawl under the furniture and refuse to come out. They may crouch in a dark corner, clasp their arms tightly over their chest, pull their hair over their eyes, and scream if anyone attempts to touch them. Some moan and whine for hours. They often say, "Nobody likes me." A few repeatedly fall asleep, anyplace, anytime, and frighten their parents and doctors because they simply can't be roused. These are the children who tend to go under the chairs when they react during provocation testing and resume normal play after their neutralization treatment. These youngsters have the "fatigue" portion of the Allergic Tension Fatigue Syndrome. (See Chapters 15, 17, and 20 and Appendix E.) They might fall asleep after lunch when they reach school age, and possibly later on at work when they are adults.

What Causes Your Toddler to Have Allergies?

Is It Your Home?

If a toddler's medical or personality problems seem worse when a child is not at home, ask why. What's different about the home that is visited? Is it dusty, moldy, filled with tobacco smoke or perfumed aerosols? Sometimes it is a food they are given to eat. Did someone change their diet? Grandmothers, relatives, or baby-sitters often feel that a mother is foolishly denying a child some special treats. They lovingly and generously give the child the forbidden nuts, homemade cookies, cake, and brightly colored beverages. These items can trigger unbelievably unacceptable behavior or sudden illness in some children. This leads to reprimands and in time, creates poor-self-image problems within the child, as well as possible in-law friction for the parents.

Is It a Food?

Remember, a toddler's favorite food is the one that is most apt to be causing food-related medical problems. Sometimes these children's diets consist of only a few favorite foods. Although parents may not be aware of it, these children may need treatment for the foods they normally crave and eat, as well as those they won't or can't eat. With appropriate allergy treatment most children will eventually eagerly ingest a reasonably normal diet without difficulty.

Is It Related to a Particular Place?

Sometimes these children feel, act, or look better when they are in a certain place. Think about why this could happen. Is your child better when you go visiting or camping? Does a newer, less dusty or moldy home seem better? What is different? You can often determine exactly why your child is ill. A temporary answer may reside in the medicine cabinet but the ultimate answer is a pencil and paper. Try to find the cause and eliminate it. Just keep records and think about them. (See Chapter 9.) Always consider molds, dust, pets, foods, and chemical odors.

Is There a Pattern?

If parents watch carefully, they can often see a definite pattern to their child's reactions to different offending items. If the child or parents can sense that a reaction is about to begin, there are a number of ways to abort an episode. Some toddlers act irritable or depressed when their ears become red or they develop dark eye circles. Others may seem a bit too quiet and have a spaced-out look. They may throw out their lower lip, begin to drool, spit, develop wiggly legs, or speak rapidly, loudly, or unclearly. At about that time if anyone says "no," "Do this," or "Put on your shoes," they will suddenly begin to race, attack, scream, or do "their thing." Parents should watch for a response that is totally out of proportion or inappropriate in a particular situation. This type of sudden unacceptable response could indicate that an allergic Dr. Jekyll/Mr. Hyde reaction has begun. Ask why.

Is It Before Meals?

If the episodes routinely occur before mealtime, talk to the doctor about hypoglycemia. If small nonsweet snacks quickly correct the misbehavior and your child is adorable in minutes, the problem could be low blood sugar (see Chapter 3).

Is It Some Other Medical Problem?

Check with your physician if your toddler's problems seem unrelated to what you've just read. Not all misbehavior episodes are related to allergy, so don't think it is the cause of all problems. Some children have emotional or medical problems affecting their behavior that are totally unrelated to allergy. Others have complex problems, of which allergy is only one factor that needs consideration.

Here is one typical example of a toddler seen in my office.

A Youngster With a Sugar Sensitivity

Karl

Karl was a darling youngster with a charming personality. His relatives had many allergies. His symptoms began during the infant period. He had thirteen "colds" in the first fifteen months of life. Most of these were ear infections, which in retrospect were possibly due to his undetected milk sensitivity. From birth on, he always had either a stuffy or a runny nose. He had dark eye circles and tended to have puffy bags below his eyes. He coughed when it was wet outside and during the damp seasons of the year, suggesting a mold sensitivity. From the age of one year on, he complained about bellyaches. He tended to be bloated, had rectal gas, and belched frequently. His mother knew that apple, grape, and orange caused intestinal problems and that milk caused diarrhea. He tended to wet his pants frequently in the daytime. His mother didn't know why.

His mother was perplexed and particularly worried about his sudden periods of aggression and hostility. His eyes seemed suddenly to become glassy and glazed when his bouts of biting occurred. He was very restless, more active than normal, and had frequent nightmares and temper tantrums. At times he tended to cling to his mother too much. The odors of certain clothing and carpet stores tended to cause his eyes to become red and puffy. He had periods when he would become wiggly and bouncy and complain that he was too tired to walk and he had to be carried. All these problems were evident by the tender age of three years.

At some point his mother noticed that when Karl ate party food or candy, his total personality quickly and dramatically changed. To check her observation, we asked that he eat nothing that contained sugar from Monday to Friday and then come to our office. We videotaped Karl as he gleefully devoured eight cubes of sugar. Just as the mother had predicted, within less than an hour he switched from a Dr. Jekyll to a Mr. Hyde. At first he stopped playing quietly and began to whine. Then he became more irritable, fussed, stomped his feet, wiggled in his chair, tossed his toys over his head, and then threw pieces of a puzzle at his mother. When he was given the correct dilution of his allergy extract for sugar, within a few minutes he was transformed back into his adorable self again. With animated expression and sheer delight he pretended to read his mother a story. She was in tears because we had confirmed what she had noticed so often. She realized she was not a bad mother and he was not a bad kid.

Our videotape confirmed exactly what Karl's mother had repeatedly told her pediatrician. (See Appendix C.) The doctor, however, had consistently reassured her that medical research stated there was no relation between sugar and her son's behavior. He was correct about some of the medical literature. Scientific studies do show that sugar quiets mice, but this is not true in the experience of ecologists in relation to sugar and children. Other studies, however, clearly document such a relationship. The repeated change in Karl's total affect and behavior after he ate sugar simply could not be denied.

Karl's mother made their home as allergy-free as possible, tried to feed her son a rotation diet, and avoided unnecessary chemical exposures. We tested and treated him for only three items, one being sugar. In only two days he had improved tremendously. His astute mother readily recognized when new sensitivities to foods or pollen developed during the next few years. These were treated with appropriate neutralization dilutions of allergy extract. Four years later he continues to be 95 percent better.

CHAPTER 6
_____

Child Allergies

Here is one youngster who had many manifestations of allergies, starting in infancy. This fourteen-year-old child's medical problems were more complex and challenging than are many patients' who have allergies. Her history was selected for discussion because it provides an ample opportunity to explain the vast array of common complaints so frequently confronting parents. Many children typically have both the classical and the less frequently recognized forms of allergy. Many of the trials and tribulations that faced Jean's desperate parents are unfortunately not unique.

A TRAGICALLY ILL CHILD WHO NEVER FELT WELL

Jean

Jean was six years old when she first came to our office. She had seen thirty medical specialists including three gastroenterologists prior to her first visit. She had been evaluated for allergies on three previous occasions.

Allergic Relatives

Jean's family was very allergic. Both parents and her brother had many of the typical, as well as the "unusual," forms of allergy.

Before Jean Was Born

Jean's mother stated that during her pregnancy the baby seemed to be unusually quiet. This is not typical of most of the patients whom we see. As noted earlier, mothers of our patients typically complain of markedly increased fetal activity or excessive hiccupping during their pregnancy.

Jean's Fussy Sleepless Infancy

As an infant, however, Jean's history was typical. She tended to be so inordinately fussy that her mother said that she was "out of it." She had intermittent periods of extreme hyperactivity, at times, alternating with excessive fatigue. She spit up and vomited much more than usual. Her mother said that carrots caused her to scream violently. There is nothing special about carrots. A variety of foods can cause this type of problem in infancy. It varies with different infants. Often parents need only to watch their infant carefully to detect which food is a problem.

As an infant Jean could not sleep. Even now at the age of fourteen she continues to have sleep problems and needs to use relaxation audiotapes. One of her parents slept with her until she was eight and a half years of age because she was constantly ill. Sleep problems are typical of many allergic infants and children.

Jean's Terrible Twos: Seasonal and Year-Round Allergies

Jean's eyes were red, watery, and itchy in the warm months by the age of two years. This suggests a hay fever problem due to trees, grasses, or ragweed pollen or molds. During the spring and fall she always had eye circles and puffy bags under her eyes. Her eye circles, however, were pink, not the typical black or blue color. Her nose symptoms continued in a milder form during the winter, suggesting that dust, mites, molds, and foods could be factors related to her complaints.

Wheezing and Coughing

Jean was only two years old when she first began to wheeze and cough. Children can begin to have this problem early in infancy or any time later on, but usually by the age of five severely allergic children have had their first bout of wheezing with infection. Her mother noticed that if she laughed, ran hard, or breathed cold air, she coughed.

She coughed much more when it was damp outside. Her cough was particularly evident when the snow melted in the late winter. These clues strongly suggest a mold sensitivity. In time her extreme mold allergy unquestionably proved to be her most challenging problem.

At the age of two years she was seen by her first board-certified specialist in internal medicine and allergy. Despite her classical allergic history, he concluded that Jean did not have allergy.

Constant Infections

Recurrent infection is frequently a problem in children who have nose or chest allergies. This certainly was true with Jean. She "never" felt well, and she "always" was ill. Her mother was so afraid that at the time I first saw her, Jean was frequently not even allowed to step outside her home. Her mother was not overprotective; she was doing the only thing she knew to help keep Jean well. She truly feared that Jean would die from her next infection. Every time Jean's nose became stuffy, she began to have another ear infection. Each time this happened, her eardrum ruptured.

Aggression and Anger

At age two Jean began to bite her brother, both parents, and even the furniture. This, again, is common in allergic children, particularly between the ages of two and four years. Discipline and hollering are of little value if a child's misbehavior is due to allergy. Asthma does not respond to a parent saying, "Stop wheezing." Similarly if the brain is reacting to an allergenic exposure, many children appear to be spaced-out, do not seem to hear, or can't respond appropriately to what their parents say. Behavior modification can be extremely helpful *after* a child's allergies respond to treatment. Before this, however, these same techniques may provide minimal, if any, benefit.

Never Happy

One of Jean's major complaints was that she was never happy. This could have been due to the fact that she never felt well and had constant daily headaches. This type of problem is unfortunately common in a vast number of children and adults. Her headaches were eventually found to be due mainly to milk, molds, and egg. After only one day of P/N allergy testing, for the first time, Jean did not have a headache. Within a couple of days her pink eye circles were gone and she was actually happy. Her mother could not recall the last time Jean had smiled and was joyful.

Dry Skin and Hives

Jean tended to have rough skin. This is true of many children who have eczema, but sometimes it also indicates a lack of the vitamins A, B_1, D, E, biotin, pantothenic acid, bioflavinoids, or other nutrients such as essential fatty acids. She also had hives at least twice a year. Records of exactly what was eaten or touched for the period of six or eight hours before a bout of hives often provides one answer. Her records indicated that soda pop was one cause of her hives. (See Chapter 9.)

Face Showed Allergic Reactions

At times she also had the typical red earlobes, red cheeks, or even a red nose tip, shortly after she ate something to which she was sensitive or drank fruit juices. Her mother soon learned that these changes in Jean's appearance provided valuable clues that helped her detect the cause of certain allergies. Because cause-and-effect relationships were evident sooner, measures could be taken to prevent a cascade to more serious symptoms.

Intestinal Complaints

Jean's abdominal symptoms were typical of many allergic children. She had pain, nausea, belching, rectal gas, bloating, and bad breath. Many times these problems were suddenly noted shortly after she ate. The fact that Jean's abdominal symptoms were associated with constipation suggested that milk, or some form of dairy might have been a problem. She also made clucking throat sounds, which again strongly suggested an allergy to milk. Milk did prove in time to be a major food problem responsible for these and a number of her other symptoms.

Itchy Rectum

Although the most common cause of an itchy rectal area is probably pinworms, many allergic children have this complaint. One other unsuspected but very frequent cause could be a possible yeast (monilia or candida) problem. This is frequently noted in allergic children after the excessive use and need for antibiotics to treat recurrent infections. Yeasts were certainly a factor in the problems of this young girl. (See Chapter 23.)

Urinary Complaints

Jean's urinary complaints, again, were similar to those of other allergic children. This problem persisted until she was placed on a rotation diet. Her need to urinate at night contributed to her insomnia. Once we began to treat her at the age of six and a half years, she stopped wetting her pants and no longer was seen rushing frantically to the bathroom. Her excessive need to urinate stopped after she was treated for an allergy to wheat.

She also complained that it burned when she urinated. This is not a common complaint of allergic children. It sometimes merely indicates that a child is not drinking enough water. Concentrated, strongly acid urine can burn.

Leg Cramps and Muscle Aches

At the age of two or three she developed the very common complaint of leg cramps or "growing pains." As she grew older, Jean developed aches in her shoulders, neck, and back of the type seen in older children and adults. These typical complaints indicated that Jean's allergy treatment needed to be adjusted and updated, and they disappeared shortly after that was done.

Chemical Exposures

Jean had obvious evidence of chemical sensitivities. Similar to others with this problem, she craved certain odors. She loved to smell fingernail polish, even though that odor made her ill. She became ill if she smelled perfume, tobacco, paint, or burning wood.

Another Allergist

When she was four and a half years old, Jean was seen by the head of a pediatric allergy department at a university hospital. He also said that Jean did not have any allergies. He did, however, reassure her mother that she was not crazy. He confirmed that Jean had reflux, or food backing up from her stomach, which then caused vomiting. As we have noted previously, food allergy is rarely suspected as a cause of reflux in infants. Beyond the toddler age many allergic children have nausea, bloating, gas, and discomfort, but only a few vomit. Vomiting is an infrequent complaint in older food-allergic children. If children tend to vomit clear mucus, however, this suggests a possible allergy.

In desperation her discouraged pediatrician urged her previous allergist to retest Jean again at the age of five years. This time he confirmed that Jean did have allergies and began to treat her. During the next year, however, she was repeatedly and definitely much worse after each injection of allergy extract. Every treatment caused her to wheeze and to have extreme insomnia. In spite of traditional allergy extract therapy for molds and pollens, her mother was disappointed because she continued to have one infection after another.

In addition her mother noticed that she tended to become moody and crabby shortly after every routine allergy injection treatment. Most traditional allergists use extracts that contain a tiny amount of a preservative chemical called phenol. Sometimes parents notice within a few minutes to a few hours after every traditional allergy injection that their child will feel fuzzy-headed, weak, exhausted, irritable, or flushed. They often develop headaches, abdominal discomfort, or aching or tingling in their muscles. If the phenol in the extract is the cause, they might have a similar reaction when they smell other products that contain phenol, such as common bathroom disinfectant aerosols. (See Chapter 15.)

The proverbial last straw occurred when she had one more bout of pneumonia. By then it was obvious to her mother that she had innumerable "untreatable" food-related symptoms. In the past her allergist had told her mother that he "would be terribly angry and not prescribe for Jean if she went to Dr. Rapp's office without his permission." Jean's mother prayed nightly for over a year that he would relent. Her allergist finally acquiesced to Jean's mother's request. He gave permission for Jean to be evaluated at our office.

Help With a Diet

Because Jean's entire family decided to follow a four-day Practical Rotary Diet, her mother quickly pinpointed problem foods for each family member. She finally found causes for many of Jean's specific problems. Apple, grape, and pear, for example, caused Jean's nose and earlobes to become their characteristic brilliant red color. If Jean had milk at bedtime, it caused nightmares. A food eaten late in the evening is commonly the cause of sleep problems or nightmares. Jean also had tenderness in the lower central area of her breastbone, in an area called the xiphoid. In time we found that milk, in particular, caused this problem. In other children, pain in this area is sometimes caused by airborne molds, damp homes, or moldy, yeasty foods. Her mother found that many of Jean's intestinal symptoms were due to eating baked goods that contained wheat or other grains, such as oats, rice, or corn.

Drug Reactions

Jean had a long list of approximately twenty drug reactions. Most of these drugs caused rashes, an inability to sleep, muscle aches, and intestinal problems. Surprisingly, codeine caused her to bite her knees. Intal powder, which contains milk sugar or lactose, is a drug commonly used to treat asthma. This caused her to become depressed. Cortisone had been needed before we saw her to control her cough and asthma. Although this drug improved her symptoms, it always caused her to develop an unnatural "high."

Answers With Allergy Testing

Before the end of the first day of testing in our office she was already remarkably improved. During that day we had tested and treated her for egg and a mold. Her mother described the improvement as "unreal and miraculous." The next week Jean's teacher could not believe the dramatic change and improvement. At that point her mother deeply regretted the forced delay of over one year before her previous allergist would sanction her decision to bring Jean to see an allergist practicing environmental medicine.

In particular we noted that whenever we tested Jean for egg, she repeatedly became exceedingly disagreeable. Her disposition changed in a similar manner whenever she ate eggs.

Allergy tests for molds repeatedly caused extreme headaches, fatigue, and stuffiness. These were the same symptoms she manifested when she was in any damp, wet area or on rainy days.

How Is She Now?

Eight years after we initially saw Jean, she continues to be over 80 percent improved. One major problem, however, persists: She continues to have periods of fatigue. This complaint is consistently relieved by repeatedly skin-testing for molds and yeast. With each visit, after appropriate retesting, she dramatically improves, often looking more alert and energetic before she leaves our office. Her improvement, however, only lasts a few weeks or months. Then she needs to be retested again. Unfortunately, some children who have severe environmental illness require frequent repeated allergy testing to stay well. The typical patient, however, only needs additional allergy testing two to four times a year at first, and fewer visits as time passes.

Jean's schoolwork is presently excellent, as is her attendance. She is no longer plagued by recurrent infections, headaches, intestinal problems, depression, and feeling ill. She can participate in normal indoor and outdoor teenage activities.

One major reason why Jean responded so well is because her parents were so caring and careful. They followed our many suggestions in an exemplary manner. Their home, and particularly Jean's bedroom, was made allergy-free and ecologically sound. Jean continues to maintain the four-day Practical Rotary Diet approximately 95 percent of the time. She tries to avoid chemical exposures as much as possible. There is no doubt that this newer, more comprehensive approach to allergy—one that includes a rotation diet, allergy extract treatment, avoidance of chemicals and pollution, yeast treatment, and improved nutrition—has helped this young lady significantly.

The personal and emotional trauma that Jean's loving parents suffered must be mentioned. Her mother was treated as if she were a hypochondriac because she kept complaining to one doctor after another that her child continued to be ill. A pediatric psychologist told her she was hysterical and that her daughter was emotionally disturbed. One physician even told her that Jean, who was only two years old at the time, "was a problem child who was trying to destroy her parents' marriage." They recommended behavior modification for Jean's inability to sleep at night. Although Jean's mother repeatedly took reference articles to her doctors suggesting that her child might have allergies affecting her brain, they repeatedly laughed at, belittled, or ignored her.

There is sort of an unwritten rule in medicine: Don't tell a doctor too many complaints, even if they are all true, because you lose credibility. If you complain too much or too often, some doctors tend to blame the patient or the parents for a child's illness.

Her Mother's Despair

At one point Jean's mother was so distraught and worried that she saw a psychiatrist. She seriously wondered if her or her children's lives were worth living. She simply could not understand how so many doctors could lack compassion and understanding. Why was she consistently rejected and blamed?

Many mothers have felt exactly the same as Jean's mother. They are directly or indirectly made to feel that if they were better mothers, their children would be fine. If your automobile does not function correctly and the mechanic says the car has nothing wrong, you don't blame the car. You find a different mechanic. Many mothers go from one physician to another trying to find someone who will listen. I personally truly believe that most doctors would desperately like to help. They simply don't know what to do because they are unfamiliar with the newer approaches that appear so effectively to resolve some unusual manifestations of allergy. I feel certain that when many young physicians find out more about these newer more effective methods, they'll be anxious to learn and adopt the philosophy of preventive allergy practiced by ecologists or doctors interested in environmental medicine. If physicians want to be eager and excited in anticipation of office hours, they need only visit the office of a specialist in environmental medicine. It truly is very rewarding in many ways for patients, as well as for their doctors.

If you don't feel comfortable with your physician, can't really discuss your concerns, find that the doctor is always too busy or that you are blamed or made fun of, maybe you need a different doctor. Unfortunately caring mothers are often ironically seen as the person at fault. At times they are ridiculed by family, friends, and co-workers because they select comprehensive environmental care for their children. Some mothers really have no choice. Jean is now well but because she was "different" in many ways, she needed "different" care. The bottom line for parents is which doctor can make their children feel better. Parents must be aware that some less well known and newer methods of health care can be beneficial (or harmful) for some youngsters. They should have the right, however, to investigate and learn as much as they can about minor variations of the usual medical forms of allergy therapy which appear to be so effective.

How Do Other Physicians Respond to Patients Who Improve After P/N Treatment

Most physicians truly care about their patients. The allergist who eventually but reluctantly referred Jean to me was so impressed by her improvement that he personally came to observe in our office. Other doctors, however, see equally dramatic improvement in children who have perplexed them for years, but show little interest in asking why. I believe peer pressure and the present-day medical literature, which does not present balanced impartial information about environmental medicine, keeps many doctors following the traditional, conservative, and secure approaches to allergy therapy.

I certainly cannot be critical because when I first began to use these newer approaches I was faced with a similar decision. I must shamefully confess that I was reluctant to change my practice even after I was certain these methods were better. It took almost two years before I fully applied them in my office. It was simply easier in many ways to practice as I had for many years. After I had no doubts that patients really responded better, and openly stated so, there were changes in the attitudes of some of my peers. I found a distinct void encircling me at our local allergy meetings. Doctors acted afraid to be seen talking to me. Longtime medical friends looked the other way at medical conferences. I was experiencing peer pressure. This exists in medicine, and is to be expected if any physician decides to use methods that are a bit different, even if they appear to be helpful. Each physician has to decide upon her or his own priorities. The choices are not always easy.

CHAPTER 7

Adolescent Allergies

The positive side of comprehensive environmental care was clearly illustrated in relation to an adolescent named Betsy. She demonstrates that unavoidable emotional outbursts are much easier not only to prevent but to accept after parents recognize that they are not to blame. They are reassured when they realize they were right all along and that their child is also not at fault. Once parents can pinpoint the specific cause of certain physical complaints and upsetting disruptions, life becomes sweeter for everyone.

A YOUNGSTER WHO TURNED IT AROUND

Betsy

We first saw Betsy when she was fifteen years old. Her parents were worried because she was depressed and suicidal each year in the late summer, when ragweed pollen was in the air in northern Michigan. Her parents had begun to dread the late summer. At the time of her first visit she appeared normal until we began to use provocative testing for ragweed. Then she crawled into the office bathtub and refused to come out. She screamed, was untouchable, and complained of so much abdominal pain that she pulled her knees to her chest and held her stomach. After we found her neutralization allergy treatment for ragweed pollen, she felt entirely normal within a few minutes. With pollen treatment, her depression did not recur that year—until the following summer, when she had to be retested. This time during ragweed testing she found an isolated corner in a dark hallway. She was untouchable and curled in a tight ball. She stated, "I want to be left alone," moaned, said her skin and stomach hurt, and screamed if anyone came near or tried to touch her. We corrected her ragweed neutralization treatment, and again in a few minutes she was normal. She remained well through the rest of that ragweed season.

Repeated School Problems

Throughout her stormy school years, Betsy had mood changes and sudden outbursts that perplexed, exasperated, and at times infuriated her teachers. Her mother never doubted that there was a plausible reason for Betsy's unacceptable, disruptive behavior. She felt sad and sorry that her child had to suffer so much, and for so long. Her mother was frustrated and puzzled because neither her doctors nor the educators could help her child. Her mother was repeatedly made to feel that if she were a better mother, Betsy would not be such a problem to raise.

Depression From Grape Skin Test

On one occasion when Betsy was seventeen years old, she came to our office and mentioned that she became very depressed if she drank wine. We skin-tested her for grape, but we did not tell her what we were injecting into her arm. A German television crew happened to be preparing a documentary in our office on that day, so her entire response was taped. Her first injection was a placebo. This caused no change in her behavior. The next injection contained a drop of a standard grape allergy extract. Her affect and personality changed totally within a few minutes. She rubbed her hands because she saw imaginary spiders. Then she curled into a ball, screamed, and frantically recoiled as she withdrew her entire body when her mother merely touched her leg. Then she said, "I don't want to live anymore if I have to live this way. I wish God would let me die." After the neutralization allergy treatment for grape, she was again a sensible, intelligent young woman.

Family History of Allergy

Betsy's parents had spent years trying to determine why she was so different. The family history for allergies was immensely positive in all immediate family members and grandparents. Neither of her brothers could tolerate milk as an infant, but the right diagnosis was made quickly because they had the obvious typical intestinal problems so characteristic of allergy whenever they drank milk. Both brothers also developed typical hay fever as they grew older. Fortunately their complaints involved classical allergy, so the right diagnosis was made quickly. Betsy was not so lucky, because her allergies were not typical. She provided a paucity of typical clues that her infant and childhood physical and personality problems might be due to milk and other allergenic substances. Her brain allergies were not recognized for many agonizing years. Although Betsy's parents and brothers recognized their own typical allergies because of Betsy, in time they became aware that they had some unusual forms of allergy too.

Betsy's Fetal Period and Infancy

Typical of allergic children, Betsy's history dated back to the fetal period. Her mother complained she was bruised from the inside with Betsy's extreme intrauterine kicking. Her mother said that when Betsy was born, "she punched her way out of the uterus."

By one week of age Betsy was already unhappy. Her mother described her as a "terror." Her parents took turns walking the floor with her, day and night. She screamed constantly as if she was in constant pain. She clutched, clawed, and scratched her skin until she bled. As soon as she could put hands on her bottle, she pushed it away with all her might. In retrospect her mother wondered if nature was telling her at that time that Betsy's milk formula was a problem. She never smiled until she was two years old. She had a red-hot "bubbly" buttock rash from the age of six months until she was four years old. If she ate cheese or oranges, her skin would suddenly become scarlet in color. Her bowel movements were either diarrhea or hard pellets, never normal.

Repeated Ear Infections and Tantrums

She began to have repeated ear infections during infancy and these persisted through the fall, winter, and spring each year until she was twelve years old.

She also began to have uncontrollable temper tantrums when she was only a few weeks old. As an infant she would arch her back, scream, and thrash about so vigorously she could hardly be held. She was seen by a neurologist early in infancy but in spite of many drugs to quiet her, nothing helped.

These intermittent episodes never stopped. As a teenager she was still unable to abate or abort them. After they were over, Betsy felt contrite and upset over her actions, but once she felt "that feeling," she knew that a tantrum was about to occur and that there was no way she could control her behavior. After her neutralization allergy extract, she could, however, prevent many of her reactions. Psychological counseling was repeatedly tried, but it was not beneficial.

Many Physical Complaints

During her childhood she had daily abdominal pain, muscle aches, and headaches. In addition she had frequent neck aches, backaches, excessive perspiration, restlessness, fatigue, irritability, easy crying, and depression. She had nightmares, a chronic postnasal discharge, seasonal nose allergies, frequent infections, itchy rashes, and conjunctivitis. Her bowels moved only once every four or five days. She coughed with exercise or laughter. She always craved foods, especially meats and cheese. She "ate constantly." She always had dark eye circles.

As is typical of pubescent females, many of her symptoms became much worse and new medical complaints were noted at that time. Her symptoms were always worse premenstrually.

Poor Schoolwork

Betsy had very well educated parents, and they always felt Betsy had above-average intelligence, but her school performance was consistently very much below par. She had great difficulty reading and was frequently frustrated trying to conform to the rules and regulations mandated in most schools. When she was seven years old, one teacher taped Betsy's mouth from ear to ear because she spoke out in class. She was a persistent school failure until her allergies were recognized and treated. After allergy treatment her academic work and demeanor in school improved dramatically. When we initially saw her, her mother said that although she was fifteen years old, she could read only at a fourth-grade level; within six months of allergy treatment her mother said she was able to read and comprehend at a ninth-grade level.

Suicidal Episodes

Her childhood and adolescence were spotted with frequent medical complaints and family crises. She would lock herself in the bathroom and threaten to kill herself with a knife. Once she threatened to hurt herself with scissors. She repeatedly sat in the middle of the street so that the cars would run over her. At times she ran into moving cars, cut her hands with glass, ran in the ice and snow without shoes, and even tried to jump into a deep gorge. Many of these episodes were preceded and possibly caused by unavoidable or accidental exposures to chemical odors such as natural gas, gasoline, fingernail polish or polish remover, fumigants, shoe dye, tobacco, air fresheners, or automobile exhaust.

Emotional Problems

Betsy's life was marked by traumatic intermittent emotional outbursts and mood changes. Frequently, she became depressed and withdrawn. She routinely started her day by stating that her muscles ached so badly, she simply could not get out of bed. She always complained of being tired. It was not unusual for her to be hostile, noisy, belligerent, agitated, and aggressive, anyplace and anytime. She would state that she could feel something happening inside her body just before she lost control. It would become "creepy and crawly" under her skin, and she would vigorously rub her arms or pull on her skin, make unusual wiggly movements, crawl into a dark corner, cover her head, and absolutely refuse to be touched. At that time it was not unusual for her to perspire, and the entire room sometimes would be satiated with a most unpleasant odor. She was distressed because in spite of bathing and washing all her clothing after these episodes, the aroma still lingered.

Sensitivity to Sound, Light, and Touch

During her strange reactions she usually complained that ordinary sounds were much too loud and lights were much too bright. During provocation testing in our office she would frantically cover her ears and rush to a secluded dark area because someone was talking. She could not stand the sound of ordinary speech. It is interesting that even as an infant she always seemed overly sensitive to noise. If her mother merely walked past the nursery, she would throw her arms in the air and scream for the next hour. Her mother wondered at that time why her response to a nuance of sound was so extreme. This characteristic of increased sensitivity to sound has been noted in many other allergic children.

Allergy Testing

Her typical behavioral changes were reproduced single- and double-blindly many times in our office during P/N allergy testing for a wide range of common allergenic items, as well as for specific chemicals and hormones. Several of these were documented on film or video-tape. Some, for example, made her sleepy, irritable, and spacey. During these reactions to single allergy tests, if she would draw, the picture would contain knives or a snake dripping with blood. After her episodes subsided with neutralizing allergy extract treatment, she would create a picture with hearts and flowers and write lovely, in-sightful poetry.

On one occasion, when she was tested for banana, she changed from a normal, quiet young lady to a "raving maniac" in seconds. She threw her book at a plate-glass window and ran out of the office and down the street before we could catch her. Our nurse had to treat her with the correct dilution of banana extract while Betsy was still in the street.

In addition to dramatic changes in her affect and behavior, we reproduced her headaches, abdominal pain, muscle aches, and several of her other physical complaints during routine P/N testing. Tests for milk reproduced the exact headache she had complained about for years.

After Betsy's initial visit in our office she confided to her mother that she was so happy. It was the first time she realized she was not crazy. She had been worried that this was her problem for years. She was relieved to know that she had a genuine medical illness. Many of her extreme psychological symptoms could be reproduced and eliminated at will during our P/N testing—it was not all in her mind. Other adolescents have had similar feelings and made identical comments.

Previous Medical Tests

The results of routine medical tests for allergy presented a mixed message. They could easily and justifiably have been interpreted as an indication that Betsy did not have a significant allergy-related illness. Her nose mucus and blood smear showed no excess of the typical eosinophilic white blood cells so characteristic of allergy. The total IgE test results were in the equivocal range. Her RAST allergy tests, however, did reveal a definite positive reaction to ragweed and eggs. RAST blood tests for other foods, however, which regularly caused reactions identical to ragweed and eggs during provocation testing, were entirely negative. In essence this means that standard current tests presently used to confirm allergy did not always provide reliable answers for Betsy, even though allergies had obviously interfered with her well-being since she was born. If her diagnosis had been based solely on the results of most of her blood examinations, she would probably have been helped to some degree with ragweed treatment. If the positive RAST ragweed test, however, was considered valid and she was treated, her depression, need for isolation, and behavior changes would hardly have been interpreted as typical complaints due to a weed-pollen allergy. Without recognition of her many food allergies it is doubtful that the course of her life could have been changed to its present positive direction.

Adolescent Independence

During the intervening years, from age fifteen to nineteen, she was usually 50 to 75 percent improved with treatment for foods and environmental factors. Similar to many adolescents, she would intermittently discontinue all her therapy and after a while her symptoms would flare up again. She would then be forced to resume parts of the recommended diet, home allergy control, chemical avoidance, or allergy extract therapy until she felt better.

Betsy as an Adult

At her present age of twenty-six this young woman now has an A average in a university premedical program. She has repeatedly proven to herself and others that she is not stupid, an impression she had been given many times by previous educators. Because of her problems with odors in the past, she tries to avoid accidental chemical exposures. She quickly recognizes potential problem situations and takes measures to distance herself from them. Because of her greater understanding and her ability to recognize when she is beginning to react to something, she can often prevent, abort, or limit her previous types of unacceptable emotional and behavioral responses. She tries to avoid or diminish any contact with known offending allergenic items as much as possible. She now not only recognizes but admits that allergenic exposures can make her moody, angry, and argumentative. When she was an adolescent, she vehemently denied that she had drastic personality changes. She continues to develop her characteristic odor on rare occasions when she reacts to some allergenic substances, especially if she is angry.

Betsy as a Mother

Betsy's food problems and allergies, in general, are much less evident since her two pregnancies. It is of interest to note that she recognized that her unborn infant would kick inside her uterus within a half hour after she ate chocolate chip cookies. This excessive activity would continue for several hours. Kool-Aid caused a similar response in her unborn infant.

After Betsy's first baby was born, whenever Betsy ate chocolate and subsequently breast-fed her infant, the baby developed diarrhea. When her pediatrician put corn syrup (dextrose) in the baby's formula, the infant screamed all day. Betsy quickly changed her infant's formula to soy without corn and the infant was content and no longer constipated and crying excessively.

Both of Betsy's children have mild allergies. We anticipate that because of their mother's superior intelligence and extensive knowledge about the diverse scope of allergic symptoms, she will be able to recognize, prevent, delay, or diminish future emotional and physical illness due to allergy in her children.

If new allergies develop in Betsy's children, she'll recognize them early, as she did shortly before and after they were born. With her understanding about better nutrition, allergy diets, ecological environmental control, and chemical avoidance, she'll be able to keep herself, as well as her family, healthier and happier.

Adolescent Allergies Are Truly Different

Although some hyperactive toddlers and children remain too active, as they grow older, they are more apt to become tired, irritable, and depressed adolescents or adults. If they were hostile and aggressive when younger, some become more gentle but others remain inconsiderate and thoughtless. Only if adolescents are truly willing to change their life-style can they be helped. Their negative attitudes and total denial, at times, can contribute to many more years of not feeling well, not being accepted, and not learning at a level commensurate with their ability.

Peer pressure is another factor that makes adolescents difficult to help. They often refuse to adhere to any diet. They want to eat whatever their friends are eating. Many work or display enough creative ingenuity to buy and eat whatever they want. They crave independence. Some are defiant. The result is that they can unnecessarily but effectively keep themselves on a seesaw displaying a wide range of emotional and physical illness. Many are reluctant to comply with either their parents' or their physician's suggestions. Betsy illustrated all of these characteristics over and over again. We often collectively worried about how *we* could cope until she matured and had more understanding.

Many adolescents will admit, after a routine initial period of total denial, that they do feel ill or act inappropriately if they eat or smell the wrong things. Unfortunately this may not deter them. When the inevitable crises arise, and they do, they run to their parents for help as they have always done. Sometimes, however, they make rash and unwise decisions during a period of unclear thinking caused by a brain-allergic reaction. Their parents must continue to be on guard so that they do not accidentally hurt themselves or others.

Maybe some of their actions are attempts to attract attention to the fact that they need help. Regardless of their intentions, efforts must be made to prevent them from being badly hurt. As these children grow older, it becomes more and more difficult to separate the purely allergic emotional responses from the secondary psychological problems created by years of not feeling well and not being accepted, often for good reasons.

Similar to Betsy, teenagers often go through periods when they refuse to take their allergy extract in spite of all the time and expense required to test and treat them. It does not matter if they understand that the treatment will improve their health and behavior. They insist on their rights to eat what they want or to go into some area that causes them to feel unwell or act strangely.

Many times their parents have given, given, and given for so long that they are exhausted emotionally, financially, and even physically. They have often had years of coping with an enormously challenging child who, through no fault of the child's or their own, has caused an unending stream of major family upsets.

The splatter effect on their siblings, who feel left out because they are "good and well-behaved," is always noteworthy. Sometimes they misbehave merely to get a little attention. Both parents often have unrecognized allergies, which causes them to have their own physical and emotional ups and downs. If their downs coincide with their children's, it can create trying situations. Some parents are on the verge of separation or divorce until the problem child is helped. Some fathers are attracted to greener, less troublesome pastures. Others have already left the frenzied family, and this in turn can lead to enormous social, emotional, and economic stresses for the mother and siblings.

After allergic teenagers are finally helped, parents often feel a peculiar blend of anger and relief. Often they had been discouraged, desperate, and simply at their wit's end until they fortuitously found a specialist who understands their child's special medical needs. The sick adolescent didn't suddenly become physically and emotionally ill. Some parents recognize that their child's problems often date back to before the youngster was born and were clearly evident throughout infancy, toddlerhood, and childhood. Older children and their parents regret and wonder why their basic medical problems were not recognized and treated earlier.

Although parents are delighted to find answers at last, they become understandably frustrated again when their adolescent child balks at the recommended treatment in spite of obvious improvement. This causes more needless anguish. Sometimes adolescents won't listen at first, but fortunately with maturity, their perception, understanding, coping skills, and acceptance improve. In time they learn that their parents cannot always be there. They find that a change in their attitude is imperative. They learn the need to recognize potential problem exposures and prevent their own illness as much as they can. They learn that they still have family support even though they are grown up. As with anyone else who has significant environmental illness, they need unconditional love, compassion, acceptance, and helpful relatives or friends. We have repeatedly been impressed with the mothers of environmentally ill children, in particular. Few parents could be as consistently understanding and loving through the thicks and thins of a challenging youngster's life.

Many intellectually capable teenagers will never graduate from college, even though they have the ability and desire, because they have never been able to sit, concentrate, or pay attention. Many have what we call brain fag. They are confused and cannot remember. Allergic adolescents often have been major discipline problems throughout their entire lives. Many have been forced to change from one school to another because of inappropriate behavior. Most parents have unsuccessfully tried behavior modification, counseling, and activity-modifying drugs repeatedly, long before the teenage years. These measures, at best, provided only partial or transient help. After these young adults, however, respond favorably to allergy care, they often need, and respond well, to the same counseling that failed before. Their self-image is often in dire need of restoration, and psychological help is imperative.

Changes in Allergic Symptoms at Puberty

When environmental illness affects adolescent youngsters, their symptoms often change, especially after puberty. In males typical allergies such as asthma, as well as unusual allergies that affect the personality, sometimes diminish after puberty. In contrast, in females, the opposite is sometimes true. Asthma and emotional moods related to allergy can sometimes become worse as girls age. Allergic adolescent girls seem to be in an especially delicate state of hormonal balance after puberty, so their monthly cycles can aggravate or intensify a diverse variety of allergies. Premenstrual young women often crave the very foods or beverages to which they are sensitive. Eating these foods can result in combined PMS and allergy symptoms. Their monthly flare-ups can lead to recurrent problems in every aspect of their young lives and can potentially last for a lifetime. Fatigue, irritability, and depression, in particular, can become extremely severe, at times almost intolerable. Sometimes they respond well to P/N treatment with hormones, as well as to treatment for typical allergic substances.[1]

Many young women have cold hands and feet, menstrual irregularities, and an inability to lose weight. Their food cravings or addictions can cause them to gain five to twelve pounds premenstrually. Although most of the weight is retained fluid, which is lost after the menses begins, some show a steady monthly weight increase. This of course leads to other problems related to their self-esteem, body image, and interpersonal relationships. Preliminary studies tend to indicate that women who have environmental illness can have mul-

1. Joseph Miller, M.D., *Relief at Last* (Springfield, Ill.: Charles C. Thomas Publishing, 1987).

tiple endocrine malfunction affecting the thyroid, adrenals, ovaries, pancreas, and possibly the pituitary gland. Physicians are only now beginning to become aware of this complex interplay. A new specialty of medicine called psycho-neuro-endocrine-immunology appears to be emerging to help these women.

In addition many allergic women appear to have a yeast problem due to an excessive intake of antibiotics prescribed for repeated infections or acne; to an overconsumption of sweet foods; and to the use of birth control pills. Sometimes their allergies surprisingly significantly diminish after their yeast overgrowth responds to appropriate treatment. In many others it is simply easier to test and treat the youngster's allergies if the yeast problem is treated first. (See Chapter 23.) We really don't know why.

Remember, not all adolescents are tired, depressed, and unable to think clearly or remember because of allergic brain fatigue. Everyone knows a few hyperactive older youngsters or adults who suffer from brain allergies. These are the ones who become workaholics. They accomplish ten times more than anyone else could do in an allotted period of time. If their excess energy is well directed, they can be most productive in their areas of interest. They can be immensely successful because of their endless enthusiasm and productivity. Unless they are so overactive that they can't complete the many projects they begin, they are envied by the more common allergic, tired individuals, who can barely drag themselves out of bed each morning.

In summary, many allergic adolescents are desperately in need of help and understanding. If they are given insight, most will listen and in time turn their lives around and amaze their parents, peers, teachers, and even themselves. If they learn a few basic facts, they can detect which foods, common allergens, or environmental factors interfere with their health and well-being. They want to decide their own future, and the recognition of their hidden allergies provides them with an opportunity to make the right and best choices.

PART THREE

How Can You Detect and Help Your Child's Allergies Quickly?

CHAPTER 8

Diets That Help Quickly

Make a list of five of your child's favorite foods or beverages. Make a similar list of your own favorites. Now look critically at your lists. Do several of the listed items contain milk or some form of dairy? Do several contain wheat or flour? You have just prepared a list of the foods or liquids most likely to be possible causes of illness in your child and yourself. Remember, most people who have food allergies are totally unaware that their favorite foods or beverages can cause any medical, personality, or learning problems. This chapter will explain how to determine whether or not the foods you listed are causing symptoms. Many investigators have conducted studies indicating that allergy diets are helpful.[1]

Most allergists believe that only 0.3 to 7 percent of the population have food allergy, although a few published reports say the incidence can be as high as 25 percent. Specialists in environmental medicine believe that 80 percent or more of the population have food allergies. Many of these, however, are unrecognized unless the following special diets are tried. The discussion in this chapter will explain how properly conducted allergy diets will possibly help your child and family in three to seven days.

---

1. D. Atherton, et al., "A Double-Blind Controlled Trial of an Antigen Avoidance Diet in Atopic Eczema," *Lancet* 1 (1978), pp. 401–403.

You've Tried Diets Before and They Did Not Help

There are many types of diets and many ways to do them. Maybe you tried the right diet but did it incorrectly. For years milk sensitivities were missed because mothers were merely told to stop milk. If cheese, for example, was not stopped when a child was off all milk, parents might be deceived into believing their child had no problem from milk products. A milk-free diet must contain no dairy *in any form* if valid answers are to be found.

An immense number of hyperactive children improved dramatically about fifteen years ago when the Feingold diet gained popularity throughout the world. Ben Feingold's first book contained his famous diet, which excluded food dyes, artificial flavors, and fruits and vegetables that contained natural salicylates. The Feingold organization offers both a cookbook and a handbook. In this cookbook, among other things, he noted that the quantity of sugar that causes hyperactivity will vary from child to child. The Feingold handbook wisely advises parents how to gradually re-add foods back into their child's diet. This helps to prevent the needless deletion of desired foods from a child's diet for prolonged periods of time when they don't cause symptoms. Dr. Feingold believed that any compound in existence, natural or synthetic, had the potential to produce an adverse reaction in any individual who had an appropriate genetic profile. He also indicated that most allergy diets needed to be tailor-made for each individual because we are all so different.

The diets suggested below may provide very specific answers very quickly. We find, in general, that ecological diets can be *much less limiting* than the Feingold diet.

In general many parents' observations are correct. They recognize that certain foods repeatedly cause their child to feel unwell or act ill. Their interpretation, however, is not always correct. For example, parents may say that wheat is a problem because bread always makes their child ill. On checking, we may find that a plain wheat cereal causes no problem. This would indicate that some ingredient other than the wheat flour in the bread is causing symptoms. Yeast, some additive, preservative, or milk are common elusive culprits. Wheat or milk in soup; eggs in mayonnaise; cinnamon in gum; a dye or artificial flavor in soda pop, toothpaste, mouthwash, or a liquid antihistamine represent a few common, typical unsuspected factors that cause illness in some children.

If you decide to follow the diets discussed in this chapter, try to do them only one time, but do them right. It will be time well spent. Many parents have quickly pinpointed major offending foods.

Common Types of Allergy Diets

There are three major diets that successfully detect allergy. Each has specific advantages and disadvantages. These diets are the:

- Single Food Elimination Diet;
- Multiple Food Elimination Diet;
- Practical Rotary Diet.

The Single and Multiple Food Elimination diets help you *detect* whether or not a food is causing some health, emotional, or learning problem. These diets provide fast, easy answers.

In contrast, although the Practical Rotary Diet can detect food allergies, it is basically a long-term "how to stay well" type diet. It is thought to help *increase a child's tolerance to many foods* that previously caused symptoms because each food can be eaten only every four days. This diet requires about a month before its benefit is apparent. It is therefore discussed later in the book in Chapter 24.

AN EXAMPLE OF HOW ALLERGY DIETS CAN WORK

Bobby

The Multiple Food Elimination diet proved to be surprisingly beneficial for one little boy named Bobby. In general if the suspect food is really a problem, it will cause similar symptoms every time it is eaten, providing it is ingested by itself and no more often than every four days. Bobby routinely reacted to many foods about fifty minutes after they were eaten.

His mother tried the Single Food Elimination Diet first and the Multiple Food Elimination Diet second. With the first diet, she confirmed her suspicion that milk affected her son adversely, and with the second diet she found several other major common foods that were not well tolerated.

What Clues Suggested a Possible Milk Sensitivity in Bobby?

Bobby's overactivity began in the uterus. His mother said she thought Bobby was going to be twins, he kicked so hard and often. She was very fond of dairy products, so she enjoyed drinking more milk than usual when she was pregnant. She wanted to create a beautiful, healthy baby. He was beautiful, but when he was only a few days old, he had a stuffy nose. He disliked being held or cuddled throughout his entire infancy. As soon as he was old enough, he tended to push away his bottle, but he ate his food vigorously. Babies give clear messages, but sometimes adults don't know how to interpret their observations. He wiggled his legs up and down in his crib and walked remarkably early. He perspired so much more than a normal infant that his clothing needed to be changed frequently each day. He never slept all night; he was always up five to six times.

By the age of eleven months his tantrums began. He screamed, kicked, hit, and arched his head backward. He always had red ears when he was having a tantrum. Nothing would console him. He had five to seven of these episodes during the day and night from the age of eleven months to three years.

As a toddler he ripped off his clothing and refused to get dressed. Unlike most little children, he had no interest in listening to a story. Abdominal pain, gas, and bad breath were frequent complaints. He tended to have one infection after another. He was totally unable to cope with any changes in his life. Something as ordinary as getting into the car to go shopping would precipitate an exhausting family crisis and turmoil.

How Effective Was the Single Food Elimination Diet?

When Bobby was three, he was placed on the Single Food Elimination Diet. Milk was removed totally from his diet because he craved milk and dairy products. Within three days his nose was dry for the very first time in his life, and his dark eye circles were gone. He no longer had bad breath. He belched less, and his rectal gas was gone. He seemed less negative, unhappy, and depressed. He ate and slept better. His tantrums decreased from five to seven a day to once a day. However, he continued to perspire more than normal.

How Effective Was the Multiple Food Elimination Diet?

Because he was better but still hyperactive once a day, his mother then tried the Multiple Food Elimination Diet. She found several other foods that contributed to his activity and health problems. After the first week of the diet she found that milk, sugar, and red food coloring caused him to become hyperactive within an hour.

This diet sometimes provides unexpected answers. During this diet Bobby suddenly began to soil his underwear. His mother had replaced milk with apple and grape juice during the first week of the diet and had fed him many raisins. If a new complaint arises during the Multiple Food Elimination Diet, it is often caused by the beverage used to replace milk. Later on, his mother confirmed that the apple and grape juice, as well as raisins, caused him to have leaky bowel movements and soil his underwear. She merely fed those foods, individually, at a four-day interval to confirm that they were the cause of this problem. In other words she used the Single Food Elimination Diet to determine the effect that each new food suspect had on him.

How Can Your Suspicions Be Confirmed?

If your child is always asking for a certain food, be suspicious. Try the Single Food Elimination Diet. It is easy, however, to be deluded when doing dietary studies. Always try to recheck any food suspect at least twice by feeding it to your child, all by itself, at a four-day interval. Repeatedly seeing the same response at a four-day period is the key to the Single Food Elimination Diet. This helps to decrease confusion in interpretation.

Remember, if your child ate some food an hour before a suspected food was eaten, and symptoms occur within fifteen minutes, you cannot be sure which of the two foods caused the symptoms. If your child feels unwell shortly after eating the second food, it could either be a delayed response to the first food or an early response to the second. The suspect food should be eaten all by itself when no other foods or beverages, including water, have been ingested for about four hours.

What Was Bobby's Response to Treatment?

After a few months of allergy extract therapy for foods, Bobby had his tantrums only once every ten days. Later on they occurred only once every two months, and when he had an outburst, the cause was usually obvious. He became pleasant, smiling, and happy. His interest in learning was intense, and his schoolwork soon was excellent. He rarely had infections, in contrast to his earlier years. His mother tried to maintain the family on a diet that rotated all foods so that they were eaten only once every four days. She kept their home as allergy-free as possible.

In time she found that several other members of the family also benefited from this special diet. After her family routinely ate different foods in a four-day pattern, she detected allergies that were previously not recognized. Prior to that diet they knew that they did not feel right at times, but they simply never thought about a possible food allergy.

What Is a Single Food Elimination Diet?

In the Single Food Elimination Diet a youngster is purposely fed a food that is thought to cause symptoms at a four-day interval. For example, if a suspected food such as milk is ingested on Monday, then the youngster is not fed *any dairy product, in any form,* on Tuesday, Wednesday, or Thursday. On Friday, when the child has *not eaten for at least three or four hours,* the youngster is fed *only* milk and cottage cheese. Similar testing for other foods can be conducted on Tuesday and Saturday for bananas; Wednesday and Sunday for oats, or a different food, and so on.

This is the first diet that a mother should try if she is suspicious that one certain food causes symptoms. Some children's food problems are more complicated than a single food, but this simple diet often relieves some medical complaints easily and quickly. If you find a spike and remove it, later on you can more easily detect the nails and the thumbtacks. This diet helps you detect one major spike at a time.

This is never to be done, however, if you already know that a food causes a devastating effect, such as collapse, body swelling, or severe asthma, for example. This diet enables you to safely check for *foods that are normally eaten* to see if they cause your child to feel unwell or misbehave. If a food has a truly terrible effect, you probably already know that it should not be eaten. There is no need to find out what that food does. The Single Food Elimination Diet helps you find hidden, masked, or unsuspected allergies. If you are concerned or unsure about any food, don't test it unless you discuss it thoroughly with your doctor first.

The Single Food Elimination Diet typically causes a child to feel unwell or become a behavior problem within fifteen to sixty minutes after a problem food is reintroduced into the diet. This method will often provide immediate clues as to the cause of chronic nose, chest, and skin allergies. In addition, it can provide specific answers about more elusive medical complaints such as headaches, muscle aches, abdominal complaints, insomnia, and behavior, activity, or learning problems.

Sometimes foods cause delayed reactions that occur within six to twenty-four hours after a problem food is eaten. These delayed medical symptoms include bed-wetting, joint tightness, leg aches, ear fluid, canker sores, colitis, and eczema. A child who has eczema, for example, may scratch immediately, or the skin in the arm or leg creases may become red at the time when a problem food is being eaten. However, the rash is typically not evident until eight to twenty-four hours later. Rarely, the rash may not appear for two or three days, making it even more challenging to detect cause-and-effect relationships.

Most food reactions last a few minutes to an hour or two. Sometimes one piece of bread or some other food, however, can cause symptoms that last for several days. The same child can have an immediate reaction to one food and a delayed reaction to another, or both an immediate and a delayed reaction to the same food.

For example, one mother of a six-year-old observed that if her son ingested any red candy, red juice, or red popsicles, he was "out of control" in a few minutes. Later that day, however, he would routinely develop diarrhea, headache, and a fever. When he ate grapes, this type of response would last two to three days.

Figure 8.1 shows a five-year-old boy's illustration after he binged on pizza, soda pop, juice, and ice cream. He could not color within the lines until two full days later, as shown in Figure 8.2. How many other children have this problem and no one has recognized that it is due to food sensitivities?

Foods You Suspect Cause Allergy

You should try to add suspected foods back into your child's diet on weekends or after school rather than in the morning, so that you can personally observe your child's response. Once again, be cautious and sensible. Check with your child's physician if any food or aspect of this diet is of special concern. *Never* test a food that you know causes a severe reaction before discussing it with your child's doctor first.

One major challenge in relation to the Single Food Elimination Diet is that the test food must be eliminated in *all* forms. Although this is simple for most foods, a few are immensely difficult to avoid because they are a hidden ingredient in so many food items. This means, for example, that if you suspect milk, your child cannot have milk, cheese, yogurt, ice cream, casein, sodium caseinate, or whey in any combination, or with any other food. This includes baked goods,

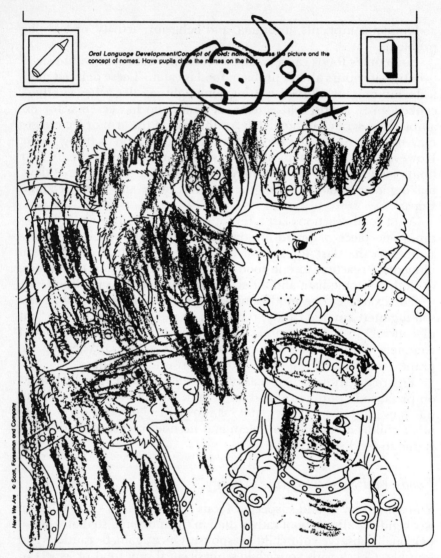

Figure 8.1. This five-year-old cannot control his drawings after he has binged on pizza, ice cream, and soda pop.

luncheon meats, soups, prepackaged food, or even some pills or capsules that use milk powder as a filler or source of bulk. Every label of every package must be read. Items that contain corn, soy, or food additives are equally common and can be difficult to avoid in all forms for the four-day testing period.[2] If a suspected food is eaten

2. See Appendix A for unsuspected sources of wheat, egg, corn, milk, and soy.

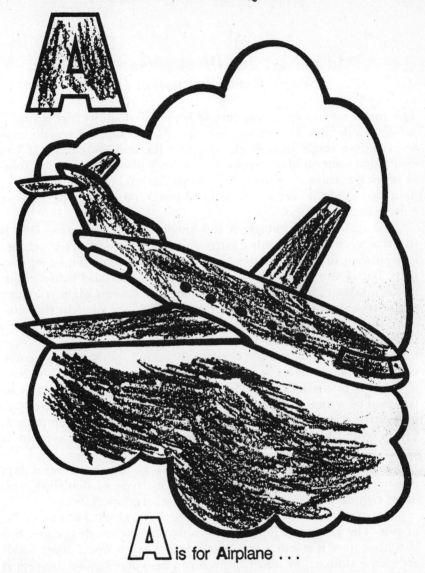

A is for **Airplane** . . .

Figure 8.2. Not until two days later, when the foods have left his system, can he color within the lines.

every day in some form and not totally eliminated, it is doubtful that the Single Food Elimination Diet will provide meaningful helpful answers. One easy way of avoiding this problem is to eat only fresh fruit, vegetables, and nonprocessed meats for the four days (see Table 8.1) before a food challenge.

Advantages and Disadvantages of the Single Food Elimination Diet

The major advantage of the Single Food Elimination Diet is that it provides a definite answer in a few days. In addition it is usually easy to exclude a single food from your diet for only four days. If you doubt that your child or you could live without some particular food or beverage, you may already have found an answer. That is the very item that might be related to some chronic common or perplexing elusive form of illness.

The major disadvantage of the Single Food Elimination Diet is that it tends to provide only a partial answer. If you have ten pebbles in your shoe and you remove one, you will still limp. This diet may help, but if you have too many other foods that also cause major problems, your child may not feel or act better, even when you have excluded a definite major problem food from the diet. In this situation the Multiple Food Elimination Diet may be the answer.

Another disadvantage is that sometimes symptoms can be worse for one to three days after certain allergenic foods are *not* eaten. Common symptoms include headache, fatigue, depression, nausea, irritability, or dizziness. If a food allergy is suddenly unmasked or revealed by a diet, it requires some determination to realize that the flare-up of symptoms is to be expected and will usually be temporary. Check with your doctor if this transitory worsening of symptoms causes concern.

On occasion a single problem food must be ingested several days in a row before symptoms are noted. This type of diet, however, often requires the supervision of a food-allergy specialist.

In summary, it must be very clear whether a child reacts to a food or not. The response depends not only on how much is eaten but also how often it is eaten and whether it is eaten when other foods are in the stomach or not. Children can be worse before they eat if they are hypoglycemic. They can be worse if they eat a food after it has been out of their diet for five to twelve days. They can be worse for one to three days if they stop eating a food to which they are sensitive—they are "addicted," they need a "fix." Sometimes they need to eat a food for several days before symptoms will gradually reappear. This is particularly true if a problem food is not eaten for several weeks. Because of the above, food-sensitive children often need a doctor who really understands how to detect food allergies.

What About Infections During Food Eliminations Diets?

If your child develops an infection during the Single (or Multiple) Food Elimination Diet, stop the diet. It is very difficult to interpret the results, especially if an infection occurs at the same time that a food is being added back into the diet to see if it causes symptoms.

One Other Way to Find Possible Problem Foods

You can also find answers by comparing "good" and "bad" day lists, when your child is physically unwell or misbehaving. For example, what was eaten when your child was a model Dr. Jekyll versus what was eaten when your child was a horrible Mr. Hyde. Cross out everything in common in both lists. One of the items left only in the Hyde list may be the cause of your child's unacceptable or impossible behavior. Each suspect food can be evaluated by doing the Single Food Elimination Diet.

How Do You Stop an Allergic Reaction From Occurring When a Food Is Added Back? Answer: Try an Alkali

A nonprescription item that can prevent and relieve allergic reactions is baking soda. In the 1940s Dr. Theron Randolph wrote that an alkali preparation of two parts sodium bicarbonate (baking soda) and one part potassium bicarbonate helped to relieve allergic reactions. It can be taken orally, and in my experience it appears to relieve about 60 percent of children's food-allergy-related symptoms within five to fifteen minutes. Unfortunately scientific studies have yet to be performed.

If a food causes an obvious reaction shortly after it was eaten, two things might help. Try to make your child vomit. Many times the child already feels nauseated, and by putting your finger down the throat, the offending food is quickly eliminated. If the food has to pass through the entire intestines and out the rectum, your child might not feel up to par for several days.

Even if your child were to vomit, however, some of the problem food is still in the digestive tract. The next step is to try one of the over-the-counter alkali preparations.

One is called Alka-Aid. It is available at most health food stores. It is a tablet and must be swallowed. Young children can take a crushed tablet in applesauce, mashed potato, peanut butter, or jelly, providing these food items do not cause symptoms.

The other is Alka-Seltzer Antacid Formula. It is available at some drugstores. This antacid preparation contains no aspirin and is a combination of sodium bicarbonate and potassium bicarbonate with a citric acid flavor. If someone is sensitive to citric acid, it would not be advisable to use it. Place it in water and allow it to fizz completely before swallowing. If taste is a problem, put it in pure orange juice or 7UP (citric acid, sodium citrate, and natural lemon/lime flavor). These mask the taste but can cause problems if someone is sensitive to some ingredient, for example orange, citrus flavor, aspartame, etc.

These preparations are normally sold to help relieve vague intestinal complaints such as heartburn. Take the time to obtain one or both of these *before* you try any allergy diet so that you have something on hand that might possibly relieve a reaction to a problem food if one occurs.

At least one or two glasses of fluid, preferably water, should be swallowed after either of these preparations is used. If this is not done, it is possible to develop some abdominal discomfort.

If you find this is helpful, carry an alkali in your wallet, purse, and car. Contact your child's physician so that a note can be sent to school regarding its use. The school nurse should be able to administer it if there is a sudden change in your child's personality, physical well-being, or ability to learn shortly after eating. Some parents say this is the best thing we ever told them.

Dosage of Alkali Preparations

The dose for a child is one-half tablet for a three-year-old, one tablet for a six-year-old, and two tablets for a twelve-year-old or adult (see Table 8.2). Persons with kidney or heart problems should check with their physician before using either preparation.

When sodium bicarbonate is given intravenously, it sometimes relieves asthma, gall bladder attacks, and even psychotic episodes due to foods within less than a half hour. The response in patients who act in a bizarre manner because of a food sensitivity can be particularly amazing. In a few minutes they can change and act entirely normal.

If some form of alkali is effective, it suggests that a food allergy is present. If an alkali proves to be helpful, immediately write down everything that was eaten or smelled within the previous few hours. Food odors also cause illness in some sensitive children. The best answer may be a pencil and paper, not one more trip to the medicine cabinet. Parents routinely and adamantly state that there was nothing unusual eaten *until they write it down*. (See Chapter 9.)

If you find you don't have any alkali preparation when you need one, you can try plain baking soda. It does not help as well as Alka-Aid, for example, but in an emergency it can sometimes be a handy blessing. Try about one-half teaspoon in a quarter glass of water, followed by another glass of plain water. Again, check with your doctor first.

One Last Caution

These preparations should not be used on a regular basis, only for emergencies. If your child accidentally eats the wrong food, see if it helps. Do not use it every day if your child insists on eating some craved food that causes daily symptoms. For that child you need food allergy extract treatment and possibly some counseling.

TABLE 8.2
Alkali Preparations

	Sodium Bicarbonate	Potassium Bicarbonate	Ratio	Citric Acid
Alka-Aid/ tablet	360 mg	180 mg	2:1	0
Alka-Seltzer Antacid Formula/ tablet	958 mg	312 mg	3:1	832 mg
Baking soda 1 tsp	952 mg	0	——	0

Adolescents are the most challenging in this regard. They understand, but peer pressure and their own independent natures and desires can make them less willing to cooperate. Even if they lose friends, can't do well in sports, or fail in school, they may insist upon eating the very foods that they know cause chaotic disruptions in their lives. A daily alkali is not the answer.

What Do These Alkali Preparations Normally Help?

These preparations were designed to relieve acid indigestion such as heartburn but they can also be helpful in preventing, treating, or proving allergic responses to foods. Sometimes they even help relieve reactions from exposures to chemical odors.

Sample of Prevention

Your child is going to a birthday party and you know that she or he can become the exuberant undesirable life of the party after eating ice cream, cake, or drinking colored beverages. Try the alkali or bicarbonate preparation *before* the party. It could prevent this response. If necessary, use it once again when your child returns home.

Sample of Treatment

Your child enters the house like a cyclone. His ears are red, his eye circles dark, and from the way he slams the door and races in, you know he is ready for action. He ate all the goodies at the school party. An alkali will often relieve the symptoms in a very few minutes, *if it is given immediately*.

Sample of Proof

If an alkali routinely prevents a reaction to a food item that you know repeatedly causes symptoms, this suggests that the alkali helped. If it relieves a physical complaint, or a behavior or activity problem, it usually indicates that some recently ingested food item was probably at fault.

Note that alkali preparations help much more than simple abdominal discomfort. An alkali can relieve food-related illness in many different parts of the body. For example, asthma, nose allergies, headache, as well as activity and behavior problems, might subside in a few minutes if they were caused by a food.

What Else Can You Do If You Want to Prevent a Food Reaction? Answer: Try Intal (Cromolyn Sodium)

Sometimes you know that a food will cause mild symptoms, but for some reason, such as an invitation to a party or dinner, you choose to eat the food anyway. An alkali and/or Intal can help.

Intal *prevents* a food allergy reaction. This is a prescription preparation. The contents of several capsules can be dissolved in warm water and taken thirty minutes before eating an offending food. However, Intal will not relieve symptoms already caused by an allergic food.

Intal has few side effects. Its biggest disadvantages are cost, and the fact that the powdered form in capsules is mixed with milk lactose powder, which can cause problems in milk-sensitive individuals. This is not true for the liquid Intal, which is available in single-dose ampoules.

Be certain to check with your physician before using this prescription drug. Food-allergic reactions often release histamine from mast cells. Intal stabilizes the mast cells so that histamine is not released. A newer, more potent, expensive form of this drug is now available in the United States, but it is designated for use in treating a problem called mastocytosis, not food allergies.

The Multiple Food Elimination Diet

The Single Food Elimination Diet helps confirm an allergy to a particular food. The Multiple Food Elimination Diet, however, provides answers in relation to several commonly allergic foods at one time. Parents can quickly detect a number of major foods that frequently cause medical, activity, and learning problems. If there are several pebbles in a shoe and only one is removed, the other pebbles will continue to cause a limp. If a person has several food sensitivities and only one problem food is removed from the diet, there may be little evidence of improvement.

Part 1 of the Diet

The Multiple Food Elimination Diet excludes the major foods that most frequently cause allergies. Do not be concerned that there is nothing to feed your child. This diet allows your child or family to eat *most* fruits, vegetables, meats, and some grains (oats and rice).

During Part 1 of the diet the following foods are omitted in all forms: milk and dairy products (yogurt, cheese, ice cream, lactose, casein), wheat (bread, cake, cookies, baked goods), eggs, corn, sugar, chocolate (cocoa or cola), peas (peanut butter), citrus (orange, lemon, lime, grapefruit), food coloring, food additives, and preservatives. No luncheon meats, sausage, ham, or bacon, or canned soups are allowed. If there is some question about a specific food, or it is a favorite, even if it is not listed, do *not* eat it. Adults must also delete coffee, tea, any other highly craved foods, and tobacco. The "allowed" and "forbidden" foods are listed in Table 8.1.

Table 8.1
Multiple Food Elimination Diet—Part 1
(read all labels first)

Allowed Cereals	*Forbidden Cereals*
Rice—rice puffs only	Foods containing wheat flour
Oats—oatmeal made with	(most cakes, cookies, bread,
honey	baked goods)
Barley	Corn
	Cereal mixtures (granola)

Allowed Fruits	*Forbidden Fruits*
Any fresh fruit, except citrus	Fresh, frozen, or canned citrus
Canned (if in their own juice	(orange, lemon, lime,
and without artificial color,	grapefruit)
sugar, or preservatives)	

Allowed Vegetables	*Forbidden Vegetables*
Most fresh vegetables except	Fresh, frozen, or canned corn,
forbidden fresh vegetables	peas, mixed vegetables
French fries (homemade)	
Potatoes	

Allowed Meats
Chicken or turkey (nonbasted)
Louis Rich ground turkey
Veal or beef
Pork
Lamb
Fish, tuna

Forbidden Meats
Luncheon meats, wieners
Bacon
Artificially colored meat or
  hamburger
Ham
Dyed salmon, lobster
Breaded meats
Meats with stuffing

Allowed Beverages
Water
Single herb or other plain tea
  with honey
Pure grape juice, bottled
Pure frozen apple juice
Pure pineapple juice

Forbidden Beverages
Milk or any type of dairy drink
  with casein or whey
Fruit beverages except those so
  specified
Kool-Aid
Coffee creamer (any type)
Soda pop

Allowed Snacks
Potato chips (no additives)
Ry-Krisp crackers and pure
  honey
Raisins (unsulfured, from
  health food store)

Forbidden Snacks
Corn chips
Chocolate or anything with
  cocoa
Hard candy
Ice cream or sherbet

Allowed Miscellaneous
Pure honey
Homemade vinegar and oil
  dressing
Sea salt
Pepper
Homemade soup

Forbidden Miscellaneous
Sugar, fructose, dextrose
Aspartame
Bread, cake, cookies, except
  from special recipes
Eggs
Jelly or jam
Jell-O
Margarine or diet spreads
  (unless no dyes and corn)
Sorbitol (corn)
Peanut butter, peanuts
Cheese
Dyed (colored) vitamins,
  mouthwash, toothpaste,
  cough syrups, etc.
Colored pills or liquid
  medicines (CONSULT
  DOCTOR FIRST)

This diet requires seventeen days. During the first week you can eat only the "allowed" foods. During the next ten days each of these omitted foods is added back into the diet, one at a time. Remember, if you know that a certain food such as egg makes your child very ill, just skip that day and *don't* try eggs. If you already know what will happen, there is no reason to evaluate that food. The purpose of the diet is to find out what you don't know or to confirm questionable suspicious foods.

Keep detailed, *exact* records in a food diary of *everything* that is eaten. Most patients who are going to respond favorably to the diet do so by about the sixth or seventh day. Improvement noted as early as Day 2 may greatly increase by Day 7. The object is to see the maximum amount of improvement that can be noted during the first seven days. If your child is better in a week or less, begin Part 2 of the diet on the eighth day. Part 2 can be started sooner if your child is *tremendously* improved in less than one week.

If you want to help your entire family, urge everyone to try the diet at the same time. Typically several family members will note improvement in how they feel or act when this is done.

The same food, for example milk, may cause the same or different problems for several members of a single family or several generations of a family. For example, milk might cause hyperactivity in one child, bed-wetting and leg aches in another, ear infections in a third, intestinal problems in a mother, halitosis in a father, nose congestion in the grandmother, and asthma in the great-grandfather.

For this reason make cooking easier by placing the entire family on the diet. A fringe benefit may be that you may relieve some emotional or "learn to live with it" health problems caused by certain foods in several family members.

If your child is *not* better within a week, carefully recheck the diet records for the initial week of the diet. Were *only* the allowed foods eaten? If your child repeatedly forgot and ate the wrong foods or drank the wrong beverages, the item that was *not* deleted or omitted from the diet may be at fault. Try Part 1 of the diet again, but this time adhere rigorously to the diet. Remember, this fast, inexpensive method of food-allergy detection can sometimes surprisingly relieve many chronic medical complaints that are due to unsuspected food allergies.

Sometimes children are worse during the first few days of Part 1 of the diet. If this happens, it could be caused by withdrawal symptoms due to food masking, as discussed in Chapter 2 and earlier in this chapter, page 166.

Another frequent cause of this problem is that an excessive amount of an unsuspected offending food or beverage was ingested. A child who substitutes apple or grape juice for milk, for example, may act or behave much worse *if* apple or grape juice are the cause of the child's symptoms. If a child is eating lots of rice or oats to replace wheat, the child will be worse if there is an allergy to rice or oats. Retry Part 1 of the diet, but stop the items that you think made your child worse if it appears that this is the cause of the problem. If that eliminates the symptoms, you may already have found one answer.

Rarely, a child who was not helped during the first week will dramatically improve with a more prolonged diet. In other words, continue Part 1 of the diet for two weeks, not one week. If Part 1 of the diet is tried and has not helped by the fourteenth day, this particular diet is not the answer for your child or your family. The child's medical problems are not related to foods, not due to the foods deleted during this diet, or are possibly due to other frequently eaten or craved food items, such as mushrooms, cinnamon, coffee, tea, and so on.

How Do You Do the Second Part of the Diet?

During Part 2 of the diet, one food is reintroduced into the diet, in excess, each day (Table 8.3). This part sometimes gives specific answers, even though the child may not have improved during Part 1 of the diet. Keep detailed records of how your child feels, before eating only the food on the top of each day on Table 8.3. Also record the effect of each food during each day. Your child should repeatedly eat the test food during the test day, preferably all by itself, and you should notice how your child feels during the next hour. At other times, the foods eaten during the first week of the diet can be consumed as desired.

Start with a teaspoon or ¼ to ½ cup of the test food item and double the amount eaten every few hours, so that by the end of the day at least a normal amount has been ingested. Do any symptoms suddenly reappear within an hour after eating the test food for that day? Do any symptoms gradually reappear as the day progresses after more of the test food for that day is eaten? If there are no undesirable symptoms during that day, during that night and the next morning before breakfast, the food tested the day before is probably all right and may be eaten whenever desired.

TABLE 8.3

Multiple Food Elimination Diet—Part 2

(Record All Foods Eaten Each Day in Appropriate Area. Read All Labels First.)

	Day 8	Day 9	Day 10	Day 11	Day 12	Day 13	Day 14	Day 15	Day 16	Day 17
	Excess milk, cottage cheese	Excess bread and wheat cereal (No preservatives)	Excess sugar (sugar cubes)	Excess eggs	Excess cocoa	Excess dyed foods, Jell-O, fruited drinks, candy	Excess corn, popcorn, whole kernel and cornflakes	Excess preservatives, baked goods, luncheon meats, soups	Excess orange, grapefruit, lemon, lime	Excess pure peanut butter
Prebreakfast					Record How Your Child Feels Before Eating Each Morning					
B R E A K F A S T					Record What Your Child Eats and When and How Your Child Feels Unwell or Misbehaves During Each Day					
S N A C K S										

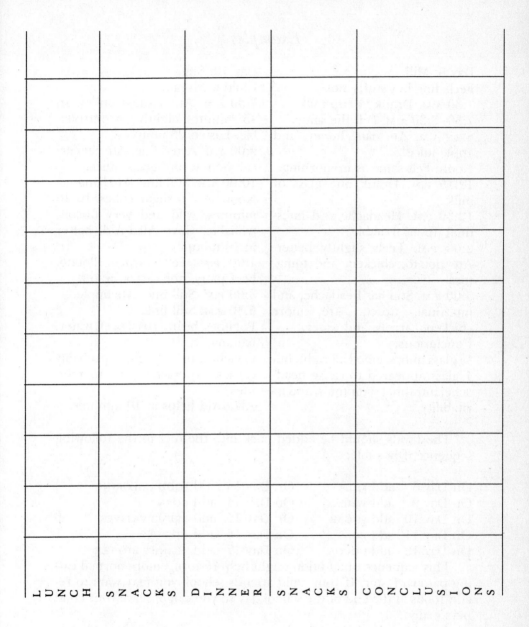

L U N C H	S N A C K S	D I N N E R	S N A C K S	C O N C L U S I O N S

Examples

Day 8: Milk
Feels fine but stuffy nose.
7:30 A.M. Drank ½ cup milk.
7:30–8:30 A.M. Felt the same.
8:45 A.M. Ate oats, honey, and apple juice.
Noon. Felt same as in morning.
12:15 P.M. Drank one glass of milk.
12:30 P.M. Headache and intestinal upset, irritable.
2:00 P.M. Feels slightly better. Ate potato, chicken, and tomatoes.
5:00 P.M. Still has headache, and intestinal upset. Ate more chicken, carrots, and water.
Conclusions:
½ glass milk seemed all right, but 1 glass appeared to cause headache, intestinal symptoms, and irritability.

Day 10: Sugar
Child a "dream"
7:30 A.M. Ate 4 sugar cubes. In 15 minutes slightly uncontrollable. Lasted 25 minutes.
9:00 A.M. Acted fine. Ate oat cereal, honey, and grape juice.
10:00 A.M. Still fine. Ate banana.
Noon. Ate 6 sugar cubes. In 10 minutes, wild and very uncontrollable. Gave Alka-Aid, better in 10 minutes.
1:00 P.M. Felt normal. Potato, beef patty, one carrot, water.
3:00 P.M. Still fine. Ate apple.
5:30 P.M. Still fine.
Potatoes, beans, roast beef, water, banana.
Conclusions: Sugar probably causes hyperactivity in 15 minutes.
Alka-Aid helps in 10 minutes.

The foods should be added back into the diet in the following sequence if possible:

On Day 8	add MILK	On Day 13	add FOOD COLORING
On Day 9	add WHEAT	On Day 14	add CORN
On Day 10	add SUGAR	On Day 15	add PRESERVATIVES
On Day 11	add EGG	On Day 16	add CITRUS
On Day 12	add COCOA	On Day 17	add PEANUT BUTTER

This sequence of addition might help restore a more normal eating pattern faster. If your child attends school, you may want to re-add foods at the end of the school day so you can observe your child personally.

At any point, if a test food causes *serious* symptoms, immediately stop eating it *in all forms* until you can secure the advice of your physician. Usually a parent will notice that the symptoms caused by a food last about an hour or so. Rarely, symptoms from a food last for several hours or days. If you are concerned about any aspect of the response to a food challenge, check with your doctor or nearest hospital.

Remember, if one of the test foods causes a reaction that is not helped by an alkali or that lasts for over twenty-four hours, *do not try* to test for another possible problem food until the previous food reaction has *entirely* subsided.

Watch closely to see what happens each day. One food might cause a stuffy nose, the next no reaction at all, the next a bellyache. Most reactions occur within fifteen to sixty minutes, others within several hours.

If you are uncertain whether a food truly caused symptoms or not, discontinue that food until the other foods have been checked. Then give your child that one suspect food again at a five-day interval, for example on Tuesday and Saturday, and see if symptoms recur.

NEVER TEST ANY FOOD WITHOUT YOUR DOCTOR'S ADVICE IF IT CAUSED SERIOUS MEDICAL PROBLEMS IN THE PAST. FOR EXAMPLE, IF EGG OR PEANUT CAUSED IMMEDIATE THROAT SWELLING OR CORN CAUSED SEVERE ASTHMA, IT IS UNSAFE TO TRY EVEN A SPECK OF THESE FOODS.

Details About Food Additions

Day 8: *The day you add milk,* give your child lots of milk, cottage cheese, and whipped cream sweetened with honey during the day. No butter, margarine, or yellow cheese unless you are absolutely certain they contain NO yellow dyes.

Day 9: *The day you add wheat,* add *plain* wheat cereal. If your child had trouble from milk, be sure *not* to give milk products. Even crackers can contain milk. Use Italian bread or kosher bread, because these should not contain milk (casein or whey), but always read labels to be sure. You can bake if you like, but you must not use eggs or sugar. Remember, your child can eat no dairy products and drink no milk if the milk day seemed to cause illness. If milk caused no problem, milk products may be eaten on Day 9.

Day 10: *The day you add sugar,* give your child sugar cubes to eat and add granulated sugar to the allowed foods. If milk or wheat caused trouble, they must be avoided or you can't tell if sugar is well tolerated. Many children feel or act differently within one hour after four to eight large sugar cubes are eaten.

Day 11: *The day you add egg,* give your child eggs in the usual *well-cooked* forms. Remember, again, no wheat, milk, or sugar can be consumed if any of these caused problems. If there were no problems, eggs can then be given in the form of custard or an egg-white frosting.

Day 12:   The day you add cocoa, give your child dark chocolate and cocoa. Only if your child had no trouble with sugar and milk can you give milk chocolate. It is best to make hot chocolate with water, cocoa (pure Hershey's cocoa powder), and honey. No candy bars are allowed because most contain corn, plus many other ingredients. Remember, milk, wheat, sugar, dyes, or eggs are not allowed if any of these caused symptoms.

Day 13:   The day you add food coloring, give your child colored gelatin, jelly, or artificially colored fruit beverages (soda pop, Kool-Aid), popsicles, or cereal. Try to give a variety of yellow, green, purple, and red items, because your child might react to only one of these food dyes. Remember to avoid milk, wheat, sugar, cocoa (cola), in all forms, if any of these were a problem. If sugar caused symptoms, use honey or sugar-free products. If milk, wheat, sugar, egg, and cocoa were tolerated, they may continue to be eaten.

Day 14:   The day you add corn, give your child a variety of corn products, such as whole-kernel corn, cornmeal, cornflakes, corn syrup, popcorn, and tortilla. Try several forms of corn because sometimes only one will cause illness. The popcorn can be air-popped and eaten plain without salt, oil, or butter. If milk, wheat, sugar, dyes, eggs, or chocolate caused symptoms, you can't give them on the same day that you give corn. If you do, and your child is worse, you won't be able to tell which is at fault. Use butter on the popcorn only if your child had no milk sensitivity.

Day 15:   The day you add preservatives, give your child foods that contain preservatives or food additives. Look for the longest list of these on the store labels. In particular, eat luncheon meat, bologna, hot dogs, breads, pastries, or soups that contain numerous preservatives and additives. If any of the above food items caused symptoms and are ingredients included in luncheon meats, etc., then the latter should not be eaten.

Day 16:   The day you add citrus, give your child a large amount of lemon, lime, grapefruit, or orange as fresh fruit, and/or as a pure juice. Avoid artificial dyes, if food colors were a problem, and citrus drinks, because of other ingredients. Avoid regular Jell-O-like preparations if sugar or dyes were a problem. Instead buy plain gelatin and make your own with pure fruit juice and honey. Use carbonated water in pure juice to create homemade pop. Do not try beverages with aspartame because the latter can also cause allergies in some children. If in doubt, check that sweetener at a four-day interval.

Day 17:   The day you add peanut butter, give your child lots of pure peanut butter without additives (Smuckers) or plain peanuts. Test for this only if it's a favorite food. Allow your child to eat the peanut butter from the spoon, or put it on Ry-Krisp crackers or rice cakes if no wheat is allowed.

If your child refuses the diet, try offering a reward. Promise a gala party if there is no cheating and if it is obvious that the child is truly trying very hard to cooperate in every way. The party should take place *after* both parts of the diet are completed. Give your child the foods that caused slight symptoms, not severe ones, and this will be a double check confirming the effect of these foods on your child. The party will probably cause symptoms if your child eats foods that caused symptoms during Part 2 of the diet. Give an alkali before the party begins if you want to try to prevent problems.

Special Tips for Following the Multiple Food Elimination Diet

The "allowed" foods in Part 1 of the diet can be selected, combined, and eaten in any quantity throughout Part 1 and Part 2 of the diet unless something causes obvious symptoms.

For a beverage you can mix the allowed fruits in the blender with spring water (from a glass bottle) or seltzer water and add honey or *pure* maple syrup if necessary.

Your child's usual medications can be taken during the diet, but if they appear not to be needed, see if your child's doctor will allow you to stop them. If your child improves, you may find that less medicine is needed by the end of the first week. If possible, try to use only white pills (crushed for small children and placed in applesauce or mashed potatoes) or colorless liquids. Most liquid medications contain corn, sugar, and dyes, which can commonly cause symptoms in some children. Check with your physician about any questions you may have. Do *not* taper Ritalin or cortisone without your physician's advice, because this can be dangerous.

Once you determine which foods cause specific symptoms, you must discuss your observations with your physician. Some foods cannot be omitted for indefinite periods of time if a child's proper nutrition is to be maintained. A dietitian or nutritionist may be needed.[3]

If your child has asthma, add each test food back into the diet with extreme care. It is possible that an unsuspected food could precipitate a sudden severe asthma attack, because *this diet reveals hidden causes of allergy.* You *must* check with your physician and have

3. Contact: Practical Allergy Research Foundation (PARF), P.O. Box 60, Buffalo, N. Y., 14223 (716-875-0398).

asthma medications on hand before you do Part 2 of the diet. See Chapter 10 regarding how to determine if a food causes asthma by using a peak flow meter. This instrument can give you an early warning that lung spasm is beginning, so measures can be taken to abort an impending asthma attack.

By the time all the foods that were *not* eaten during the first week of the diet have been added back, most parents know which major basic food items are the main troublemakers.

CHILD HELPED 90 PERCENT ON THE MULTIPLE FOOD ELIMINATION DIET

Dave

Dave was six years old when his mother initially noted that he was "completely uncontrollable, in endless motion, and constantly talking." After reading one of our books she tried Part 1 of the Multiple-Food Elimination Diet, and in one week he was 90 percent better. He was "not hyper at all, at his best again, obedient, loving, calm, and cooperative." She found that corn made him silly and wild during the second part of the diet. Dyes made him wild, nasty, and hyperactive. Milk caused him to cry and complain. Preservatives caused him to become belligerent and mean. Later on she found that soy made him nasty, hyperactive, and combative. His mother wisely suspected soy because he had to drink that during infancy to replace his milk formula. In time, Dave's mother found that more and more foods seemed to bother him. He was wonderful, but only if he did not eat. She came to see us because he was losing weight and was bored with his diet. He needed food allergy extract treatment so he could eat the basic foods that caused his allergies.

Not all children respond so dramatically to the diet as Dave, but many are helped to varying degrees. In general, if the diet helps 90 to 100 percent, most of that child's problems are probably due to foods. If the diet helps only 25 percent, other allergenic substances or medical problems have to be considered. It should also be stated that a food allergy can be missed with both the Single and the Multiple Food Elimination diets. If a child's problem is due to some favorite food not excluded in a diet, such as sunflower seeds or mushrooms, then that diet would not help even though a child had a food-related problem. Unless the problem food is eliminated from the diet and then added again at the correct interval of time, these diets would not be helpful.

Child Helped 50 percent on the Multiple Food Elimination Diet

Jon

On Part 1 of the Multiple Food Elimination Diet, Jon was 50 percent better in three to four days. He was less active and less restless. He had fewer tantrums and a longer attention span. During Part 2 of the diet two foods, milk and wheat, were major problems. When these were excluded from his diet, his mother was delighted. In a few days he no longer screamed for her to "get out of his room" in the morning. Instead she was greeted with a hug and kiss. In time we found that other factors both inside and outside Jon's home contributed to the other 50 percent of his symptoms not helped by the diet.

If you want many answers in a short period of time, with little expenditure of time or money, check with your physician and then try the Multiple Food Elimination Diet. The rewards are often rapid and tremendously gratifying. Many children's personality and physical problems stop within three to seven days. When each possible suspect food is eaten again, the answers are obvious because individual foods cause specific and often different problems.

No diet in our practice has ever been as effective for so many patients. Most patients whom we see have already tried the diet on their own prior to the first visit and already know several major foods which cause symptoms. Some find that only one food is a problem. After they check with their physicians, they can frequently eliminate it and do not need the help of an allergist.

How Can Sudden Food Allergic Reactions Be Relieved?

Let us suppose your child eats a meal and then, within about an hour, suddenly feels unwell or behaves inappropriately. What could be the cause? Think about foods first, especially if there are some intestinal complaints. Remember, however, that foods can also cause such varied symptoms as asthma, hay fever, headaches, leg aches, and changes in how your child acts or behaves. When a possible meal-related change of *any* sort occurs, make a *detailed* list of *everything* eaten. (See Chapter 9.) Do not forget, however, that dust, pollen, molds, and chemical odors might also have caused your child to change. If the problem appears to be related to a food, the following should be helpful:

1. Give your child an alkali or some form of baking soda. If this does not help within fifteen minutes or if you are concerned in any way, also give allergy medications.

2. Give both an antihistamine and asthma medicine if they are readily available and have been needed by your child in the past. A food reaction could begin with hay fever and proceed to asthma, hives, or a personality problem.

3. Try to make your child vomit to expel the problem food, if possible. If the food was eaten several hours before, however, consider giving your child a mild cathartic, such as Castoria or Milk of Magnesia (does not contain milk). The object is to help move the problem food more quickly through the intestines and out with a bowel movement.

If Your Child Already Has Food Allergy Extract Treatment

4. Give your child her/his food allergy extract if a food causes obvious physical or emotional illness. A child's specific allergy extract, however, may only help a child to eat the foods contained in that extract without difficulty. If the cause of the problem was cinnamon, and that is not in a food included in your child's allergy extract, it probably will not help. This extract can be used safely at the same time that you give your child an alkali and/or an antihistamine or asthma medicine. You can use whichever helps the most, or give them all at the same time if you are very concerned.

5. This last aid is a variant of the previous one but it helps some children so they can eat or drink some offending foods for which they have *not* been treated. If your child has had a provocation test for histamine, then the correct neutralization treatment dilution of this item can be given under the tongue

or by injection. If the medical problem is due to the release of histamine, your child's neutralizing dose of histamine should help.

This is a nonspecific way to treat an allergic reaction, similar to aspirin, is a nonspecific way to treat a headache. Regardless of the cause of a headache, aspirin often helps. When someone eats an egg, the egg antigen combines with an antibody to egg, and histamine is often one major chemical released, which causing illness in some body area. When grass pollen combines with an antibody to grass, histamine is again one of the main substances released. If it is the released histamine that is causing symptoms, treatment with the correct neutralization dilution of histamine often relieves the allergic symptoms regardless of whether the cause is egg, grass pollen, or some other substance. The neutralizing dose of an allergy extract for histamine can be used with an antihistamine. Because their mechanism of action is quite different, either or both can help relieve a sudden medical problem.

6. If you are frightened and alarmed, go to the nearest hospital or doctor and ask for an injection of adrenaline. This will help asthma, throat, or skin allergies in particular. If your child has frequent frightening food-allergic reactions, ask your physician to teach you how to give an injection of adrenaline. Keep it in your home, purse, and car for emergencies. This should be done even if you aren't trying a food diet. Allergic reactions tend to occur at inconvenient times, so be as prepared as you can be at all times. This is particularly true if you take your child on a long trip.

How Can Food Allergies Be Treated on a Long-Term Basis?

There are a number of alternative ways to treat food-related medical problems once you have found that your child is sensitive to a food. The following are three common ways to help:

1. First, try to avoid the food entirely. This is easy when the problem is a food such as squash. You usually know when you have eaten squash. It is not a hidden ingredient in prepackaged foods. Problem common food items, however, such as corn,

milk, soy, wheat, additives, preservatives, etc. can be hidden in many deceptively labeled foods, and therefore are very difficult to avoid (see Appendix A).

2. Receive a specific individualized food-allergy extract treatment, to be given either under the tongue or by injection.

You should find a physician who enjoys treating food allergies with allergy extract. After P/N testing and treatment, the usual amount of the majority of problematic foods, *but not all*, can be ingested at a four-day interval without causing symptoms.

The P/N allergy tests, however, may not reveal a food sensitivity if a food has not been ingested for several weeks or months. Sometimes a tiny amount has to be eaten the day before testing to obtain a reliable skin-test result. Check with your doctor to find out how or if you should do this.

When I was trained in allergy from 1955 to 1958, I was taught that food allergy could only be treated by avoiding an allergenic food. It took me eighteen years to find out that this was not true. Even today, although there are over twenty studies to prove scientifically that P/N allergy testing helps, occasionally poorly designed studies appear that say these methods are not helpful.[4] This is most unfortunate because learning how to treat food allergies with allergy extract has proven to be a blessing in countless ways for many children. Practically speaking, however, when a child can suddenly eat a food after treatment that has repeatedly caused illness in the past, a mother does not care about a study to prove it helps. She knows her child is better. Conservative medical scientists would justifiably say such evidence was "anecdotal." This does not mean the observation is untrue, only that it is unproven.

3. Try gradually to develop a tolerance to a food that causes allergy. Once again, check with your physician first before you initially try any food and again before each increment. The tricky part of this approach is finding the safe amount to give the first time. Some children cannot tolerate a smell or even a drop of certain foods.

The basic principle that has helped selected children so that they can eat more of a food that causes an allergy is as follows: *If your physician approves,* eat only a small quantity, or *much* less than the usual amount, of a problem food at a four-day interval. For example, three

4. See Bibliography.

glasses of milk at a four-day interval might cause terrible symptoms, but if someone drank only one-half teaspoon at a four-day interval, it might cause no difficulty at all. Then at four-day intervals gradually increase from one-half teaspoon to one teaspoon, and eventually work up to one glass a day.

It is definitely possible to treat some food sensitivities by total avoidance, without the need for any allergist. For some foods, tolerance is regained if the food is not eaten for a long period of time. This tolerance can be lost, however, if a food is eaten again in excess. By using the four-day rotation diet (see Chapter 24) and/or a food allergy extract therapy, it is often possible, in time, to regain tolerance to many foods without difficulty. This is possible even though they previously caused mild to moderate allergic reactions.

These alternatives, again, seem to be effective for foods that cause mild to moderate, rather than severe, symptoms. In time many allergic patients who cannot tolerate milk on their cereal once a day will gradually be able to increase their milk consumption to a relatively normal amount. This is most likely to happen if a child is maintained on a four-day Practical Rotary Diet and if the child's food allergies are treated with a food allergy extract. The latter is not, however, always necessary.

If your child continues to eat the foods that create illness or misbehavior every day, your child's symptoms will probably persist unless you decide to give your child drugs to subdue the allergic reactions or receive injections of food allergy extract.

See Appendix D to find a nearby physician who is experienced about this newer method of allergy testing and treatment.

Possible Food Suspects Related to Specific Medical Problems

The foods specified in Table 8.4 have been associated with the listed illnesses in the practices of many specialists in environmental medicine. Everyone is an individual, so these are only possible factors. For any person it could be any food or allergic substance causing almost any illness. Milk, for example, is so often a cause of recurrent ear problems, leg aches, clucking throat sounds, bed-wetting, hyperactivity, and nose congestion that you might find this type of information helpful, and these arbitrary groupings might provide at least a little insight to help you pinpoint the cause of your child's illness more rapidly.

TABLE 8.4

Possible Food or Other Suspects Related to Specific Medical Problems*

Nose Problems	Wheezing and Asthma	Hyper-activity	Eczema	Hives	Headache	Ear Problems	Recurrent Infection	Bed-wetting	Cystitis
Milk†	Milk†	Artificial coloring	Egg	Chocolate	Milk†	Milk†	Milk†	Milk†	Tea
Chocolate	Egg	Preservatives	Milk†	Milk†	Cheese	Egg	Egg	Juice (apple, grape, grapefruit, pineapple)	Milk† or cheese
Egg	Wheat or any grain	Sugar (cane or beet)	Chocolate	Egg	Egg	Chocolate	Corn	Egg	Orange or other fruit juice
Wheat	Fish	Milk†	Nuts	Peanut	Chocolate	Peanut	Wheat	Wheat	Sugar
Artificial coloring	Shellfish	Corn	Peanut	Peanut butter	Chicken	Peanut butter	Cinnamon or other spices	Pork	Preservatives
Yeast	Peanut	Cocoa	Peanut butter	Cinnamon	Corn	Corn	Citrus (orange, lemon, lime, grapefruit)	Tomato	Grapes
	Peanut butter	Wheat	Yeast	Preservatives	Peanut	Chicken	Chocolate	Chicken	Coffee
Dust	Cocoa	Grains	Grains	Artificial coloring or flavoring	Peanut butter	Wheat	Cola	Cola	Cola
Pollen	Corn	Egg	Potato	Seasonal: Strawberry, Melon, Tomato	Pea			Cocoa	Corn
Molds	Nuts	Apples/Juice			Bean	Dust	Molds	Onion	Nuts
Pets	Onion	Grapes/Juice	Dust	Aspirin	Cinnamon	Mites	Dust	Fish	
	Garlic	Peanut	Pollen	Penicillin	Pork	Pets		Cinnamon	Dust
	Yeast	Peanut butter	Molds	"Any" Antibiotic or Drug	Garlic	Molds		Apple	Pollen
		Tomato			Food coloring			Peanut	Molds
	Aspirin	Food additives			Shrimp			Peanut butter	Natural gas
	Tartrazine or yellow dyes	Artificial flavoring						Preservatives	Exhaust fumes
	Sulfites	Banana			Pollen			Artificial coloring	
		Orange			Molds				
	Cat	Yeast			Dust			Molds	
	Dog				Pets				
	Dust	Dust			Air pollution				
	Pollen	Molds			Auto exhaust				
	Molds				Tobacco smoke				

Muscle Pain or Weakness	Joint Tightness	Colitis	Ulcer (Duodenal)	Gall Bladder Disease	Canker Sores	Convulsions or Tics	Kidney Problems	High Blood Pressure
Perfume / Chemical odors / Auto exhaust		*Pollen / Chemical odors*			*Paint fumes / Perfumes / Chemical odors / Natural gas*			
Wheat or grains	Wheat or grains	Milk†	Milk†	Chocolate	Citrus	Milk†	Milk†	Coffee
Corn	Potato	Wheat	Chicken	Egg	Vitamin C	Egg	Wheat	Chocolate
Milk†	Tomato	Egg	Wheat	Pork	Pickles	Yeast or mold	Citrus	Corn
Chocolate	Milk†	Corn	Corn	Onion	Apples	Vitamin B	Grass	Nuts
Citrus (orange)	Beef	Cocoa	Egg	Chicken	Coffee	Chicken or any food		Peanut
Molds	Pork	Nuts	Beef	Milk†	Chocolate	Molds		Peanut butter
Chemicals	Ham	Orange	Tomato	Coffee	Potato			Milk†
Synthetic carpets	Bacon	Pork	Coffee	Orange	Nuts			Wheat
	Lard	Beef	Tea	Corn	Cinnamon			Rice
	Chicken	Chicken	Orange	Bean	Mint			Beef
	Egg	Peanut	Avocado	Nuts	Vinegar			Shrimp
	Coffee	Peanut butter	Peach		Mouthwash			Seafood
	Tea	Sugar	Potato		Mouth freshener			Chicken
	Food coloring	Molds	Barley		Toothpaste			Pork
	Molds	Yeast	Chocolate					Chemicals
	Chemicals		Grapes					Phenol
	Natural gas		Peanuts					
	Gasoline		Peanut butter					
			Spices					

*Doris J. Rapp, M.D. *Allergies and Your Family.* 1980. Practical Allergy Research Foundation (PARF), P.O. Box 60, Buffalo, N.Y. 14223-0060.
†Milk includes *all* forms of dairy: milk, cheese, yogurt, ice cream, whey, casein, or caseinate.

You Are Right—Not All Food Problems Are an Allergy or a Food Sensitivity

In particular think of allergy if a child has allergic relatives, looks allergic, and/or had repeated formula problems during infancy, but the following can be noted in any individual, allergic or nonallergic:

- Prunes and baked beans cause diarrhea and abdominal gas.
- Cheese is constipating.
- Corn can pass undigested through the intestines.
- Greasy foods can cause abdominal or gall bladder discomfort.
- Improperly chilled or canned foods can contain germs that cause illness.
- Chemicals such as tyramine and phenylethylamine in cheese and chocolate can cause headaches.
- Caffeine can cause nervousness and insomnia.
- Excess vitamin C causes diarrhea.

Some individuals have other intestinal medical problems. They can't digest milk because they lack lactase to digest the milk sugar called lactose. These individuals often have excessive abdominal gas and diarrhea if they ingest any dairy product (see Chapter 27).

Some foods naturally release histamine, so they can cause hives or asthma, for example, that are unrelated to an allergic reaction. These include cheese, lobster, shrimp, mackerel, salmon, egg white, tomatoes, pork, chocolate, tuna, sausage, bananas, and strawberries. Both pineapple and papaya can directly release histamine after they are ingested. Excess histamine released from foods can produce hives, flushing, nausea, diarrhea, and headaches.

Individuals who lack hydrochloric acid in their stomach or certain digestive enzymes can have innumerable intestinal symptoms and nutrient deficiencies. A hypoallergenic digestive enzyme supplement, with or without betaine hydrochloric acid, might be an answer. Again, check with your doctor, a gastroenterologist, or a nutritionist.

If your child has frothy, foamy, foul-smelling bowel movements; a distended abdomen; thin buttocks; a salty skin taste; and problems breathing, he or she could have cystic fibrosis. Check with your doctor.

Celiac disease, as well as cystic fibrosis, can at times be confused with a food allergy. Celiac children are pale and have bloated abdomens, diarrhea, foul-smelling stools, rectal gas, and poor growth. The symptoms appear shortly after grains are added to the diet. The culprit is a protein called gluten, which contains gliadins and glutenins. It is found in wheat and related grains such as rye, barley, and oats. This illness can be inherited. Some gluten-sensitive children are zinc deficient.

Although the immune system is involved, we really don't know exactly how or why. The only treatment is to eliminate all gluten from their diets. A few individuals can tolerate a small amount of gluten, or oats because the latter contains less gluten than the other grains. However, sometimes merely trying to eat just a little gluten can have a devastating effect on the gut.

The celiac gut can become so porous in time that larger-than-normal food particles can enter the bloodstream with the resultant development of typical food allergies in addition to the gluten problem.

It appears that many children and adults have chronic intestinal problems because they have undetected parasites that need treatment. Laboratories that specialize in parasite detection in bowel movements are very helpful in this regard.[5]

A large number of children seem to have yeast-related symptoms because of their excessive need for antibiotics in the past.

Some children have emotional problems that can cause eating or intestinal problems. Bulimia (intentional vomiting) and anorexia (refusal to eat) certainly have emotional components, but sometimes nutrients such as zinc appear to be helpful for some of these patients.[6]

Some babies have multiple feeding problems because the bottle is propped up, the nipple size is too small or large, or the temperature of the formula is not right.

You Want to Do a Diet That Gives Answers But Requires Less Time and Thought?

There are easier "no work, preparation, or think" diets to help detect allergy. Like most short-cuts, they are not 100 percent accurate because someone could be sensitive to one of the ingredients, but they surely provide some answers. At least two powdered, relatively hy-

5. Contact: Great Smokies Medical Laboratory, 18A Regent Park Boulevard, Asheville, N.C. 28806 (800-522-4762).
6. Alexander Schauss and Caroline Costin, *Zinc and Eating Disorders*. 1989. Keats Publishing, 27 Pine Street, New Canaan, Conn. 06840.

poallergenic preparations are available that are said to contain all the essential amino acids, vitamins, and necessary nutrients. If an older child ingests only these for several days and then feels magnificent, you may have found out that foods are a problem.

Ultrabalance was designed by the nutritionist Jeffrey Bland, Ph.D. Ultrabalance can be ordered through your health food store or you can write 3215, 56th Street N.W., Big Harbor, Washington 98335.

Another is Vivonex, produced by Norwich Eaton Pharmaceutical. Vivonex can be purchased at drugstores without a prescription. The flavorings in Vivonex could conceivably cause symptoms in some sensitive children.

Both preparations are tolerable; neither is delicious. They can be consumed as the *sole* food for a few days to help detect food allergy in certain children. If they help, food-related medical complaints should stop after about four to seven days. Remember that during the first two or three days after you stop eating foods that cause an allergy, you sometimes feel worse. Then, by the fourth day or so, if a food sensitivity exists, your symptoms should be significantly lessened. When you feel better again, slowly add single foods back into your diet. Add one food at each meal and notice which ones cause physical or other changes in your well-being.

Be sure to discuss the use of these nutrient liquids with your physician *before* you try them. This type of diet should be constantly monitored and closely supervised by your doctor.

One Last Easy Way to Detect a Food Sensitivity

If your child is ill for any reason, and fed only by fluids given into the veins, is there any surprising improvement in how the child acts or feels? Intravenous (IV) feeding is often needed because of a severe intestinal upset or surgery. Sometimes a child's constant wheezing, nose congestion, or unbearable behavior stop at that time, or the child's personality becomes surprisingly pleasant. Maybe the reason for this change is that the child has stopped ingesting a favorite food or beverage. Watch as craved foods are added back into the diet. You may have found an answer.

However, if a plain IV of dextrose makes a child worse, remember dextrose is derived from corn and this can cause increased symptoms in some corn-sensitive individuals.

Once You Have Found the Answer

Finding a major food that is causing your child to feel unwell or one that is contributing to your child's behavior or activity problems can be a tremendous relief. For the first time you realize that you are not a bad parent. Equally important, both you and your child will realize for the first time that your child is neither bad nor slow. You no longer have to sit back and wonder why or what you can do about it. The frustration, anger, and desperation all diminish in proportion to your understanding. For the first time many mothers shed tears of relief rather than anguish.

One Last Word of Caution

After food-allergy extract therapy *most* (not all) foods can be eaten, even if they cause symptoms. If any food, however, has repeatedly caused alarming symptoms in the past, this is called a fixed food allergy. Don't ever try to eat a speck of that food unless you discuss it with your doctor. It will probably have to be removed from the diet permanently. Examples of fixed food allergies are eggs, nuts, buckwheat, and fish because these can cause immediate, alarming medical crises in a few, very sensitive individuals. These foods can cause such extreme illness that they should not even be smelled, let alone eaten. With few exceptions, reactions of this type cannot be treated with allergy extracts. These extreme food sensitivities are most easily confirmed by an IgE-type RAST blood test, which will usually be extremely elevated. If your child has repeatedly eaten any of the above-mentioned foods in the past and not had an alarming reaction, that food probably does not represent a fixed food allergy. If there is a tinge of doubt, however, please check with your doctor.

CHAPTER 9

_____

Record-Keeping Made
Easy and Effective

How to Keep Records to Find Answers

If you want to detect the cause of illness in your child or yourself, a most effective and inexpensive way is to keep accurate records.

Before You Begin To Keep Records:

1. Buy a loose-leaf notebook and on the front write, "What Did ———Eat, Smell, or Touch?" Put your child's name in the blank space.
2. Buy some tags to be used in loose-leaf notebooks so that you can label various sectors. They are made of clear colored plastic and are attached to the sides of sheets of paper for use as subject dividers.
3. Make a list of all your child's major individual complaints. Add any unusual complaint, i.e., inability to speak clearly, clumsy, etc. (Typical common physical or emotional complaints are included in Table 9.1.)

Be sure to list each emotional factor separately because different items can cause irritability, aggression, behavior problems, fatigue, hyperactivity, or depression.

Table 9.1
Possible Major Complaints

Hyperactivity
Restlessness
Irritability
Hostility, aggression
Temper tantrums
Depression
Fatigue
Withdrawn or untouchable
Headache
Asthma
Coughing
Nose allergies
Eye allergies
Eczema, hives, or itchy skin
Intestinal problems (bloating, belching, nausea)
Diarrhea or constipation
Halitosis
Leg or muscle aches
Wets pants in daytime
Nighttime bed-wetting
Baggy eyes
Dark eye circles
Red ears, cheeks, nose tip
Wiggly legs
Can't read, write, or draw at times
Nonstop talking

4. Write each of your child's complaints on a small piece of paper so it fits into the clear plastic tag used to separate sections of your notebook. Also make an additional section for each of the other family members' major complaints. Allergies are typically a family problem, not just one child's.

5. Enter what was eaten, touched, or smelled in the appropriate section whenever your child is not well. If your child is old enough, obtain information directly from the child. Enter everything you or your child can recall in your notebook under the major symptom or complaint, and also cross-reference any lesser medical complaints in their appropriate sections.

   Suppose your child has extreme hyperactivity, a slight headache, and slight abdominal gas. You will have to cross-reference the latter two complaints. The details should be recorded only one time under the major complaint. For example, enter the major complaint, hyperactivity, with everything eaten, touched, smelled, and so on in the notebook section under "Hyperactivity." If your child is "always" hyperactive, try only to record the exceptionally bad episodes. Then under "Headache" enter the date, time, and "see Hyperactivity." Under "Abdominal Complaints" enter the date, time, and "see Hyperactivity."

   Do this each time you enter any major complaint. In this way after a while you will have four or five records under each heading. By checking for common factors, you will soon find answers.

   For example, each time the child was hyperactive, he may have had something dyed red, such as red soda pop, red gelatin, and/or a piece of red hard candy. This would suggest that red dye was a problem. Keep specific records. Writing "soda pop, gelatin, hard candy" is not enough; you need the color and, if possible, the brand names.

6. Most symptoms appear within fifteen to sixty minutes after eating or some exposure. Bed-wetting, ear fluid (otitis), eczema, canker sores, arthritis, or bowel problems, such as colitis, are more apt to occur several to many hours later. For these symptoms the records must therefore include the previous day or two.

7. Have a "Good Day" section in your notebook. This will give clues concerning what does *not* cause symptoms. If your child is fine all day long *and* the next morning, it means the foods, odors, and contacts from the day before are probably all right.

You may find that this list is immensely helpful. It will help you know which foods are "safe" for your child to eat when she or he has important exams, sports events, and so on. Such a list does not give 100 percent assurance, however, because symptoms will recur whenever the total exposure to allergenic items is greater than what your child can tolerate.

8. Use the grid in Table 9.2 or create a summary page in your notebook similar to the following:

Complaint	Probable Causes
Hyperactivity	Red dyes, sugar, milk, perfume (be specific as to brand)
Irritability	Popcorn
Aggression	Bubble gum, aspartame
Leg aches	Dairy products
Headaches	Molds, dust
Writes backward	Tree pollen, egg

The grid or this reference page will give you fast answers about possible past problem foods or offenders. Also add any clues noted during provocation testing. For example, if the test for dust produced and relieved a headache, add dust to the list of headache causes. If during the allergy test for molds your child's handwriting or ability to draw changed, add molds to the list of causes for poor schoolwork.

TABLE 9.2
Suspect Items

Medical complaints		Nose	Chest	Headache	Leg aches	GI	Aggressive	Too tired	Irritable	Depressed	Hyperactive	Writes backward	Can't color in lines
Dust				x									
Mites													

Tree pollen													x
terps													
Grass pollen													
terps													
Weed pollen													
terps													
Molds				x									
TOE or yeast													
Milk					x						x		
Wheat													
Egg													x
Chocolate													
Corn									x				
Sugar											x		
Apple													
Banana													
Orange													
Citrus													
Peanut													
Histamine													
Food dyes											x		
Bubble gum							x						
Aspartame							x						

How to Determine What Your Child May Have Eaten, Touched, or Smelled Before Some Symptoms of Illness or Emotional Change

Let's look at some typical examples or records.

When Your Child Has a Problem Between Awakening and Getting on the School Bus

Suppose your child seems fine in the morning upon awakening but by the time the school bus arrives, a headache, abdominal pain, or personality change is evident. Say to yourself, "What did my child eat, touch, or smell?" Enter the date, time, and everything you can recall. Include toothpaste, mouthwash, vitamins, medicines, even water. Include everything your child placed in her or his mouth; any odors she or he may have been exposed to, for example, personal scented items such as powder, or scouring powder; and any toys, such as crayons or chalk. Did your child play with the cat or crawl into a dusty area? If your child's pulse and breathing were normal when she or he woke up and then changed significantly, the cause of difficulty is probably some contact that occurred between arising in the morning and leaving for the bus. Think about all odors or contacts. Write everything briefly in your notebook. If the problem suddenly becomes evident every day for one to four weeks in the warm months, think about outside pollen or molds. If the symptoms are noted when the weather gets cold, think of dust, indoor molds, or possibly an early infection. If the complaints occur only on rainy days, after a winter snow thaw, or after being in a damp basement, think of molds. Think about anything new or different in your home.

When Your Child Has a Problem Between Leaving Home and Arrival at School

Let us suppose that your child left for school and was fine but the teachers complained that the child was ill or misbehaving by the time of his or her first class. Think back again: It could be a delayed reaction from breakfast. List *everything* eaten. Or it could be some odor on the school bus, for example, fumes, tobacco, perfume, odors of fabric softener, and so on. It could be some food or snack shared with another child on the bus. Try driving your child to school if you suspect the odors on the school bus.

Asthma (think of molds, dust, pets, and foods in particular)

11/20/90—Sudden severe asthma at 8:30 P.M. (This child's peak-flow meter [PFM] routinely ranges between 275 and 300. To find your asthmatic child's usual range, check it several times a day for three to four ordinary days. For example, if the PFM falls from 280 to 200, try to determine what caused the drop or subsequent asthma at 8:30 P.M.)

Ate	Smelled	Touched/Activity

Dinner at 6:30:
  Spaghetti
    (Brand X)*
  Apple
  Milk
	Bedroom furniture
	cleaned with
	lemon furniture
	polish
		Played games in
		damp basement
		family room

11/23/89—Severe asthma at 5:00 P.M., *before* dinner.

Ate	Smelled	Touched/Activity

Snack at 4:00 P.M.:
  Apple juice
    (Brand X)
  Peanut butter
    (Brand X)
  Grape jelly
    (Brand X)
  Natural bread
PFM fell 275–210
about 20 minutes
later
		Raked wet, *moldy*
		leaves
		Slight drizzle out-
		side
		PFM fell 276–220
		about 30 minutes
		later

11/27/89—Severe asthma at midnight.

*Specify exact brands of products eaten whenever possible.

Ate	Smelled	Touched/Activity
Snack at 10:00 P.M.: *Apple*sauce Milk PFM 280 before eating, down to 225 about 20 minutes later Glass of water just before bed	Hair spray in bathroom at 9:00 P.M. PFM not checked	Helped take clothes from dryer in *damp* basement PFM not checked

Common suspects on 11/23, 11/27 are: *apple* and *moldy* basement.

Confirmation:

1. Eat apple and drink pure apple juice at a four-day interval. Watch for a drop in PFM.

2. Check PFM before and again after purposeful exposure to moldy basement for 15 minutes. This will help tell if basement mold is a problem. Remember, more than one allergenic item can cause asthma.

Headache (often due to a food, pollen, mold, or dust)

10/8/90—Okay until shortly after breakfast, at 7:00 A.M.; 10 minutes later, headache over left eye.

Ate	Smelled	Touched/Activity
Milk *Oatmeal* Sugar Fresh *orange juice* Vitamin (Brand X) Toothpaste Water Aspirin	Dad's tobacco	Chased sister around house

10/9/90—9:00 P.M.—Slight headache—see "Hyperactivity" cross reference for details. Records show *orange* Jell-O was eaten 30 minutes before headache and increased activity.

10/14/90—Okay until after school; 10 minutes after a snack, headache over left eye.

Ate	Smelled	Touched/Activity
Snack after school: *Orange* Nutrition bar with *oats*	None	In classroom, draw- ing backward

10/20/90—Okay until after lunch; 10 minutes later, headache over
left eye.

Ate	Smelled	Touched/Activity
Orange juice (Brand X) Egg salad sandwich Mayonnaise (Brand X) White bread (Brand X) Egg, salt, pepper *Oatmeal* cookie	Odor in cafeteria	Played outside at noon recess

Suspects on 10/8, 10/9, 10/14 and 10/20 are: *orange* and *oatmeal*
cookie.

Confirmation: Try eating each item, one at a time, at a four-day
interval to see which causes a headache over the left eye.

Hyperactivity (think, in particular, of sugar and red dyes)

10/11/90—Okay from 3:00 P.M. after school until about 7:00 P.M.,
then became hyperactive and developed red ears and abdominal gas.
(Because of abdominal complaint, think first of something the child
ate or drank.)

Ate	Smelled	Touched/Activity
Snack at 4:00 P.M.:	Used crayons	Did homework
Corn chips		Played with Legos in
(Brand X)		family room
Lemonade		Watched TV
(Brand X)		
Dinner at 6:00 P.M.:		
Beef patty		
Baked potato		
Carrots		
Lettuce		
Tomato		
Mayonnaise		
(Brand X)		
Red candy		

10/14/90—Awakened late; okay until forty minutes after breakfast, then very hyperactive with red earlobes.

Ate	Smelled	Touched/Activity
Breakfast 9:00 A.M.:	Sister's hair spray	Watched TV
Red lollipop	(Brand X)	
Donut		
Oatmeal		
(Brand X)		
Milk		
Sugar		
Toothpaste		
(Brand X)		

Suspect on 10/11 and 10/14 is: *red food coloring*

Confirmation: Feed child some red-dyed item after no food or beverage for four hours. Be sure no red-colored food, beverage, or medicine is ingested for four days before this food challenge.

Leg Aches (think of foods, milk or dairy in particular; and chemicals and molds)

10/7/89—Awoke at 4:00 A.M. with leg aches.

Ate	Smelled	Touched/Activity

Dinner 6:00 P.M.:
  Fried chicken
  Paprika
  Baked potato
  Peas
  Banana
Bedtime 10:00 P.M.:
  Banana
  Milk
Toothpaste (Brand X)
	Leaky gas heater in basement
	Odor in bathroom from scented bath soap (Brand X).
		Played card game
		Used computer
		Did homework
		Took bath

10/8/89—Leg aches again at 4:00 P.M.

Ate	Smelled	Touched/Activity

Lunch at 12:00 P.M.:
  Bread (Brand X)
  Peanut butter (Brand X)
  Strawberry jelly (Brand X)
  Tomato soup (Brand X)
  Milk
	Played near heat duct
	Gas furnace malfunctioning	

10/19/89—Leg aches at 2:00 P.M. See cross reference records under "Headache," this date. (Check for gas exposure.)

11/4/89—Leg aches at 7:00 P.M.

Ate	Smelled	Touched/Activity

Dinner 5:30 P.M.:
  Tunafish (Brand X)
  Salad dressing (Brand X)
	Stood next to Dad while putting *gas* in the car at 6:30 P.M.	

Egg (hard-boiled)
Potato (boiled)
Carrots (boiled)
Toast (Brand X)

Suspects on 10/7, 10/8, and 11/14 are: *natural gas* and *gasoline*

Confirmation: Find a gas kitchen stove and light all the burners as if cooking. Sit next to the stove and read to the child for thirty minutes. Notice if leg aches occur that evening or night. If they do, recheck again and then discuss with a specialist in environmental medicine if you detect a consistent cause-and-effect relationship.

When Your Child Has a Problem Between First Class and Lunch

Perhaps your child is all right by the first class but before lunch there is a physical, behavioral, or learning problem.

Ask which classes the child attended in the morning. Could it be the odors of marking pens in art class, molds in gym, a dusty auditorium, some exposure in chemistry class, cooking odors, the home-room pets, or the new carpet in the cafeteria?

What rooms was your child in? Were there any unusual odors of paint, varnish, or cleaning solutions in the hallways or classrooms? Did the teacher or other student smell of perfume, tobacco, hair spray, mothballs, fabric softeners?

Did the child go into the lavatory? Was there an aerosol or tobacco odor there? Did your child become ill shortly afterward? Did your child have a snack, chew some gum? Record all that your child or the teacher can recall in the appropriate section of the book.

Caution:

If the medical or behavioral problems are routinely evident at 10:30 to 11:30 A.M., consider the possibility of hypoglycemia. Such youngsters often *demand*, rather than *request*, food. If your child last ate at 6:00 or 7:00 A.M., it may be low blood sugar that is the problem. If this is true, your child may also be tired, irritable, short-tempered, or upset on a daily basis, between 2:30 and 4:00 P.M., or whenever she or he has not eaten for three to four hours. Your doctor can order a glucose tolerance test if you are suspicious (see Chapter 3).

When Your Child Has a Problem Within One Hour After Lunch

Again, enter into your notebook everything eaten, smelled, or touched.

Because the change in attitude, behavior, or well-being is evident *after* lunch, think of foods first, in particular if your child has any associated digestive or abdominal complaints. Do not, however, discount the odors in the cafeteria (sterno heaters for food, etc.). The odor of fish or peanut butter from other children's lunches can certainly be a problem, particularly for some asthmatics.

Remember, consider each classroom separately. What is unusual or different about each room or teacher? You may have to go to the school and discreetly follow your child from place to place to detect the source of difficulty. New synthetic carpets, the chemicals in the pool, rooms that smell moldy or dusty, or portable classrooms often cause children to become ill in school.

When Your Child Routinely Has a Problem in the Late Afternoon at School or Upon Arriving Home

Again, ask what was eaten, touched, or smelled. List classrooms and exact times of physical or personality changes. Was a snack eaten an hour or so before the personality change? If so, it could be the cause of the difficulty. Call the teacher. Did your child's writing change? Was your child thinking and acting normally late in the afternoon? Were the windows open when the lawn was sprayed? Was the inside of the school cleaned with an odorous item? Was an insecticide used inside the school? If your child was all right before the school bus ride and then became a problem, think about contacts in the bus or try a possible snack on the way home. If food relieves the symptoms, the cause could be hypoglycemia.

When Your Child Is Worse After Dinner and Before Bed

Record under the major symptom all foods eaten and cross-reference the other complaints. Think about foods first if the symptoms are related to digestion. Was your child worse before or after the bath? Could odors in the bathroom be a factor? Did your child play directly on a dusty old or a new synthetic carpet? Which rooms was your child in—a moldy basement, a dirty attic? Did your child snack on popcorn? Did your child play with anything unusual? Did your child use a new toothpaste?

When Your Child Is Okay at Bedtime But Terrible During the Night or Upon Awakening the Next Morning

Think about delayed reactions to bedtime or midnight snacks first, or possibly a late response to dinner. Think about activities or hobbies engaged in during the evening before bed that had an odor or caused direct contact with dust or molds. Think about the bedroom—was it cleaned the day before? Does the vacuum cleaner spew dust when it is used?

Consider:

- polish, waxes, or sprays used in bedroom or bathroom;
- freshly dry-cleaned clothes or mothballs in the closet;
- new sheets, clothing, or bedclothes;
- new laundry soap, fabric softener;
- the odor of scouring powder after bath;
- toothpaste or mouthwash;
- any personal body or hair lotion, cream, powder, oil, and so on.

You cannot always detect the cause, but many children have distinct and consistent patterns to their illness or inappropriate behavior. By spending time and thought you can often find the answers. *No one knows your child the way you do.* With a little time and effort you may be able to find many answers that perplex the most astute and critical doctor or observant teacher.

How to Evaluate Your Child's Progress

Enter all the symptoms you listed on the reference tags in your record-keeping notebook on a piece of lined paper as shown on the Symptom Monitoring Sheet illustrated in Table 9.3. Along the left side of the paper you can place the symptoms and all the medicines you use. Along the top you can write the date of your entry.

Whenever possible try to put a number after each item listed. For example, next to bed-wetting put "4x/wk" or "4/7," next to headache

TABLE 9.3
Symptom Monitoring Sheet*

	Conclusion (Probable Suspects)	Recheck at a four-day interval	Milk	Most foods
After 20 Days on Rotation Diet			0	1+
1 Week After Allergy Diagnosis			0	1+
Gave Away Pets			1+	1+
Clean Bedroom, New Mattress/No Rugs			1+	1+
Bought Air Purifier			1+	2+
After Peanut Butter			1+	3+
After Citrus			1+	2+
After Preservatives			1+	3+
After Corn			1+	3+
After Food Coloring			1+	3+
After Cocoa			1+	2+
After Egg			1+	3+
After Sugar			1+	2+
After Wheat			1+	3+
After Milk			3+	3+
After Diet/Part 1			1+	1+
Before Diet			3+	3+

Your Child's Symptoms

Date

Nose symptoms

Cough

	1	2	3	4	5	6	7	8	9	10	11	12	13	14	15	16	17	Trigger
Peak Flow meter	150	190	80	75	100	70	120	80	70	80	100	80	120	140	160	190	205	Most foods, dust, pets
Eyes	2+	1+	2+	2+	1+	2+	3+	2+	3+	2+	2+	2+	2+	1+	1+	0	0	Dyes, corn
Wet bed	7/7d	2/7d	0	0	0	0	0	0	0	0	yes	0	0	0	0	0	0	Citrus
Bellyache	5/7d	1/7d	1+	1+	3+	1+	1+	2+	3+	1+	1+	1+	1+	1+	1+	0	0	Egg, corn
Headache	6/7d	2/7	3+	1+	1+	1+	1+	1+	2+	1+	1+	1+	1+	1+	1+	0	1+	Milk, corn
Muscle ache	2/7d	0/7	1+	3+	1+	0	0	0	0	0	0	0	0	0	0	0	0	Wheat
Behavior	poor	good	poor	poor	OK	poor	OK	poor	OK	good	OK	OK	good	good	good	good	good	Milk, wheat, egg, cocoa, corn
Temper tantrum	8/d	4/d	6/d	6/d	7/d	5/d	7/d	7/d	3/d	3/d	2/d	3/d	3/d	2/d	2/d	1/d	1/d	Most foods
MEDICINES Nose	3/d	2/d	3/d	3/d	2/d	3/d	2/d	3/d	2/d	2/d	2/d	2/d	2/d	2/d	2/d	1/d	1/d	
Asthma	4/d	4/d	4/d	4/d	2/d	2/d	2/d	4/d	4/d	3/d	3/d	3/d	3/d	2/d	1/d	1/d	1/d	
Allergy extract use																3/d	3/d	
Percent better		70	30	30	50	50	50	30	30	30	40	40	75	80	85	90	90	

Percent on rotation diet													80	
Best day of 4 day rotation													1	
Worst day of 4 day rotation													4	
Percent of home changes completed								60	60	70	80	80		
Percent chemical avoidance done													80	

*For a free blank copy of the Symptom Monitoring Sheet, send a self-addressed stamped envelope to: Practical Allergy Research Foundation (PARF), P.O. Box 60, Buffalo, N.Y. 14223-0060.

"2x/day" or "2/d," next to tantrums "6x/day" or "6/d." Next to each specific listed medicine put "3x/d" or however often your child uses it. If your child has asthma and uses a peak flow meter, enter the typical reading, for example 150, indicating the level your child can blow.

If a complaint such as stuffiness or irritability can't be quantified with a number, then use a 1+ to 3+ scoring system. The simplest gauge is to mark the symptom 1+ if it is very mild. Mark it 3+ if it is extremely severe. Anything in between is called a 2+. Then merely note the intensity of each symptom and mark it in the appropriate square.

If a treatment is helping, your child should have progressively fewer complaints each day or week and should use less medicine. If the asthma is responding favorably, the PFM should show significant increases even though less asthma medicine is needed.

If a major change occurs, write it in as indicated on the record. Note such items as an infection, heavy chemical pollution in the air, damp weather, playing in wet leaf piles, extensive house cleaning, moving to a new house, starting a rotation diet, making the bedroom allergy-free, problems with the furnace, playing with a dog, and so on. If your child is always worse on Day 4 of the rotation diet, note it. This may provide a clue that some food eaten repeatedly on that day is a problem.

If records of this type are kept before the Multiple Food Elimination Diet is begun and again at the end of one week, you will readily see that common foods can affect your child. Then if you keep detailed daily records as you add each food back into the diet every day, you'll see which medical complaint is related to which food item. For example, you may see that the stuffiness goes from 3+ to 1+ at the end of the first week of the diet. This suggests that one of the foods taken from your child's regular diet affected your child's nose. Then, after you add milk back into the diet on Day 8 of the diet, the stuffiness increases again to 3+. That suggests that milk is contributing to the nose symptoms.

CHAPTER 10

_____

What Else Can You Do?

Peak Flow Meter to Detect Causes of Asthma

A peak-flow meter (PFM) is a plastic tube that has a numeric gauge on it.[1] When your child uses this or similar instruments, they enable you to tell how much air your child can forcibly blow from his lungs when he breathes out as hard as he can. Children over five years of age can easily use this instrument. After taking a very deep breath they put their lips *tightly* around the mouth end of the instrument and then expire or blow out as hard and as fully as possible. A short, fast, forced expiration is more effective than a long-drawn-out attempt to blow the air slowly from the lungs.

These instruments provide superb help for parents and adult asthmatics who want to detect exactly what is causing lung spasm or asthma. For example, if your child blows 200 before she eats a meal and only 150 about twenty minutes later, you should ask why. Then each food item eaten should be checked separately to find out which food causes lung spasm.

If your child blows 300 before and after a ride in Dad's car, but a drop of 50 points always occurs after a ride in Mother's car, ask why. What is inside Mom's car that could be causing difficulty? Is the smell of perfume, gas fumes, the plastic upholstery, or a moldy odor from the air conditioner causing spasm?

If a child blows 200 before bed, and the first thing in the morning routinely blows only 125, ask why. Could it be the scented laundry detergent or fabric softener used on the bed linen or bedclothes? Is it the dust in the mattress or the feather pillow? Is it the snack eaten just before bedtime? With a little thought the answer can be found. When you find the answer, eliminate the cause, and if you can't or

1. See Appendix B.

are concerned, check with your physician for advice.

Many parents can learn to detect an early infection or recognize a brewing early asthma attack because their child's routine PFM readings suddenly drop significantly from 275 to a consistent 200. The normal daily variation in PFM readings should be about 10 percent, at most 20 percent. A significant drop should enable an experienced knowledgeable parent to abort or decrease the intensity of some incipient asthma attacks. Prompt treatment should lessen the severity of asthma, and earlier recognition of a problem means that cause-and-effect relationships should be easier to detect. If the cause of the sudden PFM fall is not evident, the expertise of a specialist in environmental medicine might prove helpful.

Other common causes of sudden drops in a PFM reading which last for days or weeks could include the onset of a pollen season and damp weather in mold-sensitive children. A drop could detect a dietary change or pattern, for example, such as when a child repeatedly eats too much of a particular problem food on one specific day of a Practical Rotary Diet. If the PFM reading consistently falls after an allergy extract treatment, the extract may need adjustment (see the record sheet for PFM and pulse in Table 10.1).

ALLERGIES DETECTED WITH A PEAK FLOW METER

Theresa

When Theresa first came to see us, she wheezed so badly each morning that she needed to use her vast personal array of asthma medications as soon as she woke up. She lived in a very old, moldy and dusty home, but the family could not afford to move. I asked that she use the PFM instrument to measure how well she could breathe in each of the different rooms in their home. I suggested that she sleep in one room after another and compare her capacity to breathe before she went to bed with her ability to breathe the following morning. In this way we hoped to determine which room would be best for her to use as her bedroom. Much to our surprise, Theresa found that she could breathe remarkably better in the morning if she slept in one particular room. When we questioned her mother, she readily provided the answer. This bedroom was built as an add-on in the middle of their home because they needed another room. Because it had a separate heating unit and the door was always kept closed, it was less moldy and dusty than the rest of the house.

TABLE 10.1
How to Use the Peak Flow Meter (PFM)*

The aim of these records is to reveal what causes your child's breathing or pulse to change significantly. If a PFM reading of a quiet child consistently drops 50 points or more or more than 10 to 20 percent and the pulse increases 20 points or more, this can provide a significant clue that can indicate why some child is not well. If your child does not have asthma, there is no need to do PFM readings.

Is Your House a Problem?

Before	PFM	Pulse	After	PFM	Pulse
8:00 A.M.			8:00 P.M.		
Bed			Arising		
Kitchen			1 hour later		
Bathroom			1/2 hour later		
Family room			1 hour later		
Living room			1 hour later		
Basement			1 hour later		
Bedroom #1			1 hour later		
Bedroom #2			1 hour later		
Vacuuming			1/2 hour later		
Dusting			1/2 hour later		
Furniture polish			1/2 hour later		
Laundry bleach			15 minutes later		
Fabric softener			15 minutes later		
Floor wax			15 minutes later		
Bathroom aerosol			15 minutes later		

Basement			15 minutes later		
Carpet play			15 minutes later		
Air conditioner			15 minutes later		
Furnace blower			10 minutes later		
Paint odor			10 minutes later		
Church odors			10 minutes later		

Are Your Personal Items a Factor?

	Before	PFM	Pulse		After	PFM	Pulse
Toothpaste				15 minutes later			
Mouthwash				15 minutes later			
Deodorant				15 minutes later			
Hair preparation				15 minutes later			
Powder				15 minutes later			
Cosmetics				15 minutes later			

Is Outside the House a Problem?

	Before	PFM	Pulse		After	PFM	Pulse
Outside air				15 minutes later			
Backyard				15 minutes later			
Garage				15 minutes later			
Long car rides				15 minutes later			
Grocery store				15 minutes later			
Clothing store				15 minutes later			

Are Chemicals a Problem?

	Before	PFM	Pulse		After	PFM	Pulse
Filling gas tank				15 minutes later			
Lawn spray				15 minutes later			
Pesticide or termiticide				15 minutes later			
Perfume				15 minutes later			
Tobacco				15 minutes later			
Aerial sprays				15 minutes later			
Hobby odors				15 minutes later			

Is School a Problem?

	Before	PFM	Pulse		After	PFM	Pulse
Before school				End of school day			
School bus				30 minutes later			
Gym				30 minutes later			
Homeroom				30 minutes later			
Lavatory				15 minutes later			
Library				30 minutes later			
Swimming				30 minutes later			
Art class				30 minutes later			
Chemistry				30 minutes later			

Is Work a Problem?

	Before	PFM	Pulse		After	PFM	Pulse
A.M. Work days				8 hours later			
A.M. Days off				8 hours later			
P.M. Work days				8 hours later			
P.M. Days off				8 hours later			
Lavatory				15 minutes later			
After air purifier at work				8 hours later			

Are Foods a Problem?

	Before*	PFM	Pulse		After*	PFM	Pulse
Breakfast—Day 1				20 minutes later			
Lunch " "				20 minutes later			
Dinner " "				20 minutes later			
Breakfast—Day 2				20 minutes later			
Lunch " "				20 minutes later			
Dinner " "				20 minutes later			
Breakfast—Day 3				20 minutes later			
Lunch " "				20 minutes later			
Dinner " "				20 minutes later			
Breakfast—Day 4				20 minutes later			
Lunch " "				20 minutes later			
Dinner " "				20 minutes later			

*Record what was eaten. If PFM falls 25–50 points or pulse increases 20 or more points, then eat each food eaten at that meal separately to determine which one caused the change.

Are Your Medicines a Problem?

Before	PFM	Pulse		After	PFM	Pulse
Asthma Med #1			20 minutes later			
Asthma Med #2			20 minutes later			
Antihistamine #1			20 minutes later			
Other meds			20 minutes later			
			20 minutes later			
			20 minutes later			
Allergy extract medicine* #1			20 minutes later			
Allergy extract medicine* #2			20 minutes later			
Allergy extract medicine* #3			20 minutes later			
Allergy extract medicine* #4			20 minutes later			

*By injection or under tongue

Miscellaneous

Before	PFM	Pulse		After	PFM	Pulse

*For a free blank copy of a record sheet for PFM and pulse, send a self-addressed stamped envelope to: Practical Allergy Research Foundation (PARF), P.O. Box 60, Buffalo, N.Y. 14223-0060.

Where Can You Buy a Peak Flow Meter?

One brand is Standard Mini-Wright. It can be purchased by anyone from Keller Medical Specialists (see Appendix B). Depending on the type of insurance coverage you have, the cost may be covered if your doctor writes a note that requests your child to use this instrument to help detect causes of asthma or in an effort to abort potentially severe wheezing episodes.

The major advantages other than the monitoring of lung function are that the Standard Mini-Wright instrument is easy to hold, compact, has removable and disposable mouthpieces, and registers up to 800 liters per minute. The major disadvantage is that it is made of breakable plastic.

Another type of DX Peak Flow Meter is made by CDX Corporation. They provide one instrument for young children, and another for older children and adults (see Appendix B).

The peak flow meter or pulse record in Table 10.1 illustrates how accurate records can be used to detect possible causes of physical health, learning, or behavior problems in your child. If hypertension is a problem, merely add another column to record blood pressures.

Pulse Changes—
To Detect Unsuspected Allergic Reactions

One easy way to detect a possible allergic reaction is to learn to take your child's pulse. Any medical friend or the nurse at your doctor's office or at a hospital would be pleased to teach you.

It is easy to take a pulse. Merely place your right palm under your left wrist. Curve your fingertips about the outer edge of the left wrist and press gently. You should easily feel the pulse beat with your first three fingers. However, be sure to take the pulse only when your child is relatively quiet and not crying.

If your child is very small, you can purchase a stethoscope for about ten dollars at any medical-supply store. Be sure to purchase the right-sized earpieces so that the stethoscope does not hurt your ears. Just press the instrument directly on the bare chest about an inch inside and one inch below the left nipple. You should easily hear the heartbeat. Merely count the number of beats for a full minute.

To take a pulse, you need a watch or clock with a second hand. Count the beats for a full minute—don't count for fifteen seconds and multiply by four. This method may be efficient, but accuracy is more desirable until you are much more experienced.

A nonallergic child's pulse rate is similar to an adult's. It is usually about 80 beats per minute, with a range from about 65 to about 85. (Some people, especially athletes, normally have lower pulses.) An infant's pulse is about 110 until the age of six months, and 100 between the age of six and twelve months. In time you will know the usual range of your child's pulse. If you check it before and twenty minutes after meals, car rides, visits, school, church, unusual contacts, and so on, you may find that your child is a pulse indicator. A significant increase of 20 or more points during the night may indicate a sensitivity to something in the bedroom or be related to a bedtime snack. Some children's pulses increase 40 points or more in various areas of a house or after an exposure to some item to which they are sensitive.

Sometimes you can detect that an allergy extract, drug, or antibiotic is not right for your youngster because of a significant pulse increase. Place a pill you are concerned about on your child's tongue for about three or four minutes. Do not let your child swallow it. See if the pulse alarm goes off. The pulse of some sensitive children can suddenly increase more than 20 points or at times become irregular within ten to thirty minutes after certain allergenic exposures or contact with an offending medicine or substance. If such problems arise, do not allow your child to swallow that pill but instead check with your doctor.

During P/N testing we monitor children's pulses every seven minutes between every skin test. The pulse often increases by 20 to 30 points (85 to over 100) after we begin to test for certain items. When the neutralization dose is found, the pulse frequently drops to about the 65-to-75 range. It may not always increase, but when it does, this is considered to be one more indication of a probable sensitivity to the item being tested.

PULSE CHANGES DURING P/N TESTING IN A FOUR-YEAR-OLD BOY

Mark

Mark first saw us at the age of four years. His behavior was violent and extreme. Until he came to see us, he would have two or three very violent episodes a day, which lasted as long as two hours. Then he would remain nasty for the next forty-eight hours. On her own his mother tried the Multiple Food Elimination Diet and detected his major problem foods. Milk, wheat, and corn caused him to become mean, aggressive, and unpredictable. During the next few months his mother tried to avoid these foods, but every time an error was made, he would explode. She knew that the odors of marking pencils, bleach, bus fumes, and perfume could cause similar periods of uncontrollable behavior, but as soon as Mark was taken away from the odor, he quickly returned to normal. She came to see us because he needed treatment for his food problems; avoidance was simply not practical or possible.

His mother sobbed as she related how often he would kick his siblings and her. Mark would not listen. No one would baby-sit. They could not take him anyplace without being embarrassed. His grandparents urged his parents to hit and discipline him. This darling boy looked and acted like an angel and then suddenly he would become totally impossible. His mother learned to be wary if she saw his earlobes and cheeks become red. The typical glassy, glazed eyes quickly followed, and then he was out of control.

His behavior, however, was not his only challenging problem. His mother was worried and concerned about his schoolwork. She desperately wanted to help him. After she learned more about allergies, she noticed that whenever he ate corn, he could not differentiate symbols such as circles and triangles. If he did not eat corn, he could easily recognize them.

He had been seen by a well-trained, board-certified allergist about three months before we saw him. His parents were told that there was a controversy about foods and behavior and were told that this was not their son's problem. They were told to "liberalize his diet" because his prick or scratch allergy skin tests showed no food or other allergy. The allergist suggested that he be seen by a pediatrician specializing in behavioral problems.

At about that same time he was also seen by another specialist in environmental medicine. He became wild and violent during allergy testing. He kicked, scratched, screamed, and cried during the milk and corn provocation allergy tests in particular. His neutralization allergy treatment seemed to make him better at first, but then he seemed worse after each treatment. Because of this, that doctor referred Mark to our office.

When we tested him, he drooled, whined, yelled, and cried during the test for milk. During the provocation allergy skin test for milk his pulse rose from 64 to 84. His pulse fell to 64 again when we found his correct milk neutralization treatment dosage. With the corn

TEST WITH MILK ALLERGY EXTRACT
Changes in Drawing of a 4 Year Old Boy

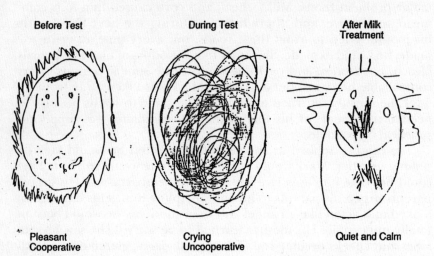

Before Test   During Test   After Milk
Treatment

Pleasant
Cooperative   Crying
Uncooperative   Quiet and Calm

Figures 10.1–10.3. Changes in drawing of a four-year-old boy during a milk allergy extract test

TEST WITH SUGAR ALLERGY EXTRACT

Changes in Drawing of a 4 Year Old Boy

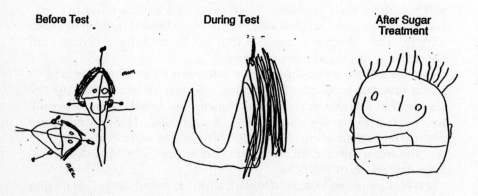

Before Test   During Test   After Sugar
Treatment

Figures 10.4–10.6. Changes in drawing of a four-year-old boy during a sugar allergy extract test

test he frowned and wanted to leave the office. His pulse rose from 68 to 88 and then fell to 64 again after he was given the right dilution of corn. At that point he felt normal again. Figures 10.1–10.6 clearly illustrate how well he drew before and after his P/N tests for milk and sugar. It is truly amazing that a weaker drop of sugar allergy extract would cause his ability to draw to change so drastically.

One of his most violent reactions occurred during the yeast test. He drooled, took off his shirt and shoes, cried, whined, yelled, said his feet itched and hurt, developed a headache, and acted terribly. When we found his treatment dose of yeast extract, his personality totally changed and he kissed his mother. His pulse was 64 before the test, 96 during his reaction, and it fell to 64 again after we found his treatment dilution for yeast. Routinely after we found the right neutralization dilution for each food that was tested, he acted calm and normal.

One day, shortly after we had begun to test Mark, his mother could not believe the change. That night they had gone out to dinner. He was unbelievably pleasant! They actually enjoyed each other's company. This had never happened before. She said he had improved 80 percent. His Conner's Hyperactivity Score decreased from an abnormal high of 24 before the allergy diet to 15 after the first week of the Multiple Food Elimination Diet.

After only one day of testing in our office this score fell to an extraordinary normal level of 1. This pattern is somewhat typical. Children often improve initially because of the P/N testing and treatment. On a long-term basis they are better because of the home, diet, and nutrient changes.

Unfortunately Mark's improvement was very short-lived. On our extract he was fine, but again only for about two weeks, just as he had been with the previous ecologist's treatment. If his pulse rose shortly after he received his extract, it indicated he could no longer receive that particular allergy treatment, even though it had helped in the past. His mother found that if she sharply limited his diet, he acted fine. However, he also appeared to be unable to tolerate relatively hypoallergenic vitamins and nutrients that he needed, or his allergy extract. Frequent retesting was impossible because the family lived so far away.

The first night after his family moved into an environmentally safe home, he slept all night, and this pattern has continued since then. Prior to the move it was most exceptional if he slept three nights a week. His nose symptoms of allergy stopped and his violent episodes decreased in frequency. He continues to flare up with certain chemical exposures.

Our present challenge is to determine why he cannot tolerate allergy extract neutralization treatment. We're investigating the non-food components in allergy extracts to see if treatment for these will resolve his difficulties. In the meantime he remains 80 to 100 percent better, but his diet is very limited. We must find a way to treat him before he becomes allergic to the few remaining "safe" foods he can presently eat without difficulty.

After more retesting, he definitely improved but his extracts needed to be rechecked frequently.

A Food-Coloring Sensitivity Detected With Pulse Changes

Derrick

Derrick's mother thought he was allergic to food coloring. He was tested for this possible sensitivity by placing one drop of red, blue, and yellow food coloring under his tongue. Within a few minutes he became hyperactive and his pulse increased from 84 to 128. Within ten minutes after he was given the correct dilution of dye under his tongue, his pulse decreased to 76 and his activity level returned to normal. His pulse change helped to confirm that we had found the correct neutralization dose for food coloring. In the future when his mother had to give him a colored medicine, she also gave him his neutralization dose for dyes. He no longer became hyperactive as he had in the past from this item.

Some allergic children have a marked pulse elevation whenever they are exposed to certain items such as dust, molds, pollen, foods, pets, or chemicals. The pulse acts like a silent smoke alarm. It often increases by 20 to 50 points in response to certain food exposures or contacts that cause children to feel unwell or act inappropriately.

A Mold Sensitivity Detected With Pulse Changes

Nicky

Nicky came to see us from upper Canada when he was about two years old. His mother noticed that when he was home, his pulse tended to range around 140. When he was in Buffalo, however, his pulse was typically about 80. In time we found that his pulse increased whenever he was inside his home, which happened to be extremely damp and moldy. When the family moved to a different home, his pulse decreased to 80, as it was whenever he was in Buffalo. The increase in pulse gave us the clue that something in his home environment was causing a silent alarm in his little body.

Allen

Allen came to see us when he was nine years old. He stated he felt much better in Buffalo than when he was home in New York City. We found his pulse ranged in the eighties in Buffalo, but he was routinely about 100 or above when he was at home, or after he reacted to testing with an allergy extract. His mother took his pulse in an airplane. She found that after he had been in the air for three hours, his pulse dropped from over 100 to the mid-seventies. In both New York City or Los Angeles, the pulse rose back over 100 shortly after the plane landed and it stayed elevated until he left these cities. His personality and behavior deteriorated dramatically in each of these cities.

Do Doctor's Agree About the Significance of Pulse Changes?

They certainly do not. Dr. Arthur Coca, a distinguished allergist, wrote about the importance of pulse changes in the detection of allergy in 1956. In his book entitled *The Pulse Test* he discusses how pulse changes can vary if someone is sensitive to water, foods, pollen, molds, dust, pets, chemicals, tobacco, alcohol, lipstick, and so on. He repeatedly showed that certain exposures or contacts caused consistent pulse increases. These changes often provided clues that helped him to relieve a wide range of illnesses. He said that the maximum normal range for the human resting pulse was only 16 points. He believed that a deviation greater than that indicated a possible allergy. It is unfortunate that the majority of physicians today continue to disbelieve that the pulse can provide a valuable clue to the cause of some illnesses.

When I studied allergy in the late 1950s, I was taught that the pulse was of no value in the diagnosis of allergy. I was therefore amazed when I initially learned to do P/N allergy testing. It was not uncommon for many children repeatedly to have significant pulse changes during testing for some, but not all, allergenic substances.

We found that their pulses routinely dropped to the normal range at the same time that the other symptoms diminished after we found the neutralization treatment dose.

Many patients' mothers have now learned to check their child's pulse, and I am continually impressed by their ability to pinpoint specific causes of their child's illnesses or behavioral problems. We frequently find that new patients have pulses in an elevated range until their allergies respond to treatment. Then their pulses remain in the normal range unless they need retesting or are exposed to some item for which they have not been treated. Our bodies are truly amazing and magnificent. They give us so many nonverbal answers. We only need to pay closer attention.

High Blood Pressure and Other Cardiac Problems

Joseph Harkavy, M.D., and William Rea, M.D., in Dallas, Texas, both studied many cardiac patients.[2] They scientifically documented that the heart and blood vessels of some allergic individuals can react in a wide variety of ways when they are exposed to various allergenic substances, including chemicals. The latter can cause the blood pressure of some patients to increase. Others develop a rapid or very slow heart rate, an irregular heartbeat, angina (heart pain due to blood-vessel spasm), or blood clots in their blood vessels. Once again a bit of thought may provide answers to some chronic problems. The clue may be what was eaten, touched, or smelled just prior to the first indication that the heart was not functioning normally. Once again, if the cause of the cardiac problem can be found, maybe drug therapy or surgery will not be necessary. By feeling the pulse, it is easy to spot some irregularities.

The specific cause of hypertension or high blood pressure in children or adults can sometimes be due to allergies or food or chemical sensitivities. Dr. Rea's studies have shown that the blood pressures in a group of fifty-three patients he studied were initially in the range of 173/104. The levels fell to the normal range of 121/77 after appropriate comprehensive environmental care. Prior to therapy his patients all needed blood pressure medication, while after an envi-

2. See Dr. William Rea's reference articles listed under Vascular Disease in Bibliography; Joseph Harkavy, *Vascular Allergy and Its Systemic Manifestations*. 1963. Butterworth's, 7235 Wisconsin Avenue, Washington, D.C.

3. Gerald Ross and William Rea, "Environmentally Triggered Hypertension, Part II," Environmental Health Center—Dallas Treatment Experience, presented at the 8th Annual International Symposium on Man and His Environment in Health and Disease, Dallas, Tex., February 22–25, 1990.

ronmental evaluation only 8 percent needed antihypertension drugs. As Dr. Rea's studies have indicated, sometimes cardiac medicine can safely be decreased or discontinued, or bypass surgery can be prevented if the cause of a vascular-type allergy is detected and eliminated.[3] *Again, get the advice of your personal physician.*

Of course all food-related hypertension is not allergy. Obesity and the use of tobacco are commonly recognized factors. Foods, however, such as chocolate, coffee, bananas, and citrus contain natural substances that can increase the blood pressure. Sometimes natural toxins and chemical additives can cause similar changes. Quite often an elevated blood pressure is caused by an unsuspected magnesium, essential fatty acid, or other nutrient deficiency. Hypertensive adults tend to have significantly more toxic chemicals in their blood than do normal control groups.

AN ENTIRE FAMILY AFFECTED IN DIFFERENT WAYS BY THE SAME FOOD

The Hammond Family

The Hammond family clearly demonstrated that the same food item could cause a variety of symptoms in individual members. If Marion ate chocolate, she developed red cheeks, an unpleasant personality, and difficulty learning. Her mother repeatedly developed a heart irregularity called premature ventricular contractions shortly after she ate chocolate. Her grandmother developed sudden tachycardia with a heartbeat over 200 during the night if she ate her favorite chocolate dessert for dinner. Both the mother and the grandmother found the cause of their heart problems because of Marion's chocolate sensitivity.

In summary, although there are many causes and factors related to asthma, pulse changes, and hypertension, you can become a detective and often find answers on your own. The causes are at times revealed by simply learning to use a peak flow meter or learning to take your pulse or blood pressure. Once you find an answer, discuss the need for your present medications with your doctor. We all need to spend more time determining why we are ill and what could possibly be causing our medical problems. Drugs are not necessarily the only or best answer.

CHAPTER 11

Allergies Due to Factors Inside Your Home or Child's School

Since 90 percent of each day is usually spent indoors, and only 10 percent is spent outdoors, the contents of the inside of our homes, schools, or work areas contain critical health-related factors. There is about ten times more pollution inside homes than outside at the present time. Over 350 different indoor air pollutants have been identified. Increased interest in air quality was generated because of the energy crisis a few years ago, which helped create more energy-efficient, but progressively "sicker" homes. Since then publicity about the "sick-building syndrome" and knowledge about delayed harmful health effects from formaldehyde, asbestos, and radon have raised everyone's awareness. Other factors that also need consideration are irritating substances, allergic contacts, toxins, and potential causes of cancer.

What Factors Inside Homes or Schools Can Cause Illness?

- allergenic substances, such as dust, mold, and pets;
- sources of heat (gas, oil, kerosene, wood, benzene, etc.);
- modern chemical cleaning agents and construction materials;

- chemicals, especially formaldehyde, toluene, xylene, phenol, trichloroethylene, and so on;
- pesticides, termiticides, or fungicides;
- sources of bacteria and viruses in old used sleeping cots, mattresses, carpets, and so forth;
- hidden contaminant toxins or pollutants, such as lead, radon, fluorescent lights, asbestos, and electromagnetic energy from TVs, computers, microwaves, and so on;
- poor ventilation leading to an increased humidity or temperature that enhances mold, dust, mite, and chemical contamination;
- the use of chemicals, odorous substances, or tobacco in unventilated confined spaces.

Which Clues Suggest a Possible "Inside" Problem?

Many children and adults find that they feel fine when they are not home. This suggests a possible problem related to the inside of the house. This can be noticed when someone remains outside, for example when camping, on vacation, or when hospitalized. On those occasions sometimes physical illness or undesirable personality changes subside within a few hours or days. Such common symptoms as hay fever, asthma, eczema, headaches, muscle aches, fatigue, hyperactivity, joint pain, depression, and irritability can routinely disappear within a few hours or days each time someone leaves her or his home. If something inside a home is a problem, however, these symptoms become apparent again within minutes to a few hours after returning home. Remember, a person's symptoms are not as much related to *how much* exposure as to *how sensitive* that person happens to be. Those with exquisite sensitivities need only negligible exposures to cause major illness.

Unfortunately leaving your home will not always resolve every child's home-related problem. For example, if the family dog is causing your child to wheeze and you take the dog along when you camp and visit, your child will not seem better even though you left your home. If the place you visit is as moldy or dusty as your own home, you may notice no improvement if molds and dust cause your child's allergies. In contrast, if the place you visit is pristine pure, some allergic children feel wonderful in a few hours and remain well until shortly after they return home.

Another clue relating illness to inside the home is provided by noting the time of the year that your child seems ill. Does your child seem worse mainly during the winter months, when more time is spent indoors and the windows are closed? Is your child always better during the summer, when the home is aired out and your child plays outside for prolonged periods of time? This type of pattern strongly suggests a possible problem within the home.

Be wary, however, because some food allergies can also appear to be worse during the winter months for reasons we do not fully understand. For example, some children who cannot tolerate a glass of milk in the winter can eat ice cream and drink milk in the hottest summer months without difficulty. This was noted over fifty years ago by Dr. Albert Rowe, and since then by many other observant physicians and parents.

Clues in the Bedroom

This is the room where the most time is spent in a twenty-four-hour period. It should be an allergy-free oasis. Common causes of allergy-related illness include

- dusty, moldy carpets;
- particleboard furniture that outgasses formaldehyde;
- old dusty cotton mattresses (which contain dust, molds, germs, and formaldehyde as a flame retardant) or mattresses made of foam rubber or polyurethane;
- synthetic mattress covers—plastic or polyester;
- synthetic bedding—Perma-Press (formaldehyde), or polluted with chemicals found in fabric softeners or certain laundry soap;
- feather, foam, or urethane pillows;
- synthetic blankets;
- heating blankets (plastic-coated wires emit odors when heated);
- floor wax or furniture polish;
- dusty closets, bric-a-brac, lamps, shelves, tables, floors, venetian blinds, curtains;
- plastic shades;

- pet hair, dandruff, and saliva;
- synthetic stuffed toys;
- plastic-smelling toys;
- chemical-smelling clothing;
- synthetic odorous clothing, raincoats, sweatshirts with plastic or rubberized imprints;
- clothing with odor of dry-cleaning fluid (tri or tetrachlorethylene);
- moldy, dusty wallpaper;
- forced-hot-air outlets that emit dust and molds when furnace blower is active (Some also leak natural gas or exhaust fumes.);
- moldy air-conditioners;
- cosmetics, fingernail polish, or remover;
- scented candles or incense.

What Should an Allergy-Free Bedroom Contain?

- Solid wooden furniture, no plastic;
- 100 percent cotton mattress that is not chemically treated;
- 100 percent cotton mattress cover or one that is entirely encased in heavy-duty aluminum foil, shiny side up;
- 100 percent cotton pillow or 100 percent cotton pillowcase stuffed with 100 percent cotton towels;
- 100 percent cotton or wool bedding;
- 100 percent cotton curtains;
- enclosed bookcases or storage toy box;
- electric space heater and air purifier;
- heating ducts closed and sealed with heavy-duty aluminum foil;
- no pets, mothballs, cedar odors, or odorous furniture polish;
- no odorous toys;
- 100 percent cotton stuffed animals;
- damp-wiped walls and floors;
- no feathers;
- no storage of odorous personal or other items.

Clues to Look for When You Move to a New House

Commonly a move to a new home seems to make allergic children either better or worse. The response depends upon what is inside the home you are moving into, in comparison with what was inside the home you left. If you have an ill child, think back. Did your child's problems begin within a month or two after a move to a new home?

The process of moving can itself make many allergic individuals temporarily worse because of the stirred-up dust and use of cleaning-related chemicals that are associated with this type of change. Sometimes it is helpful if an allergic child can live with a relative during the period just before and after a move.

A BOY WITH SENSITIVITIES TO A NEW HOME

Dave

Dave's allergy problems began in infancy. By the age of only nine months Dave had had so many ear infections that he needed surgery to place tubes through his eardrums. This strongly suggested a possible food allergy, particularly to milk. A red-colored medicine used to treat one of his ear infections caused him suddenly to bounce all over the car, laughing and screaming at the same time. His mother avoided red-dyed foods, beverages, and medicines from then on.

When Dave was three years old, they moved from an all-new electric home to an old, dusty, moldy, gas-heated home that had previously contained dogs. The very first morning in that home, as soon as he got out of bed, Dave began to run around "like a madman," making weird noises. He actually took a door off its hinges.

Unfortunately his "new home behavior" became typical. From early every morning until late each day, he was hyperactive and uncontrollable. He did compulsive things such as repeatedly writing on the walls and taking things apart. His parents' increased knowledge and awareness eventually enabled them to detect that whenever they stayed in homes in which they cooked with gas stoves or heated with gas, he became hyperactive. The hydrocarbons found in gas heat often cause sensitivities of this type.

In a few years his parents noticed he was also much worse on rainy days or when the pollen counts were high. This indicates that outdoor or indoor molds and pollen had become a problem. The dust and gas heat in their home were other possible suspects.

This child clearly illustrates a common pattern noted in allergic children: The allergies first become evident early in life because of food sensitivities, and then indoor and eventually outdoor environmental factors become prominent factors, creating an ever-increasing variety of physical and behavioral problems.

Clues to Look for at School or Work[1]

One classic clue that points to something inside a school or work area as a cause of illness is when the medical or personality problems tend to become progressively worse as each weekday passes, peaking by Friday afternoon. Slowly on Saturday and through Sunday the child or adult feels better, and then the pattern starts again. This type of history indicates that the school or work area needs to be investigated.

If symptoms occur only on a particular day, at a specific time, this often indicates a cause-and-effect relationship. Try to figure out why. What was eaten, smelled, or touched that was different? Is that the day the cleaning is done? Is it the day that an odorous mimeographed paper is distributed? Sometimes parents can narrow the problem down to one room that smells of molds, chemicals, a teacher's perfume, or a colleague's aftershave. If the symptoms are related to one room, a room air purifier that removes pollen, molds, and odors might solve the problem.[2]

Some children always become ill when they return to school after a holiday. The cause is usually related to special renovations, spraying, or cleaning done inside the school building prior to the children's return.

Each fall frantic mothers call because their children have been told not to return to school because of their impossible behavior. Although the most common reason is a seasonal weed pollen and mold allergy, the cause can also be a moldy or dusty school building or classroom, a new heating system, the smell of paint, or other refurbishing materials used in the school during the summer. Other considerations are scented personal items used by teachers or pupils, the lingering aroma of dry-cleaning fluid (trichlorethylene), tobacco (benzene), or fabric softeners (formaldehyde) in clothing.

Although a child's previous teacher may have understood a child's health problems in relation to molds, dust, and chemical odors, new

1. Irene Wilkenfeld, *How Environmentally Safe Are Our Schools?* 1990. Heal of Michiana, 52145 Farmington Square Road, Granger, Ind. 46530.
2. Contact: AllerMed, Air Purifier, 31 Steel Road, Wylie, Tex. 75098 (214-442-4898).

teachers may have to be informed each school year.[3] If educators learn how to detect and prevent illness in one particular child, this knowledge will in turn help that teacher to recognize and help other children who have similar problems.

A Boy With Sensitivities to His School

Peter

One eight-year-old boy, Peter, routinely started his school day with difficulty remembering, thinking, and completing his work. His first teacher, who taught arithmetic, smoked heavily and smelled of a strong perfume. Some days she complained that he could not add 2 plus 2. Peter seemed to improve gradually during the morning when he had another teacher who did not smell of either tobacco or perfume. At 1 p.m., however, after he ate lunch in the cafeteria, which contained the combined aromas of the perfumes worn by several aides, and of cooking and chemical odors from the kitchen, his ability to learn and concentrate deteriorated again. He also routinely developed an afternoon headache. These complaints persisted throughout most afternoons. We wondered if the symptoms were due to what he ate, or smelled, or both.

His problem was easily resolved. We requested that he be given ten minutes of oxygen, at the rate of three or four liters per minute, as soon as he arrived in school, and again immediately after lunch. This enabled the youngster to learn well throughout the day. His teachers could easily detect the progressive deterioration in his scholastic ability and behavior on the occasions when he forgot to receive his oxygen. It is difficult to treat for chemical sensitivities with an allergy extract, but this easy inexpensive solution was very helpful for Peter. His grades and performance improved dramatically throughout the rest of that school year. The next year, he had an air purifier in his classroom and his teacher did not smell of perfume or use tobacco. He no longer required oxygen and his schoolwork was again outstanding.

Clues to Look for in Motor Vehicles

If a child has a change in behavior, acts ill in some way, or seems to be unable to perform at a level comparable to her or his usual ability

3. Doris Rapp, M.D., *The Impossible Child*. 1989. Practical Allergy Research Foundation (PARF), P.O. Box 60, Buffalo, N.Y. 14223-0060.

upon arrival at school, think about the fumes on the school bus. Some are very old, but even the new ones can smell of construction chemicals or exhaust fumes. During the long ride, when they pick up one student after another, the drivers leave the engine running with the result that the bus fumes enter the bus through the open door. If your child is affected adversely by the ride to or from school, you may have to make arrangements to drive your child back and forth each day. If this resolves the problem, you can either assume that chore or you can speak to the school about the possibility of your child riding on a different, less chemically contaminated bus.

Some children also can become ill or change in mood or attitude because of the odors inside the family car. Many cars smell moldy as soon as the air-conditioner is put on. If you complain to the car dealer, a perfumed chemical is often added to the ventilation system. This can compound the problem by circulating a toxic perfumed chemical that masks the odor of the molds as it helps inhibit their growth.

Many allergic children wheeze; misbehave; develop headaches, dizziness, nausea; wet their pants; or develop other symptoms due to chemical odors and/or molds. One mold inhibitor commonly used to treat car air conditioners contains methylenebis-4 chlorophenol and triclorethane. It cautions that "it is a hazard for humans," and "repeated exposure can damage the nervous system." It clearly states that it is toxic and that the container should be disposed of in a sanitary landfill. The automobile mechanic who uses the spray should wear goggles and a mask. When your car is returned, you may not smell the molds, but your family is still breathing this chemical. We should not have to choose between having an allergic reaction from the molds and being poisoned by a toxic mold inhibitor.

Other cars smell moldy all the time because the car windows were left open during a rainstorm. Once the upholstery has been contaminated with molds, it is very difficult to eradicate the odor. Cleaning with special mold retardants, using baking soda, and placing Nature's Odor Guard[4] under the car seats should help safely decrease mold contamination. Newer ozone-generating machines also appear to be helpful to decrease the mold content in some cars.[5]

It has also been said that pollen can build up in car air conditioner filters so that after these units are turned on, pollen can circulate through the car and precipitate sudden symptoms. If this happens, it should be obvious. Affected individuals feel worse or act differently

4. Contact: The Living Source, 3500 MacArthur Drive, Waco, Tex. 76708.
5. Contact: N.E.E.D.S., FMC 110 Odor Control Unit, 527 Charles Avenue 12-A, Syracuse, N.Y. 13209 (315-446-1122 or 800-634-1380).

each time the air conditioner is turned on. Car air purifiers help diminish this problem by removing pollen, molds, and dust. Some remove chemicals as well.[6]

Another common cause of sudden illness or emotional outbursts in a car is related to the smell of gasoline while the gas tank is being filled. Some sensitive children lose total control or develop headaches, nausea, drowsiness or even wet their pants shortly after the car door or window is opened at a gas station. If unsure, purposely allow your child to stand nearby as you fill your gas tank. If the odor creates a problem, it will be obvious within a few minutes.

Common car-related health complaints include drowsiness, nausea, dizziness, headaches, and behavior problems. If these occur during car rides, the cause can be due to the odor of exhaust fumes that enter the car while it is being driven. Auto exhaust, gasoline fumes, and outdoor pollutants routinely enter cars when the vents labeled "Fresh Air" are open. If the car has a button labeled "Recirculate," it means that only about 20 percent of outside air pollutants enter the car.

Some children are sensitive to the smell of recent undercoating, new upholstery, or car trim. Genuine leather, as well as synthetic fiber seats in a car, emit or outgas chemical odors that make some individuals ill. Some chemically sensitive patients cannot ride in a new car for months without becoming ill because of the strong chemical odors inside the car or the sealant and rust-inhibitor odors that permeate the automobile. For the above reasons they tend routinely to purchase older cars, which have fewer chemical odors, or if they decide to buy a new car, they air it outside for weeks or months before they attempt to drive in it.

In summary, if your child routinely becomes ill or misbehaves during short or long car rides, you can try one or more of the following:

- Powder the inside contents of the car with baking soda overnight to help decrease the mold content. The residue can be vacuumed and removed the next day.
- Place some open trays of charcoal under the front car seats to help remove some of the odor. Change the charcoal monthly.
- Cover the upholstery entirely with heavy-duty aluminum foil to seal in odors emitted from it. Then cover the aluminum foil with a thick blanket made of 100 percent cotton.

6. Contact: AllerMed, Autoaire II, 31 Steel Road, Wylie, Tex. 75098 (214-442-4898). Also see Appendix B.

- Install a car air purifier, which can be attached to the cigarette lighter, to remove odors, molds, and pollen (see Appendix B).
- Rent an ozone-generating machine from some ecological supply houses. Attach it to the inside of the car for several hours; it can remove mold and tobacco odors.[7] Be careful to follow the directions regarding this machine exactly.

A BOY WITH SENSITIVITIES TO THE FAMILY CAR

Chuck

Chuck came to see us when he was six years old. He had several types of personality changes associated with exposures inside automobiles or buildings.

Routinely when he went for a car ride, his symptoms progressed through several distinct stages. At first he made mouth noises, then he became bouncy, jabbed at the other children, tapped on the windows, and refused to quiet down. During the next stage he punched his own face and hit his legs. Then he would say, "Let me out, I want a truck to run me over." These symptoms were all worse in the family diesel car than in the other car, which used gasoline. Diesel fumes are usually worse than gasoline fumes. His neutralization treatment with a histamine allergy extract helped, but he could not remain in the car. If he did, he was better for only a few minutes and then he began to make noises, pound his legs again, and coil his body into a ball.

When he was exposed to one brand of furniture polish, he told his mother he wanted to "jump off the roof." After he was away from the smell for twenty minutes, he returned to normal. He obviously has multiple chemical sensitivities.

Clues That Explain Why an Entire Family Is Ill

Sometimes illness strikes an entire family. Everyone may be well and content, and then one after another the family becomes ill with similar complaints. If these complaints include congestion, fatigue, irritability, aches, or depression, the cause could be a viral infection. If these

---

7. Contact: Practical Allergy Research Foundation (PARF), P.O. Box 60, Buffalo, N.Y. 14223-0060.

complaints persist, however, an aware parent might suspect the cause is something in the home environment. Again, the key question is what is new or different inside the home? It could be a new synthetic carpet, a new or faulty furnace, a new cleaning material, furniture polish, floor wax, fresh paint, new construction, a pesticide or termiticide, a flea or ant spray, a flooded basement, a leaky ceiling, a new or shedding pet, a new potted plant with moldy soil, new plastic curtains, a plastic shower curtain, synthetic drapes, new insulation, a new mattress or pillow, different furniture, a new bathroom or kitchen aerosol, or a recent oil spill in an attached garage. These are the types of things that have to be considered. Ask yourself the following questions. When did my family begin to show symptoms? What was different in the few days or weeks before the illness? What was purchased? What changes occurred in your house at that time? You may have found an answer.

A Family Who Repeatedly Became Ill From Gas Exposures

The Milon Family

In the winter of 1980 Mrs. Milon noted severe weakness and tingling in her arms and legs. She had several extensive medical evaluations by a number of specialists in a hospital, but no cause was found. She was too weak to work, even part-time, that winter, but in the summer she was energetic and could work full-time without difficulty. No one understood why.

Her husband also seemed to be worse during the winter months. His major problem was persistent headaches, and he needed 50 to 100 Tylenol a week to control his pain. He also had dark eye circles and tended to be irritable.

Their son, Aaron, developed headaches, congestion, depression, and trouble with his memory whenever the weather became cold. His symptoms became progressively more evident as the winter continued. During the warm months he was always much better.

Linda, the youngest child, had recurrent infections and headaches, again mainly during the cold months. Her major complaint, however, was severe leg aches. Every evening for years her parents had to rub her legs. She also had nosebleeds, easy bruising, and even vaginal bleeding at times. Repeated medical evaluations did not provide any answers.

Eventually it was found that many of each member's medical

complaints were related to leaks of natural gas or chemicals within their home.

At first the parents could not notice any relationship between the family's illnesses and anything in particular. Then, in 1984, a gas odor was noted in the kitchen. After the family changed to an electric stove, they were all pleasantly surprised. In three days Aaron stopped having temper outbursts and his disposition was remarkably better. Linda's legs amazingly stopped aching at about the same time. For the first time in five years Linda did not cry with leg pain at night!

When the weather became cold, the Milons realized that many of their past medical complaints seemed to get worse each winter after the gas heat was turned on. The parents therefore installed a heat pump in 1984, which meant that they would have electric heat during most of the winter, with a gas supplement during the coldest months. Within one week after the new furnace was installed, the entire family felt better.

This gas-health connection was confirmed on many subsequent occasions. Once while visiting a relative over a period of several days, Linda noted the odor of natural gas in that home. After the first night there she wanted to stay in bed because she again developed such severe leg and joint pains. In addition, her fatigue, depression, and easy crying returned. She developed black-and-blue marks on her body. She began to act groggy, cried, and said everyone was "picking on her." This continued to be a recurrent problem every time she visited her aunt until she bought a new gas stove in 1987.

After their new heat-pump furnace, the family continued to feel unusually well for several months until the fall of 1984, when Mrs. Milon noted that she felt dizzy and had difficulty waking up in the morning. She thought she had the flu. In a while the entire family seemed tired and sick to their stomach. One morning as Mrs. Milon dragged herself out of bed at 11:00 A.M., she fortunately noted a peculiar hissing sound downstairs. She called the fire department and discovered that the water heater was leaking natural gas and that their new heat pump was leaking freon gas. The family found that their unexplained nausea, fatigue, and flulike symptoms subsided when they remained outside their house or if they breathed oxygen from a portable oxygen tank.

The next summer the family felt well. The winter of 1985, however, proved to be another challenge. The family remained well when the winter was mild and their house was totally heated by electricity. When it became unusually cold, however, the electric heat pump automatically was supplemented with gas heat. At that time, their symptoms returned. Because of a peculiar odor in the basement, the gas company was called. They said that it was hazardous for them to remain in the house and they must evacuate. The heat pump had not been vented correctly and the fumes generated from the sudden supplementary need for natural gas heat were not being exhausted correctly through the chimney. Once again, after it was repaired, the family felt better.

When the children had P/N allergy testing for hydrocarbons or gas, we could reproduce the type of headaches and abdominal pain noted previously when they were exposed to gas fumes. The day after that test we were surprised because Linda developed the characteristic black-and-blue marks on her knees and ankles. Her repeated history of bruising associated with gas exposures suggests that some change routinely occurred in her blood vessels or blood platelets after she was exposed to hydrocarbons.

At the present time Mr. Milon rarely needs Tylenol, and his wife does not have weak extremities or extreme fatigue in the winter months. The children's symptoms are much less evident. However, they all seem to be much more sensitive to odors now than they ever were before. (See Chapter 13.)

One must wonder why an entire family would be affected by so many forms of allergy. There must be some genetic weakness in their immune systems. The multiple inadvertent chemical exposures, however, in all probability also contributed to their immune weakness. Their efforts to decrease their total allergenic load by making their home more ecologically sound, adhering to a rotation diet, avoiding chemicals, using allergy extract, and improving their nutrition should help diminish future symptoms. Hopefully these measures should directly or indirectly also strengthen their immune systems.

Rapid Onset Clues

Sometimes the onset of an illness is very fast. You put up the Christmas tree and your child begins to wheeze, becomes congested, or has a total personality change within a few hours. You remove the tree and your child feels well or acts normal in a few hours. That type of situation is quite easy to recognize and confirm.

Another example of a cause of rapid onset illness would be a heating problem, such as the use of a kerosene heater, which could cause some family member to feel ill within a few hours. The use of fingernail polish, airplane glue, or marking pens often precipitates rapid illness in some individuals. The first time a previously used air conditioner is turned on in the summer, the initial moldy odor can quickly cause asthma or other symptoms in a mold-sensitive person.

A Girl Who Developed Asthma From Moldy School Books

Kathy

Fifteen-year-old Kathy had not wheezed for years. Her mother no longer worried about her asthma because she had been well for so long. When she went to school in the fall of 1989, however, they passed out some extremely moldy social studies books. Within an hour she began to wheeze. She improved that evening, but the next day, in the same class, she wheezed again. She needed emergency hospital care within two weeks. She returned to our office so that her mold allergy extract treatment could be adjusted. By the time she left the office, after her updated mold neutralization allergy extract treatment, her breathing had improved remarkably. We requested the school either to stop using those books or to excuse Kathy from that class. They changed the books, and she has stopped wheezing again.

This young lady illustrates that asthma rarely goes away. Asthmatics can be well for years, and then suddenly, after some unusual exposure or an infection, the problem recurs. Sometimes recurrences are self-limited, but if the cause is not eliminated, the problem can certainly persist. Wheezing can recur anytime, even if years have passed without an attack. The temporary answer is effective antiasthma medications. The long-term answer is to detect and eliminate the cause of the wheezing.

Insidious Gradual Onset Clues

Molds

Insidious symptoms are those that gradually become evident over a period of months. For example, if a basement has been flooded after a storm or a roof leaks, the mold contamination in affected areas can gradually spread throughout a home. Initially a child may have symptoms only in the basement. Later on, if the house has registers or a blower in the forced-hot-air heating system, molds can circulate through the entire house. In time a mold-sensitive individual can have symptoms in any room.[8]

More subtle causes of some children's problems are damp, moldy sneakers, shoes, boots, and socks. Each time these items are touched, molds directly contaminate the hands of the child, and indirectly can affect a child's nose or lungs because of the odor. Many sensitive youngsters make themselves ill by merely removing their moldy shoes or socks.

Sometimes busy mothers leave the wet laundry in the washer after the cycle is completed. Such clothing develops a moldy odor, which can persist even after the clothes have been thoroughly dried. This can be an unsuspected cause of rashes, hay fever, asthma, or personality problems.

Chemicals in Personal Items That Can Cause Illness

- Strong odors such as perfume, cologne, toilet water, aftershave, fingernail polish or remover, incense, scented candles;
- any perfumed body soap, lotion, cream, deodorant, lipstick, powder, or aerosol hair or body spray;
- hair dye, lightener, mousse, spray, or oil;
- scented facial or toilet tissue;
- sanitary napkins, douche materials, or prophylactics of various types, for example condoms;
- tobacco in any form (Inhaling the tobacco smoke of others is known to be one cause of increased chest and ear infections, as well as decreased lung function in some asthmatic children);
- preservatives, additives, artificial colors, and synthetic flavors in toothpaste, mouthwash, and so on;
- new clothing, which often has a characteristic odor. The odor of the rubbery plastic designs on T-shirts, for example, gives off a chemical odor that causes some children to become ill or misbehave;
- freshly washed or dry-cleaned clothing (carbon tetrachloride);
- phenol, used as a preservative in most allergy extracts or as a disinfectant in common cleaning products or aerosols.

8. Mold plates can be purchased to identify and quantitate the types of molds found in damp areas of a home, school, workplace, or car. Contact Northeast Center for Environmental Medicine, 2800 W. Genesee Street, Syracuse, N.Y. 13219. 315-488-2856.

Chemical Factors Inside Your Home, School, or Work Area That Can Cause Illness[9]

- Mattress or furniture stuffing made of foam rubber or polyurethane (phenol). Formaldehyde is also used as a fire retardant in mattresses.

- Soft, odorous plastic of the type used to cover furniture, for example vinyl, Naugahyde, plastic-coated mattresses, mattress covers, shower curtains or window shades. The odor is more intense if the plastic item is near a source of heat.

- Adhesives, caulking material, and sealants.

- Carpeting, carpet pads, and carpet sealers. Many schools are now carpeting cafeterias, halls, and classrooms. The cost is approximately twice the cost of asbestos tile and five times less than that of wood floors. This is creating problems related to dust, mites, molds, and sanitation (due to bleeding or vomiting on the carpet). Even more important may be the numerous chemical exposures due to the content of the carpet, the "antimicrobial" agents used in the carpet, and carpet adhesives.

   It is of interest to note that the Environmental Protection Agency (EPA) installed new carpeting in their agency in 1987–88.[10] About 124 of their 2,000 employees developed eye, nose, and throat irritation, breathing problems, headache, nausea, problems thinking, fatigue, and an increased sensitivity *to other odors*. A few employees had to leave the EPA, and some had to work in different areas or at home. They did not remove the carpet! The culprit was the 4-phenylcyclohexene used to bind the carpet to the fabric.

- Foods or beverages stored in plastic. When you drink such water or other beverages, the plastics can enter your blood and then can be stored in your fat if they can't be excreted.

- The smell of plastic toys, plastic lunch boxes, pencil or book bags, or loose-leaf notebooks. This can cause some children to develop asthma, personality changes, or learning problems. Phenol is only one problem chemical found in plastic.

9. Furnace/air-conditioning units that absorb toxic odors and gases from the air in homes are available through Thurmond Air Quality Systems, P.O. Box 23037, Little Rock, Ark. 72221. 501-227-8888 or 800-AIR-PURE.
10. Nicholas Ashford, Ph.D., J.D., and Claudia Miller, M.D., *Chemical Sensitivity—A Report to the New Jersey State Department of Health.* 1989. New Jersey Department of Health, John Fitch Plaza, CN 360, Trenton, N. J. 08625.

- Chemicals in wrapping products. I recently saw an elderly man who complained that whenever he held a colorless sandwich bag in his hand for about twenty seconds, he would suddenly develop a seizure and drop the bag. He said this happened repeatedly and he was very upset because after this type of exposure he always developed a severe headache. His wife then handed him an ordinary sandwich bag and he promptly had a seizurelike episode. He had had a similar response when he was seen by another doctor in the office. This type of response is certainly uncommon, but that it exists at all is cause for concern.

- Soft rubber products such as rubber bands, mattresses, or pillows. Children in particular need 100 percent cotton mattresses. Those used by other children, especially if they were ill, could harbor harmful bacteria or viruses. This can lead to recurrent infections in some youngsters who use older hand-me-down mattresses.

- Various items routinely kept under the kitchen or bathroom sink, in the garage, and in the basement. These factors often contribute to chemically related illness.

- Strong disinfectant odors from cleaning compounds or aerosols. These are used in bathrooms, hospitals, schools, and hotel rooms. Fresh pine or other "clean"-smelling disinfectant-type solutions, for example, contain phenol.

- Floor polish or wax (turpentine, chloroform, and carbon tetrachloride).

- Insecticides (ants), pesticides (roaches), or termiticides (termites).

  —Insecticides contain chloroform, DDT, formic acid, and kerosene.

  —Pesticides contain over six hundred active ingredients, and the EPA has reviewed only four for safety. Ninety-one percent of American homes use pesticides that contain benzene, lindane, malathion, and formaldehyde. Pesticides or organophosphates, organochlorides, and carbonates are found on and in many ordinary store meats, fruits, and vegetables.[11] When chemically contaminated foods are cooked, it is not unusual for chemical odors to be obvious in the kitchen, as well as in the taste of the food.

—Pesticide use has increased tenfold in the past twenty years. It is estimated that only 1 percent of the tons used ever reach any insect. Prophylactic use can in time potentially create pesticide-resistant strains of insects. Biological forms of pesticides are certainly preferred, and everyone should insist upon their use.[12]

—Termiticides contain organophosphates, organochlorides, chlordane, and heptachlor.

- Various alcohols in tinctures, solvents, antifreeze. The rubbing alcohol used for massage, sprains, or muscle aches.

- Glycerol in sweeteners or preservatives. This is also found in cosmetics, inks, glues, cements, medicines, or suppositories.

- Menthol in perfumes, candles, candy, tobacco, liquor, and in cold or sprain medications.

- Newspapers, magazines, or books. It may be only certain ones, or specific sections of one particular newspaper, for example, that cause symptoms. The colored sections and shiny paper in books seem to be particularly offensive. Although it is usually the ink, the paper can also be at fault. Some people are so sensitive that they can read only books or papers that are enclosed within a glass reading box.

- Scented fabric softeners, laundry detergents, dish soaps, or window cleaners.

- Furniture, metal, or shoe polish.

- Paint, turpentine, or shellac.

- Chlorine in scouring powders, bleaches, or cleaning products. Some sensitive individuals even have problems whenever they drink chlorinated water, others with water-softened water.[13] Some soft drinks and even milk can contain chloroform.

- Chemicals in art class, vocational shops, science labs, teachers' lounges, cafeterias, print shops, home-economics rooms, pool areas, locker rooms, and portable classrooms. These areas can all cause problems for some sensitive students.

12. For further information, see: "Recognition and Management of Pesticide Poisoning." Write EPA, 540/9-80-005, 26 W. Martin Luther King, Cincinnati, Ohio 45268 (513-569-7931).

13. Doris Rapp, M.D., "Water as a Cause of Angio-Edema and Urticaria." *JAMA*, 221 (1972): 305.

- Coal-tar roofing materials, pine paneling, plywood, vinyl floor covering, and sealants.

- Wood-burning stoves and fireplaces emit hydrocarbons and formaldehyde plus other potentially offending chemicals into the air.

- Gas, oil, benzene, or kerosene sources of heat. Over 12 million kerosene space heaters are used in the United States. The EPA safe levels for nitrous oxide are elevated in 50 percent of the homes using this type of heat. For sulfur dioxide, 71 percent exceed the EPA standards.

- Heating systems should be enclosed so that there is no possibility of inside-home contamination with combustion products. They should not be housed inside a home. Furnaces must also be properly ventilated so that there is minimal backdrafting.

- Natural gas in gas kitchen stoves, hot-water heaters, clothes dryers, and furnaces. These are probably one major unsuspected cause of home pollution causing headaches and arthritis in particular.

- Gasoline or oil spills. These contain hydrocarbon petrochemicals or coal-tar derivatives.

- Automobile, school bus, or truck exhaust fumes. Be sure that the buses that are standing in the school lots with their motors running are not parked near the air intake of the school, or the fumes can be circulated throughout the school.

- Odors from hobbies or work such as photography, ceramic glazes, oil painting, glues, dyes, etc. Of eighty-one different art materials used in ten surveyed schools, only twenty were certified safe.[14]

- Odor from crayons. Nonodorous crayons are available from Toys "R" Us.[15]

- Scratch-and-sniff stickers, Play-Doh, rubber cement, glues.

- Naphthalene mothballs, sprays, or cedar. These are used in closet or storage areas.

- Sterno heaters in cafeterias or restaurants.

- Treated wood in log cabins can be contaminated with molds and is routinely treated with chemicals.

14. Irene Wilkenfeld, *How Environmentally Safe Are Our Schools?* (See Bibliography.).
15. See Appendix B.

Studies indicate that sickness is significantly increased in air-conditioned buildings, in contrast to those with natural ventilation.

Special Problems

Studies have shown that there are certain forms of home and school pollution that can endanger everyone's health. A few major ones are discussed below.

Perfume

The FDA has said that fragrances cause 30 percent of all allergic reactions. About 72 percent of asthmatics develop respiratory symptoms when exposed to perfume. About 95 percent of all ingredients in fragrances are synthetic. Some contain as many as 100 chemicals; a portion of these are known to cause cancer, birth defects, and problems with the nervous system.

Formaldehyde

Urea formaldehyde foam insulation (UFFI) tends to cause slowly developing symptoms over a period of weeks to months. When the sun warms the insulation on the sides of a building during the hot months, sudden medical illness can definitely become apparent. New homes present increased formaldehyde exposures due to particleboard, subflooring, paneling, synthetic carpets, and polyester fabrics. (see Table 13.6, page 292). It is used extensively in portable classrooms. Desk tops and classroom cabinets, for example, made of fiberboard can outgas formaldehyde for over twenty years.

Irritability, vague aches, dizziness, lack of energy, eye irritation, respiratory problems, coughing, and difficulty remembering are common complaints. Fortunately this is no longer being used as insulation, but great caution must be used not to purchase a home in which it was previously installed.

Pesticides

Some entire families have gradually become ill over a period of weeks or months after a home is pesticided or termiticided. One family used more than the advised amount of ant spray on the wooden beams in their new log-cabin home. Shortly after this was done, their one son developed incapacitating joint pain and his younger brother developed periods of weakness, extreme dizziness, and heart irregularity. Innumerable sensitive families, reported by Dr. William Rea, have developed multiple nervous-system symptoms after the use of chemicals to control home infestations.[16]

Ask for the safety-data sheet in relation to any chemicals that are to be used inside or in the vicinity of your home or your child's school. Sometimes it is not only the pesticides but also the "inert ingredients" that can produce illness. Pesticides are routinely used in many city and school libraries, as well as in apartment buildings. The pollution can penetrate walls, so the chemicals a neighbor uses can affect your apartment and you.

Lead Poisoning

The majority of homes constructed before 1940 used paint that contained lead. The dust from lead paint is not removed by ordinary vacuuming. Lead pipes continue to be a problem in many homes. Some ceramic glazed dishes also release lead. It can also be found in rubber, plastic, and gasoline. Lead and other heavy metals, such as cadmium, can interfere with the function of the brain and nervous system. Poisoning can cause fatigue, headaches, bone aches, and muscle aches.

Asbestos Poisoning

Asbestos was used for many years in fireproofing, thermal and acoustic insulation, for reinforcing roof and floor products, and as an insulation around pipes in homes and schools. This material gradually disintegrates so that asbestos dust contaminates the air. This can lead to lung disease and cancer, which usually occurs years after the original exposure. If this is a potential problem in your home or child's school, be certain that it is removed professionally so that the removal does not lead to further contamination.

Radon

Everyone has heard about radon, the newly recognized colorless and odorless indoor air pollutant that causes cancer. It is a gaseous radioactive decay product of the uranium series. It is now known that geologic and soil information is of no value in predicting which homes

16. William J. Rea, M.D., "Pesticides and Brain Function Changes in a Controlled Environment," *Clinical Ecology* #2 (1984):145–149; William Rea, M.D. *Chemical Sensitivities*, Lewis Publishers, Inc., 121 S. Main St., Chelsea, Mich. 48118 Available in 4/91.

are most apt to be in danger. It leaks from the soil into a home through cracks in walls or pipes that enter from below a house.

The harmful effects of chronic low-dosage exposures were not appreciated or recognized until recently. Children appear to be at more risk than adults. The rate of cancer is proportional to the amount and duration of the exposure. Schools, public buildings, work areas, and homes must be monitored.

In 1983 naturally occurring as well as unacceptably high radon or ionizing radiation was found in a few homes clustered in the eastern United States, areas that happened to be situated over granite or crystalline formations. These areas were later designated as "hot spots." In 1988 one study of one thousand homes in Minnesota revealed that 44 percent had elevated radon levels.

The Environmental Protection Agency (EPA) has outlined how you can determine if this is a problem in your home and what you can do about it. They have designated the normal safe level to be below 4 pCi/L. Call 1-800-505-RADON. They also published a booklet in 1988 entitled *Radon Reduction Techniques in Detached Houses*.[17] In addition, they have suggestions for preventing this problem in future construction.

Information about charcoal radon detectors can be obtained through your local health department. With these, homeowners can determine whether their homes are contaminated with radon or not.

The final answers are not easy, not always available, and sometimes not known. Persons who have ecologic illness, in particular, must be careful not to replace one problem with another in an attempt to limit radon exposure. Certain polyurethane sealants for wall cracks emit toxic fumes that can be harmful. If less toxic silicone sealers are used, they may be ineffective in excluding the entrance of radon.

The air pressure between the outside and the inside radon-contaminated houses must be balanced. At times this can be a major challenge. If this is not done properly, pressure differentials can either suck more radon into the house or can backdraft exhaust from appliances into the house, causing problems with hydrocarbons. Pressure inequities can also cause excessive condensation on the outside walls of a home, which increases home deterioration. Other pressure problems can impede the proper exhaust of moisture when the laundry is being dried. This can lead to increased indoor mold contamination, which in turn leads to innumerable mold-related allergy symptoms.

17. Contact: Environmental Protection Agency, 625/5/86-0/9, 26 W. Martin Luther King, Cincinnati, Ohio 45268 (513-569-7931).

Electromagnetic Energy

Electromagnetic energy is another potentially harmful environmental factor that is less obvious. Some people are adversely affected by exposure to 60 hertz or other low-frequency electromagnetic fields. It can interfere with normal biological body functions. Some families tend to become ill after they move near a television transmitter, radio tower, high-power tension wires, power transformer, or microwave tower. All of these emit electromagnetic radiation. A few exquisitely sensitive individuals feel different or ill if they simply walk in front of a microwave machine, work on a computer or in a computer pool, sit too close to a television, or drive under high-power electrical wires. Electric blankets, electric razors, and other common household appliances can bother some individuals. A few electrically sensitive people have seizures or lose control, in some manner, during electrical storms. Affected individuals feel much better if they ground themselves by walking barefoot directly on the soil. A new book, entitled *Cross Currents*, by Dr. Robert Becker, explains the risks related to the electromagnetic world that surrounds us.[18] Fortunately it is the rare individual who is affected. The evidence is accumulating, however, that nervous system problems, and cancer in particular, can unknowingly be related to certain electromagnetic exposures in some people. With increased awareness, perhaps more related illnesses will be prevented or at least recognized earlier.

Fluorescent Lighting

Studies by John Ott have indicated that not only children but plants as well are sensitive to the emanations of fluorescent lights.[19] In Germany this form of lighting is banned in schools. Some radiation-shielded full-spectrum fluorescent lights are available in this country, but they are quite expensive. Ordinary incandescent light bulbs appear to be better tolerated by some hyperactive children.

18. Robert Becker, *Cross Currents* (Los Angeles: Jeremy P. Tarcher, 1990).

19. John Ott, "Influence of Fluorescent Lights on Hyperactivity and Learning Disabilities." *Journal of Learning Disabilities*, 9 (1976): 417–422.

An Adult With Seizures Due to Electromagnetic Energy Emissions

Mark

Mark was an engineer in his mid-twenties. His seizures were being discussed at an environmental medicine conference. During the presentation of his history he was standing near the podium. At that time a physician's beeper happened to go off. Instantly Mark had a seizure and was on the floor. Later on, at that same conference, I happened to be sitting behind Mark. Another physician from London turned on a machine that emitted electromagnetic energy. Again Mark had an immediate seizure. Fortunately there may not be many individuals who have this type of illness, but we must wonder if Mark's response does not represent the tip of an iceberg. More and more patients are gradually finding their way to certain physicians who have more understanding about these types of problems.[20]

Cancer and Home Chemicals

Attached garages that may not be sealed properly from the rest of the house are another common home problem. If your car is warmed in a closed garage, the auto-exhaust fumes can leak into your home. A gas leak from your car can cause benzene fumes to permeate your home. Benzene is known to cause leukemia, as well as heart irregularities.

Smoking is another source of cancer. Tobacco contains many carcinogens, and these can cause asthma, heart problems, cancer, repeated lung infections, and other chronic lung disease. Tobacco affects *not only those who smoke but also those who breathe the air that contains tobacco smoke.*

Para dichlorobenzenes are also carcinogens, and these are found in bathroom air deodorizers and moth-killing preparations. Tri- and tetraclorethylene, found in recently dry-cleaned clothing, causes cancer in animals, so it would be best to ventilate all dry-cleaned clothes outside for a while before placing them in your closets.

---

20. Two physicians who are knowledgeable about this type of illness are Dr. William Rea in Dallas, Texas, and Dr. Allan Lieberman in Charleston, South Carolina.

Help for Those Who Are Ill From Indoor Pollution

Parents must try to make their home as free of known allergenic substances or chemicals as possible. Every allergic child or adult should have an environmentally safe bedroom where he can go and know that there is *nothing* in that room which causes him to have allergic reactions. The relative humidity should be maintained at 30 to 40 percent, and the ventilation must be adequate. Both dehumidifiers and humidifiers must be monitored regularly to decrease both mold and bacterial contamination. Air purifiers, which remove chemicals, as well as dust, molds, pollen, and pet hair, can be immensely helpful. This type of sanctuary certainly can abort or relieve certain sudden allergy-related episodes.[21]

The key facts to remember are that most "inside" problems are worse during the colder months, or are related to a move to a different home or to changes inside a home. With a little thought you may find some obvious answers that will benefit your entire family.

21. David Rousseau, William J. Rea, and Jean Enwright, *Your Home, Health and Well-Being.* 1989. Hartley & Marks, 3663 W. Broadway, Vancouver, B.C., Canada V6R 2B8, and Natalie Golos and Frances Golbitz, *Coping With Your Allergies,* (New York: Simon & Schuster, 1986).

CHAPTER 12
_____

Allergies Due to Factors
Outside Your Home

We often see children who obviously have difficulty mainly when they are outside. Most of these children are worse when tree, grass, weed pollen, or mold spores are in the air. For example, those youngsters who are worse a few days before certain trees develop leaves are sensitive to that tree pollen. Trees with large flowers, such as horse chestnut, are insect-, not wind-pollinated, so they are less apt to cause allergies than the trees that have such tiny flowers that you've never even noticed them.

Each variety of tree tends to pollinate at a slightly different time. It is sometimes easy therefore to pinpoint the fact that elm trees, for example, rather than maple trees, are causing a particular child's hay fever or asthma because the elm trees have obvious tiny leaf buds and flowers, while the maples look exactly as they did in the winter months. Although tree pollen can blow for many miles, it is usually the type of trees near your home or your child's bedroom window that are causing symptoms in the early spring. Allergists can examine special glass slides that have been exposed to the air and roughly gauge the number and the type of pollen or molds in the air at any particular time.

Youngsters who are worse when grass needs to be cut are often sensitive to grass pollen. If the odor or contact of freshly cut grass causes symptoms, then grass terpines or molds on the grass are probable factors that need to be considered. Lawn sprays also cause medical symptoms after they are applied, especially if the child is in close contact with the grass shortly after the spraying. Notice if you or your child feel unwell in any way as you walk down the street shortly after the lawn care chemical truck has left your neighborhood.

Children who are worse in the late summer or fall are probably reacting to ragweed or other weed pollens, as well as to mold spores that are in the air at that time. Rarely do ecologists see an allergic child who is not sensitive to both.

Mold-sensitive children also complain of more symptoms on damp, rainy days in the spring in particular, or when they are exposed to moldy basements or bathrooms. Damp areas in buildings, such as near school pools, showers, or locker rooms, often trigger allergies.

Some children are always ill in the late winter after the snow has melted but before the trees have begun to pollinate. These children tend to improve after they are treated for the molds found on decayed grass and vegetation.

Many parents notice that their children initially have more allergy symptoms during the winter when children stay inside their homes most of the time. These winter complaints can occur year after year during the colder months. At that time allergic children tend to be ill and prone to recurrent infections because of sensitivities to dust, molds, and household pets. As toddlers grow up, however, their winter symptoms typically tend to become worse in the spring, summer, and fall months. This indicates that in addition to their year-round allergies they have developed the typical seasonal flare-ups due to tree, grass, and/or ragweed pollen, as well as to molds. Their symptoms are certainly not confined to hay fever and asthma. Any of the medical complaints that are discussed in Chapter 3 may also be seen.

Sometimes parents assume that pollen is causing a problem because their child has difficulty every summer *at the same time*. You can check with your health department or a local allergist to ascertain exactly when certain types of pollen are in the air in your area. Sometimes, however, a child's symptoms do not correlate to the time when specific pollen or molds are prevalent. Some children are worse simply because they are drinking more carbonated pop or juices than normal. They can be sensitive to some ingredient in their favorite beverage, for example aspartame, dextrose, food dyes, or artificial lemon flavoring. Other children who have repeated non–pollen-related seasonal symptoms are ill because they ate large amounts of seasonal foods such as corn, tomatoes, peaches, melon, cherries, or berries. If children seem worse on the days when crops are harvested, the culprit can be molds, yeast, or fungi that are released in the air at that time.

Much can be learned by paying close attention. One asthmatic girl has no difficulty in Puerto Rico, but as soon as she gets off a plane in her hometown, she starts to wheeze. The problem is not due to something inside her home but to the outside air pollution in the town were she lives.

Another six-year-old child was exposed to fireworks and a bonfire during the same evening. He began to cry for no apparent reason and continued to cry for three hours before he finally fell asleep. He had had similar episodes of this type in the past from the same chemical exposures.

INCAPACITATING HEADACHES PARTIALLY DUE TO OUTDOOR FACTORS

Valerie

The following patient illustrates how you can find the answers even when some complaints initially appear to be elusive and complicated. Valerie began to have headaches at the age of twelve years. She came to my office when she was fifteen because her headaches were so incapacitating that she had been unable to attend school for the previous six months.

She had many allergic relatives, and her personal allergy history dated back to infancy. As an infant she could not tolerate evaporated milk. Her excessive vomiting improved after she was changed to a Similac formula. Between the ages of one and five years she had recurrent ear infections. These did not subside until her tonsils and adenoids were removed. The ear infections so early in life, combined with the fact that she loved milk and ice cream but hated cheese, strongly suggested that she might have had an undetected milk sensitivity.

She coughed with exercise and laughter, suggesting she was beginning to have lung allergies. Since the age of twelve years she had daily nose wiggling and rubbing, stuffiness, and throat clearing. She tended to have a sore throat each morning from a postnasal drip, and her ears frequently felt plugged. Her eyes watered more than normal. She also felt nauseated after she ate. She tended to cry easily and seemed at times to be more tired, irritable, and depressed than normal.

Her parents took her to one specialist after another. Most of them said she had a psychological problem. They believed she was fearful of school, although Valerie insisted she enjoyed her studies. Her parents repeatedly asked if her headaches could be due to allergies, but they were reassured that it was an unlikely cause. Eventually she was also seen by an allergist who did sixty scratch allergy tests. These revealed no sensitivities, so he concluded that her headaches were unrelated to allergies.

1. Headache Related to Foods Craved Premenstrually

Valerie had two distinct types of headaches. Her first headache always occurred just before her menstrual period. She craved chocolate at that time. This suggested to us that cocoa, milk, or corn syrup might be a factor, because premenstrual women often crave the very foods that cause their allergies. The other possibility was that Valerie had a hormonally related PMS headache that often responds well to P/N allergy extract dilutions of progesterone.[1]

Her premenstrual headache was intermittent and had been present since the age of twelve years. It was located behind her right eye and usually made her sick to her stomach. The headache would recur each morning and disappear each evening. No matter where she was, this headache seemed to go with her. This suggests that it was due to a food. If it had been related to her home, she should have felt better when she left her home for several days.

2. Headache Due to Outdoor Pollution in Her Hometown

At the time we initially saw her, Valerie had developed a distinctly different excruciating headache, which made her unable to attend school; however, she appeared to be extremely anxious to return to school in time to take her final examinations. She described this headache as daily, incapacitating, constant, behind both eyes, and so severe that she was unable to read. It was intensified by exercise. Her teachers, similar to her physicians, thought that she did not want to come to school and that her problems were entirely emotional.

She came to see us from a small town that is several hours from Buffalo. She found that when she stayed out of her hometown for one to two hours, she felt a bit better. If she was out of town for twenty-four to forty-eight hours, her most severe headache disappeared entirely. We therefore asked her to return home *but to stay outside for two hours before entering her home.* When she did this, she developed her excruciating headache within thirty minutes. This told

1. Joseph Miller, M.D., *Relief at Last* (Springfield, Ill.: Charles C. Thomas Publishing, 1987).

us that it was something in the outside air that caused this headache. Our next challenge was to find out what.

Her hometown had a cheese factory that at that time contaminated the air so much that it smelled of cheese. The environmental division of Air Pollution Control for the State of New York kindly agreed to help us. They attached impingement paper filters in such a way that the air from the city could be blown through them. This enabled us to collect whatever was in the air on the special filter paper. We then prepared an allergy extract from this paper. When we tested her with this, we could provoke or reproduce her exact headache with the most concentrated solution. In addition, her mother noted during testing that her bubbly, friendly disposition changed. She became quiet and withdrawn, even angry. The headache disappeared completely within ten minutes after we injected one drop of a dilute solution of allergy extract made from her hometown air. Her personality also returned to normal as soon as she received the correct neutralization treatment.

We cultured the filter paper used to make the allergy extract of air and it grew a number of molds. When she was tested for these molds, we could again reproduce her headaches. This meant that the molds in the air in her town, possibly from the cheese factory, were one cause for this headache.

Her air treatment extract always relieved this headache within a half hour, and she remained well for a full twenty-three hours. If she was one hour late for her treatment, her headache recurred.

She gave us permission to confirm the effectiveness of the allergy extracts she used to prevent or relieve her two different headaches.[2] On one occasion she was delighted to eat an excessive amount of chocolate. She developed her right-eyed nausea headache. Her parents were given three coded identical bottles to use for treatment. Only one contained her correct allergy extract neutralization dosage for cocoa. She had no difficulty determining which bottle contained her treatment dose for milk and chocolate because that extract relieved her headache in less than ten minutes.

Repeated diets and single-blinded provocative allergy skin testing also confirmed that milk and chocolate caused her premenstrual headaches.

In a similar manner on one occasion she allowed herself to develop her hometown air–related intense headache. She correctly and quickly determined which of the three coded bottles contained her

2. See Doris Rapp, M.D., "Double-blind Case Report of Chronic Headaches Due to Foods and Air Pollution," Abstract 13, *Annals of Allergy* 40 (1978), p. 289.

neutralization allergy extract treatment for the air in her city, because only one relieved that headache.

Until we resolved her hometown air problems, Valerie had to live with relatives in a nearby city. However, she initially had problems inside their home until we determined that the fumes from the gas heater were the cause. Again she was better when her bedroom was heated solely with an electric heater. In time we also found that she repeatedly developed headaches after visiting other homes heated with natural gas or after long automobile trips because of exposure to automobile exhaust. The hydrocarbons found in natural gas and gasoline were one more probable cause for her headaches.

As with many allergic children, her symptoms were eventually found to be due to a combination of a few foods, to items in the air she breathed, such as molds, and to chemicals, such as gas heat.

We were able to check with her thirteen years later, when she was twenty-eight years old. She still has headaches three to four times a year. They are usually caused by eating an excessive amount of chocolate, but she no longer craves this food before her menses. Her family now lives in the country and they no longer smell the cheese factory. She completed college without difficulty and feels well.

I anticipate that this young lady will continue to be careful about her diet and particularly about exposures to yeasts, molds, and chemicals in the future. With her present knowledge and personal medical expertise, she should be able to prevent future environmentally related illness. If she does become ill, she should be able to recognize and pinpoint the cause quickly.

SOMETIMES WE KNOW THE CAUSE, BUT IT IS DIFFICULT TO TREAT THE CHILD

Dave

Dave lived in the South. His home was lovely with its lush greenery, but the humidity in the river valley presented special problems for some very sensitive individuals. Dave literally became "wild" if he was allowed outside for a few hours after school or on weekends in the damp weather. If he was kept indoors and ate only the foods that did not bother him, he was wonderful. His parents felt guilty, however, because he simply could not play outside like other eight-year-old boys.

Five months after neutralization treatment for his mold and other allergies, his parents said he was "excellent" and 75 percent better, "but only when it is dry and cool outside." He was far from perfect when it was damp and warm outside. When molds and large amounts of pollen were in the air, he was only 25 percent better. This indicates that P/N allergy treatment cannot relieve symptoms if the exposure is too great. When the mold and pollen counts in that area were extremely elevated, Dave's mold and pollen treatment could not compensate for the exposure. It is rarely necessary to ask a family to move to a different area of the country, but this youngster appeared to be a child who would probably feel and act better if the family lived in a dry, rather than wet, moldy city.

In general, after our treatment he could eat most foods in the usual amount without difficulty. They noted, however, that when he ate an excessive amount of chicken, he still becomes "hyperactive and mouthy." He also cannot eat party or restaurant foods. He continued to need 20 milligrams of Ritalin on school days. His parents were pleased because they learned which foods cause their son to become ill or misbehave. If a mistake was made, they could pinpoint what caused him to act in an unacceptable manner and take steps to avoid future exposures.

TABLE 12.1
Outdoor Factors Causing Seasonal Illness

Spring
    Early tree pollen
    Grass pollen
    Mold spores
Summer
    Late tree pollen
    Grass pollen
    Mold spores
Fall
    Weed pollen
    Mold spores
    Odor of burning leaves
Winter
    Odor or fumes from burning wood or other forms of heat
    Molds on vegetation, burning wood, or other forms of heat
    Molds on vegetation after the snow melts

In desperation his family moved to New Mexico. He did not improve for about two or three weeks. Then each week was better than the last. He could tolerate foods such as chicken, but he remained on a four-day rotation diet of organic foods. He became a normally active, happy child who could play outside at any time, even on rainy days. He no longer required Ritalin or allergy extract. Best of all, he commented that he liked New Mexico because he no longer was "bad."

TABLE 12.2

Possible Outdoor Factors Causing Illness *Anytime*

Aerial spray

Airport odors

Asphalt (fresh)

Asphalt sealers

Bus odors

Diesel fumes

Lawn sprays

Outdoor home insect sprays

Factory odors

Fertilizers

Sewer fumes

Paint smells

Fire smoke

Traffic odors

Trash incinerator fumes

Natural-gas furnace odors

Petroleum refinery odors

Burning rubber tire odors

Chemical spills, any type

TABLE 12.3
Symptoms Associated With Outdoor Air Pollution

Headache

Nausea

Asthma or bronchitis

Irritability

Hyperactivity

Blurred vision

Depression

Tremors

Heart irregularities

Digestive upsets

Chemical Factors Outside Your Home

Other common outside factors that cause problems at special times or any time are listed in Tables 12.1, 12.2, and 12.3. Many children are worse from outdoor chemical pollution of various types. Even fresh paint or a running lawn mower can create smelly odors that cause symptoms in some chemically sensitive children.

Is your child suddenly unable to learn or behave if the windows are open at the time when the school lawns are sprayed or cut? Maybe pollen or chemicals are factors that need consideration. Some studies indicate that not only lung and heart problems increase when outdoor pollution rises but psychiatric problems also become more evident.

Some mothers notice their children repeatedly become ill if they pass certain factory polluted areas on the way to our office. Other parents sometimes notice that they feel well if they are twenty miles outside their hometown, but they routinely become ill the closer they are to the pollution in their own city. Unfortunately, these patients represent a gradually enlarging sector of our society.

C H A P T E R 13
_____

More About
Chemical Pollution

This is unquestionably one of the most important chapters in this book. The impact of the global total disregard for our environment affects all of us. The problems of worldwide chemical pollution can no longer be ignored by the public, physicians, educators, or legislators. We must insist upon measures to protect the health and well-being of this and future generations, even if the price is a temporary economic loss. We can no longer remain oblivious of the increasing pollution of our air, water, soil, food, clothing, and homes.

Look at any newspaper or magazine or listen to any radio or television news program—almost always you will hear reports about chemical exposures that have caused illness and devastation somewhere. This will become more and more evident as everyone becomes more knowledgeable about and aware of the devastating effects that our progressively efficient high-technology world has produced. Everything lasts longer, but there is a price for the longer shelf life of baked goods and groceries; the convenience of lightweight, unbreakable plastic bottles, the strength of nonbiodegradeable garbage bags; and the durability of synthetic carpets and clothing.

Some children and adults are already ill, but many are totally unaware that a chemical is at fault. Whether your family is ill at the present time or not depends upon their degree of exposure, level of sensitivity, heredity, and nutrition. This chapter will discuss the kinds of medical symptoms that chemicals can cause. It will explain some simple precautions your family can take to possibly delay or prevent the development of chemically related health problems. If someone in your family unknowingly already has this type of illness, it is hoped that the information that follows will provide some practical pointers to enhance her or his health and well-being.

As a resident in training in pediatrics, and later in allergy, it was obvious to me that asthmatic children arrived in the emergency room in clusters. Sometimes it was at the peak of a pollen season or when it was very damp outside, so airborne pollen and molds were most likely at fault. I clearly recall, however, that pollution from a large fire in Buffalo caused many asthmatics in that locale to rush into the hospital emergency room for care. That was not an allergy but an irritation from toxins or chemicals created during the fire, which caused twitchy, asthmatic lungs to go into spasm.

Later on, when I was in practice, I often wondered why the youngest and the sickest asthmatics and eczema patients came from nearby highly industrial neighborhoods where toxic chemical pollution was prevalent. Some mothers in one localized area commented that they would rush to take their asthmatic children inside their homes as soon as certain chemical factories released their characteristic noxious fumes. They knew which smell would mean a visit to a hospital emergency room.

Just How Serious Is Our Chemical Problem?

There are over 300,000 toxic and hazardous waste dumps in our country. Every day 50 billion gallons of liquid hazardous wastes are deposited in disposal sites. Unfortunately, 85 percent of these are said to be located above our aquifers or water-storage areas. We have no federal, but some state regulations about pesticide contamination of the ground water. Over 500 billion pounds of hazardous wastes are improperly disposed of each year. As many as 90,000 land disposal sites may be contaminating surface ground water. Every year 100 billion gallons of liquid hazardous wastes are absorbed into our ground water. There are some 800,000 underground waste-storage tanks, and about a third are considered to be structurally impaired, which means that they leak. This spilled waste can eventually contaminate the ground water, which in time becomes our drinking water. Very few of these priority sites have been cleaned up by the EPA.

Our sewage plants are not all at peak efficiency, and some discharge raw sewage, along with germs and parasites, into our lakes, streams, and rivers. *Safe water must become everyone's concern.*

The EPA has set standards for only about *seven* of the currently used 70,000 toxic chemicals. In New York State, 87 million pounds of toxins were released into the air in 1987. About 40 percent of these were emissions from cracks in valves, pipes, and so forth, which are totally unregulated. The remaining 60 percent came from industrial smokestacks. These chemicals in essence cause a low-grade poisoning. Some of the released pollutants are known to cause various toxic reactions, as well as cancer, miscarriages, deformed infants, and sterility.

In time, our fat stores can become saturated with the smorgasbord of chemicals that we breathe, eat, drink, or absorb through our skin. Some chemicals cannot be completely broken down and removed by means of our expired air, perspiration, saliva, urine, and bowel movements. We must wonder how long our bodies, as well as those of our children, can handle our progressively increasing chemical overload.

How Can You Tell If a Chemical Causes Illness?

Notice if your child or you tend to feel fine until some odor is smelled. Ask yourself if the problem can be related to some odor outside your home, inside your home, or from some personal item that you use. Notice how your family feels when the prevailing winds bring factory-contaminated air toward your home? Does the neighbor's chemical lawn spray bother your family? Which outdoor odors affect your family? If you are unsure, purposely notice the next time your child is exposed. Compare how your child felt both before and during the next few hours after some unavoidable exposure. If this repeatedly causes the same symptoms, you may have confirmed which chemical causes your child's illness. Take the time not only to smell the flowers but also to critically smell the pollutants in the air that your family breathes.

Even after I entered the field of ecology, I sincerely believed that Dr. Theron Randolph had carried his suggestions to a ridiculous degree when he recommended that some patients remove *all* gas appliances and gas heat from their homes. I believed what he said about foods, but as a well-indoctrinated traditional allergist, I thought it foolish and inappropriate to believe that the slight odor of hydrocarbons leaking from a gas kitchen stove could cause illness.

Sometimes the Lord makes us believers in odd ways. When we had a sudden accidental gasoline and natural-gas leak in our home, one member of our family developed a serious cardiac irregularity overnight. Fortunately, because of my awareness and with the help of Dr. William Rea, in Dallas, the home and health problems were quickly remedied. The gasoline spill was cleaned up, and the gas stove and gas heat were both replaced with electric. Had I not been knowledgeable, the cardiac problem could easily have persisted and not been relieved as quickly and completely as it was.

Basic Concepts Needed to Understand Chemically Related Illness

There are three key basic principles that help in our understanding of chemical sensitivities.

1. Some Odors Make You Feel Better

Similar to patients with food or drug addiction, some persons with chemical sensitivities have odor addictions. It is called masking when recurrent exposure to an odor makes an individual feel better. This could be illustrated by the painter who is on vacation. Because he begins to feel unwell or not right in some way, he finds someplace that has been freshly painted. The odor of fresh paint temporarily makes him feel better. He "needs" to smell the paint to get his "fix," like the heroin addict who must have one more shot to feel better. The relief, however, is only temporary. Other common odor addictions are found in those who crave the smell of gasoline, perfume, or even the aroma of funeral parlors.

Many affected individuals do not recognize they have a sensitivity to an odor. They only know that they like a certain aroma. They may not even realize that some smell makes them feel better and that without it they don't feel right. If any family member has an extreme craving for a particular odor, this could indicate a sensitivity to that item.

The symptoms of withdrawal or need for a "chemical or food fix" are similar. Either can cause the type of illness illustrated in Table 13.1. Many complain of headaches, muscle aches, stomach cramps, nausea, confusion, depression, sluggishness, fatigue, or irritability. These symptoms can last for one to four days and usually begin within a day or two after the individual has not smelled the favorite odor or eaten the craved food. These temporary symptoms are to be expected but not to be feared. Once they pass, it is possible to break the addiction. However, most individuals weaken and are inclined to relieve their potentially temporary symptoms with just one more exposure. Thus the vicious cycle starts again, which leads to progres-

TABLE 13.1
Typical Chemical Sensitivity or
"Sick-Building Syndrome" Symptoms

Headaches
Lethargy
Dizziness
Malaise
Weakness
Nausea
Flushing
Eye itch or irritation
Dry eyes
Blurred vision
Stuffy or watery nose
Dry throat
Arthralgia or joint pain
Skin problems
Cough and asthma
Numbness and tingling
Muscle weakness
Muscle cramps
Weight loss
Insomnia
Confusion
Loss of memory
Poor concentration
Edema
Moodiness
Depression
Fatigue
Increased perspiration
Hyperactivity
Loss of voice or laryngitis
Hearing loss
Irregular heartbeat

sively more severe illness. To demonstrate a chemical or food sensitivity, it is often necessary to have no contact with the offending smell or food for about four days. This unmasks the sensitivity so that the next exposure will cause obvious symptoms. If this basic principle is not understood, it is easy to be deluded into believing that you do not have a sensitivity, when one truly exists.

2. Some Odors Make You Feel Worse

At a different stage of the same chemical or food sensitivity, certain individuals can feel worse shortly after they smell or eat an offending item. These individuals are just as sensitive as those who have masked allergies. These are the people who complain bitterly about feeling unwell after exposure to some smell that others insist is not even present. The irony is that sometimes the addiction is so powerful that informed adults still cannot resist certain odor temptations. They crave the smell of gasoline, for example, even though they know it makes them giddy or causes a personality change. Once again, it is similar to the chocoholic who eats the candy even though it causes hives or a headache. We must wonder if the present sniffing craze in our youths could in part have a similar basis. (See below.)

If odors are neither particularly disliked nor intensely liked by a particular individual, it is doubtful that he or she has a chemical sensitivity. This is especially true if the person does not have the types of medical complaints listed in Tables 13.1 and 13.2.

Table 13.2
Serious Potential Long-Term Effects of Some Chemicals

Sterility
Reproductive problems
Miscarriages
Infants with birth defects
Cancer
Liver disease
Kidney disease
Heart disease

A Special Problem of Great Concern

It appears that up to 30 percent of the children, aged ten to fifteen years, for example, in certain large cities in Texas, are presently sniffing various substances.[1] They apparently sometimes start sniffing correction fluid, glue, felt-tipped pens, fingernail polish remover, nonstick pan aerosol, and in time, even paint thinner. The chemicals sniffed usually include benzene, toluene, xylene, or methyl ethyl-ketones or hydrocarbons. These can cause a wide range of symptoms, the most serious being permanent brain damage. *Some of these children will spend the rest of their lives in institutions because they cannot think or function in a normal manner.* Less severe symptoms include an irregular heartbeat, moodiness, slurred speech, a loss of memory for recent events, and various behavioral or psychological problems. These chemicals can also damage the liver, kidneys, and immune system.

Every effort must be made by parents to become aware of this type of problem. If you find your children seem to crave or have an unusually intense desire to smell certain odors, be suspicious. If there is evidence in the child's bedroom that sniffing odors might be a problem, it is important to try to help your child as soon as possible. Look in the wastebasket for evidence of products that could be inhaled.

There is a special Inhalant Screening Panel that can identify and document if a child has an excessive amount of any of the common chemicals found in odorous substances. This test is available through Accu-Chem.[2]

How Chlorine Affected One Youngster

Linda

One of Linda's most dramatic chemical problems was related to her sensitivity to chlorine. Initially this problem was noted when she was about four years old. Her mother observed that shortly after Linda swam underwater in a chlorinated pool, she would cry much more

1. John L. Laseter, M.D., "Monitoring of Aromatic and Chlorinated Solvents in Blood Following Inhalant Abuse in Juveniles." Presented at the National Inhalant Abuse Prevention Conference, San Antonio, Tex., March 13–16, 1990.

2. Accu-Chem Laboratories, 990 North Bowser Road, Suite 800, Richardson, Tex. 75081. (214-234-5577).

easily than normal and would complain of a headache and leg cramps. Even though she was very bright in school, she could not follow the simplest instructions during swimming class. She eventually had to discontinue her swimming lessons. This was the first clue that chlorine could interfere with her personality or thinking.

Linda did not have difficulty from chlorinated tap water because she didn't drink it. The family drank only purified, glass-bottled water, and Linda seldom drank water outside her home because she did not like the taste.

When she was thirteen years old, five years after an accidental exposure to a malfunctioning gas furnace, her chlorine problems recurred. This time they were precipitated by a *minute exposure* to the odor of chlorine bleach. She was doing her homework in her brother's room, and as she wrote her composition, both the content and her penmanship suddenly began to deteriorate, as indicated in Figure 13.1. Linda then became extremely irritable and tearful. When her mother checked, she found that there was a direct duct leading from the laundry room into the area where Linda was writing. At the time when Linda suddenly could not write well, her mother had just used chlorine bleach in the basement. The trace of chlorine odor in the bedroom affected Linda's brain. Her personality and ability to think and write changed. When her teacher saw her composition, she sent home the note in Figure 13.2. This family's awareness of the role of chemicals in relation to health helped Linda's grades, and school performance remain at an optimal level. More details about this child's earlier history are provided in Chapter 11 and Appendix E. (See also Bill, Appendix E.)

3. Some Chemicals Make You Sensitive to Other Chemicals

After a prolonged or massive chemical exposure many individuals typically find that minute amounts of *many* other chemical odors can cause progressively more severe physical and emotional symptoms. Linda clearly illustrates "the spreading phenomenon." She and her parents and brother became more and more sensitive to smaller and smaller exposures of many other chemicals after an unfortunate ac-cidental gas exposure in her home. Her history indicated that chem-icals were a factor related to some of her earlier medical complaints, but recurrent leaks of natural gas and combustion products greatly magnified her original chemical sensitivity.

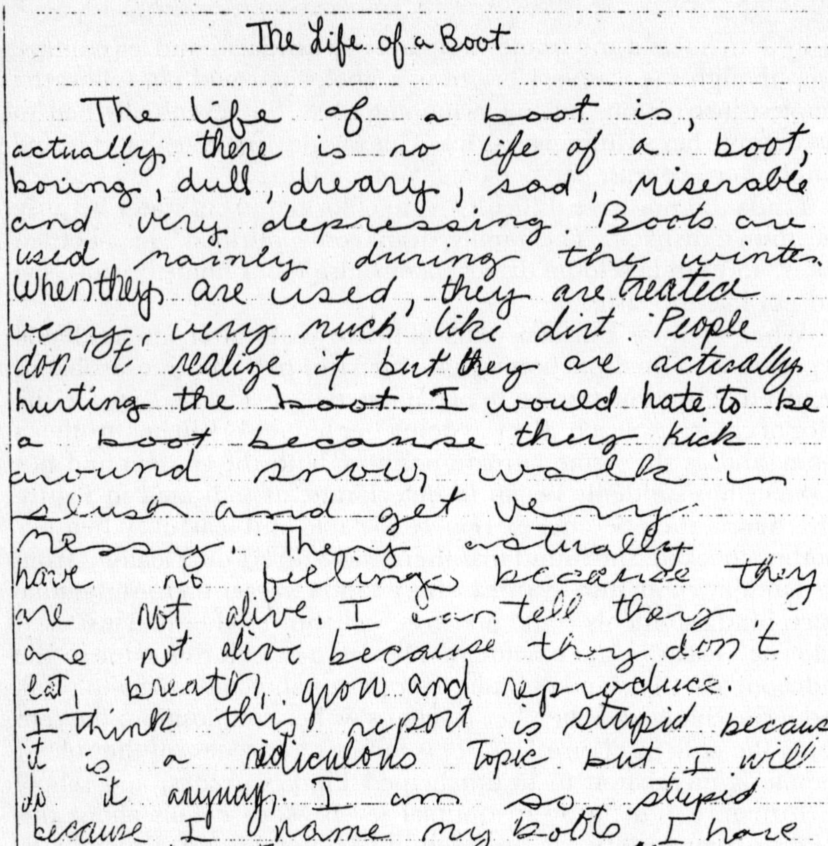

The Life of a Boot

The life of a boot is, actually there is no life of a boot, boring, dull, dreary, sad, miserable and very depressing. Boots are used mainly during the winter. When they are used, they are treated very, very much like dirt. People don't realize it but they are actually hurting the ~~boot~~. I would hate to be a ~~boot~~ because they kick around snow, walk in slush and get very messy. They actually have no feelings because they are not alive. I can tell they are not alive because they don't eat, breath, grow and reproduce. I think this report is stupid because it is a ridiculous topic but I will do it anyway. I am so stupid because I name my boots I have many ~~boots~~ so I name all of them. My blue boots are called bluey and my green boots are called greeny. I know you are glad to know the names of my boots. I know naming my boots is pretty childish but at least I have an imagination. Most boots have a friend to talk, communicate with and share its feelings.

Figure 13.1. Linda's penmanship deteriorates from exposure to the pungent odor of chlorine bleach.

Response of Teacher to Youngster's Handwriting Change
Noted After Chlorine Exposure

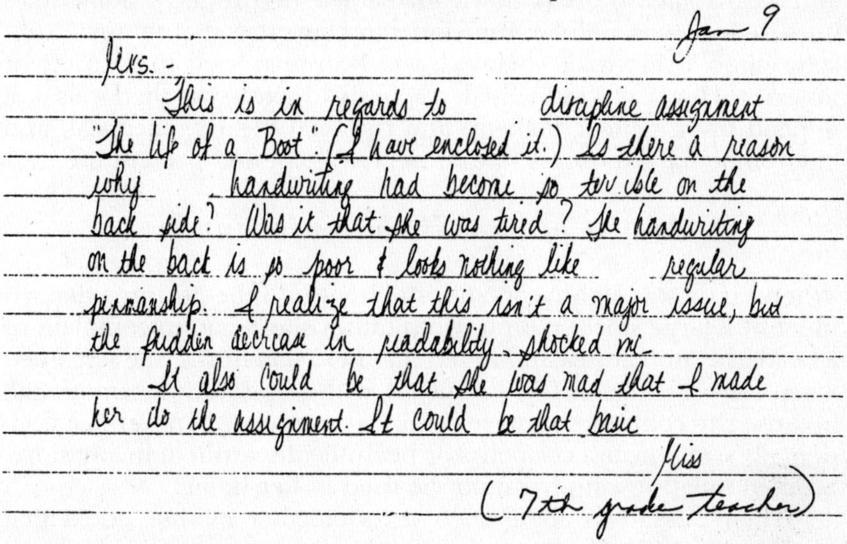

Jan 9

Mrs. -

This is in regards to   discipline assignment "The Life of a Boot". (I have enclosed it.) Is there a reason why   handwriting had become so terrible on the back side? Was it that she was tired? The handwriting on the back is so poor & looks nothing like   regular penmanship. I realize that this isn't a major issue, but the sudden decrease in readability shocked me.

It also could be that she was mad that I made her do the assignment. It could be that basic

Miss

(7th grade teacher)

Figure 13.2. Linda's teacher noticed the change in content and penmanship and notified her parents.

The Spreading Phenomenon
Associated With Odor Sensitivities

Chronic small or single large exposures can cause similar chemical sensitization. Once this happens, the spreading phenomenon is often noted. This means that the tiniest exposure to almost any new chemical odor, such as a whiff of perfume, tobacco, exhaust, or incense, can immediately precipitate a sudden change in how a previously sensitized child or adult feels or acts. This happens even though these odors never caused problems before. These people are the first to smell an odor. In time this increased sensitivity can spread not only to other chemicals but also to foods, dust, molds, and so forth. They seem to develop a heightened sensitivity to smaller and smaller amounts of an ever-increasing number of potentially offending items of all types.

It is thought that part of this enhanced sensitivity is due to bodily biochemical changes in response to certain chemicals. Chemicals can damage our immune system and interfere with normal cellular functions, such as metabolism and detoxification. Formaldehyde breakdown, for example, requires folic acid. If a child uses up all the available folic acid in her or his body because of certain excessive chemical exposures, this can lead to a lack of folic acid in the future and an inability to break down formaldehyde properly. Sometimes impaired normal cellular function can convert a slightly toxic substance into a very toxic chemical, which in turn leads to a variety of illnesses. How each individual responds to excessive chemicals will depend upon genetic makeup and the total dietary, chemical, and environmental exposures in that person's past and present life.

More Chemical Problems for Linda

When Linda was eight years old, she went into the perfume department of a large store. Within two minutes she began to complain of a headache and nausea and stated that her "skin hurt." She screamed when she was touched. We doubt that this episode was emotional, because she continues to have similar symptoms whenever she accidentally strays near a cosmetics or perfume department in any store. Scented toiletries simply cannot be used in her home.

When Linda was about nine years old, her mother noted that Linda's disposition became disagreeable whenever they visited one of her grandmothers. This personality change recurred with each subsequent visit until her mother recognized the cause: Her grandmother's home smelled of mothballs. When these were removed from the closets, Linda's pleasant disposition was no longer affected by these visits.

At about the same age Linda complained about a daily headache after the ride home on the school bus. Combustion fumes from gasoline often cause this problem in children. You might ask why she didn't have the same problem when she went to school. It is possible that a child can tolerate going to school on the same bus without difficulty because it is early in the day. After the cumulative, daily multiple chemical or other allergenic exposures that occur throughout the course of a normal school day, however, she might tolerate less on the way home. When Linda's total allergenic load was lowered, she could ride the bus home without difficulty.

Linda's problems definitely improved after her bedroom was made significantly more ecologically sound with a ceramic floor, air purifier, and scant furnishings made of natural fibers. Her total twenty-four-hour exposure to offending items was decreased below the level that caused symptoms. Her "barrel" was no longer overflowing. If a child breathes clean air for eight hours at night, for example, increased unavoidable or accidental contacts with allergenic items can be better tolerated during the day without causing symptoms. (See Chapter 2.)

Be Careful, You Can Be Fooled

Martin

Ten-year-old Martin's mother said that recently, whenever her son swam in a pool, he became grumpy, surly, irritable, and hyperactive. His drastic personality change seemed to happen late in the day with a tantrum and extreme negativity, but only after his swimming class. His personality change often lasted throughout that night and the next day. His mother jokingly stated that she was "ready to let him be adopted." He swam only in chlorinated water, so my initial impression was that he was probably sensitive to the chemicals used in pools. His complaints, however, happened to occur at the hottest time of the year, when the local water had a characteristic taste of algae. We tested him for both chlorine and algae and he appeared to be sensitive to both items. Much to our surprise a delighted mother returned two weeks later. If he took only his neutralization allergy extract therapy for algae before he swam, he had no change in disposition. His response after swimming appeared to be due to the chlorphyll-containing plant called algae and not to the chlorine chemical so commonly used in pools.

One other patient was always ill after swimming, which again suggested a possible sensitivity to pool chemicals. A careful history revealed, however, that after each swim he always ate popcorn and drank soda pop. The corn caused his symptoms, not the chlorine, algae, or soda pop. The key to finding answers is often a detailed history. *What did the individual drink, eat, smell, or touch before a sudden change in physical health and personality?*

The symptoms caused by foods, molds, pollen, dust, yeast, pets, chemicals, toxic metals, nutritional deficiencies, hormone imbalances, and stress can all be similar. Your physician must be able to evaluate all these factors to determine what is causing modern-day illness. The body has a rather limited number of ways in which it can react to a wide range of harmful substances. In other words, a headache, fatigue, and irritability could be caused by any of the above factors, as well as by a multitude of other medical illness. The challenge for physicians is to determine exactly what is causing each individual complaint.

Tips to Help You Detect Chemical Sensitivities

The following are some tips to help you recognize chemical sensitivities. Children and adults who are ill or incapacitated because of this problem characteristically have certain complaints in common. Let us review the major clues.

- Do you become sleepy or nauseated, do you vomit, or do you develop headaches when you travel in cars, buses, or planes?

- Do you smell odors before anyone else? Our bodies really try to protect us. At first we tend to adapt to smells, so we may not even notice the odor. With continued or excessive exposure, we often become supersensitive. It is as if our bodies have sent out larger antennae. At that point certain individuals may recognize that their obscure illness appears to be caused by a chemical. Cause-and-effect relationships are apparent. If the noxious exposures persist for a prolonged period of time, however, there can be a total loss of smell in some sensitive individuals. Our bodies seem to give us an ample early warning at first, but eventually the alarm system fails or becomes exhausted. At that point chemically sensitive people are usually incapacitated and potentially in grave danger. They can no longer smell odors and they therefore become progressively more ill because they can't avoid them.

- Do you crave or detest certain chemical smells, such as paint, marking pencils, perfume, gasoline, or aerosols?

- Do you commonly complain of any of the symptoms listed in Table 13.1? Chemical odors can cause any combination of the listed complaints, for example dizziness, irritability, fatigue, depression, insomnia. Unexplained periods of hostility and temper outbursts are also characteristic. Sometimes affected children or adults cry easily or find they are unable to think clearly or remember. Although they are fatigued, rest may not revitalize their energy level. Did the doctor diagnose your child's vague complaints as a viral infection, yet weeks later your child was still acting tired and weak? Sometimes these complaints are due to chemicals.

- Do you tend to have muscle aches, especially in the region of the neck, upper shoulders, or legs? Older children and adults complain of burning feet or calves, especially after walking on synthetic carpets or in plastic-lined shoes.

- Do you tend to have five-to-ten-pound fluctuations in weight during a single day or two? Some individuals notice swelling of different body parts. For example, the fingers can swell so much that on certain mornings a wedding ring can't be worn. Chemical and food sensitivities commonly cause this type of problem in adolescent or adult females. Think about odors and your favorite foods.

- Do you have sudden excessive perspiration that is unrelated to exercise? The perspiration may even smell of a chemical or have an unusual odor or color.

- Are there drastic changes in some family member's speech? Is the voice too high-pitched at times or the speech unclear or too rapid? Some children or adults who are affected stutter; others can't speak at all or can only whisper.

If any of these complaints is combined with a racing pulse, trembling inside the body, and a feeling of anxiety, it could be interpreted as a panic attack. Not infrequently, however, exposures to chemicals, molds, or food sensitivities, in particular, can cause such episodes.

Typical Medical Symptoms of the Sick-Building Syndrome

If several individuals develop similar medical complaints when they are exposed to certain chemicals in a new building, one must wonder about the health effect of something used in the construction or furnishings of that building. (See Table 13.1.) The diverse multiple substances that outgas odors within a new or refurbished home, school, or office building can sometimes cause certain susceptible individuals to become ill at about the same time. Although a building may be beautiful, the pervasive accumulation of chemicals may insidiously cause a wide range of symptoms. This can be noted shortly after a new modern building or school begins to be used. Within a few hours, weeks, or months certain susceptible individuals will act like canaries in a coal mine. Boys and women are more apt to be affected than girls and men. They complain of feeling unwell in some way. Small chemical exposures tend to affect the nervous system and short-term memory first. Long-term chemical exposures can totally incapacitate some sensitive individuals so that they can no longer work or function at a level anywhere near their previous degree of efficiency.

Of the 49,000 commercially used chemicals, toxicity data are available for only 20 percent. New office buildings contain approximately ten times as many hydrocarbons as older ones. This means that the newer the building, the more likely it is that there will be an excessive chemical exposure. In general, the more humid and warmer a building, the more likely it is that chemically related health problems will be evident. Air-conditioned energy-efficient buildings also create more health problems than those that have more conventional ventilation, for example windows that open.

A few of the major chemicals in buildings that are most apt to cause illness include: formaldehyde, nitrous oxide, ozone, carbon monoxide, and hydrocarbons such as toluene, xylene, benzene, trichloroethylene, perchlorethylene, and styrene. Carpet chemicals can emit odors of formaldehyde, toluene, xylene, benzene, tetrachlorethylene, and styrene, to name only a few. Another common indoor chemical is vinyl chloride. This is found in plastics, toys, computers, and indoor furnishings.

Sick-Building Syndrome in One School

In 1979, while dyslexic children were on a three-week Christmas holiday, their school carpets were cleaned with petrochemicals and the area was sprayed with a pesticide. After the vacation the children and the staff developed fever, nausea, and respiratory illness on a daily basis by 10:00 A.M., and after returning home, their symptoms subsided. Some children's ability to learn and write deteriorated. The reading and comprehension of some children fell by two or three grades.

Drs. Hardman and Lieberman therefore conducted a double-blind study. They found that 76 percent of the thirteen children who were tested for the specific chemical malathion or for the general category of chemicals called petrochemicals or hydrocarbons reacted adversely. The affected children had deterioration of their perception, learning, and/or behavior. Forty-six percent of the affected children reacted only to the malathion and 46 percent reacted only to petrochemicals. Malathion exposure caused changes that could have been interpreted as emotional disturbances.[3]

3. Published with permission of Allan Lieberman, M.D. Allan Lieberman, Patricia Hardman, and Patricia Preston, "Academic, Behavioral, and Perceptual Reactions in Dyslexic Children When Exposed to Environmental Factors—Malathion and Petrochemical Ethanol." 1981. Copies of this article are available through Dyslexia Research Institute, Inc., 4745 Centerville Road, Tallahassee, Fla. 32308 (904-893-2216).

A Few Specific Chemicals That Cause Illness

There are a large number of chemicals that are virtually impossible to avoid. Industrial exposures are obvious but there are some less obvious ones found in our water, air, meat, fish, homes, and gardens. A few are also in our automobiles. The major categories can be divided into organic and inorganic chemicals. Inorganic chemicals include heavy metals such as lead, mercury, etc. Common organic chemicals include pesticides, herbicides, hydrocarbons and solvents, polychlorinated biphenyls (PCBs), chlorinated and nonchlorinated phenols, and formaldehyde. If you are concerned about a possible exposure, contact your physician, who can order a test from Accu-Chem, as they have panels to test for certain categories of contamination in a patient's blood or urine.[4]

Pesticides and Insecticides[5]

As of 1986, there were 46,000 pesticides on the market. In California, in 1980, 268 million pounds of pesticides were applied to food crops. Of these, 7.8 million pounds were known to cause cancer in animals. Over a billion pounds were applied across the United States in 1984, almost double the amount used in 1964.[6]

It has been said that of the two billion pounds of pesticides used on food crops, 99 percent never reach a pest but they do enter our soil, water, and food chain. About 20 percent to 25 percent of all toxic pollutants of the Great Lakes come from polluted air. Some of these chemicals can kill birds, pets, and people. For more information, write Citizens Against Pesticide Misuse, P.O. Box 670608, Dallas, Tex. 75367-0608.

Two major groups in this category are called chlorinated hydrocarbons and organophosphates.

Chlorinated Hydrocarbons

The common (not commercial or chemical) names for chlorinated hydrocarbon pesticides are:

4. Accu-Chem Laboratories, 990 North Bowser Road, Suite 800, Richardson, Tex. 75081 (214-234-5577).

5. Contact: National Pesticide Telecommunications Network (800-858-7378).

6. Joseph Beasley and Jerry Swift, *The Kellogg Report*. 1989. The Institute of Health Policy Practice, The Bard College Center, Annandale-on-Hudson, New York, N.Y. 12504. For a copy of publication, write to 221 Broadway, Suite 301, Amityville, N. Y., 11701.

- Aldrin, dieldrin, for termites
- Endrin, for crops
- Lindane, for seeds, beetle control in wood, and termites
- Chlordane, for gardening, seeds, and termites
- DDT and its derivatives. Sixty percent of the population has this chemical in their bodies due to the extensive use of this chemical prior to 1971. It is presently brought into this country from Mexico and is found on produce from foreign countries. It is still legally used in this country in some pesticides.
- Hexachlorobenzene is present in the blood of 55 percent of the population studied. It is used as a fungicide.
- Endosulfan has been found in about 35 percent of the population. It is used in agriculture.
- Mirex is used to control fire ants in the South and West. It can adversely affect reproduction, the blood, and cause cataracts.
- PCBs, or polychlorinated biphenyls, are used in insulating coolants in electrical transformers, paints, varnishes, lubricants, plasticizers, and flame retardants. Unfortunately, these are so stable that they will remain a persistent environmental problem.

Chlorinated hydrocarbon pesticides accumulate in various organs, especially in the fat tissues, but the primary acute effect is in the nervous system and muscles. The half-lives of these chemicals in the soil can be in excess of twenty years. Even though many of these chemicals have been banned by state and federal agencies, large quantities still exist around homes, waste sites, and storage areas. Also, several may be used by special permit to control agricultural pests in limited situations.

Check the ingredients of the lawn-care or garden chemicals stored in your garage. You and your family may be exposed and not realize it.

Organophosphates

Dursban, parathion, and malathion are typical organophosphate-type pesticides. Once they enter the ground, these chemicals remain active in the soil for over one season. The chemicals disrupt the nerve function in insects, animals, *and humans*. Dursban is absorbed through the skin. It can cause giddiness, blurred vision, and headaches at first;

later on nausea, vomiting, cramps, chest pain, tingling, and twitching. Some individuals notice a loss of coordination or balance. It has caused death when used on a golf course.

These organophosphates can markedly alter the ability of the brain to think, concentrate, or remember. Both personality and co-ordination can be affected. Studies by Dr. Satoshi Ishikawa have documented that aerial malathion spray, for example, can cause se-vere and long-term visual problems in those who are exposed. The pupil and the optic nerve both can be affected.[7] The aerial malathion spraying in California is tragic. It is unbelievable that the authorities advise people to cover up their cars to protect the paint, but they spray little children's sandboxes and contaminate the soil with mal-athion. They appear to be more concerned about protecting the crops when they spray to control the Mediterranean fruit fly than they are about the people. Somehow, someone's priorities have become very mixed up.

If you are concerned, ask your child's school officials or the city health department to supply safety data sheets for all the chemicals used on or near your child's school. Similarly, check the ingredients in any aerial spraying near your home. Remember that golf courses, playgrounds, school lawns, etc. can also be contaminated.

Herbicides

Common names are Chloroxone, Dinoxol, Verton 2D, Weedar, Wee-done, Weed-B-Gon, Weed & Feed, and Inverton 245. The defoliant Agent Orange contained some of these herbicides. We have direct contact through contaminated edible plants, livestock, and water as well as from exposure to various aerial and lawn sprays.

Hydrocarbons

Dr. Theron Randolph warned of the dangers of these chemicals in the forties, but few listened. These chemicals include gasoline, fuel oils, ketone solvents, aromatic and aliphatic solvents, and halogen-ating solvents (see Table 13.3). They are routinely used to supply heat from fossil fuels such as oil, coal, gas, etc. They are routinely used in hundreds of industrial processes. The solvent wastes from such industry subsequently contaminates our water supplies. Typi-

7. Satoshi Ishikawa et al. in "Evaluations of the Autonomic Nervous System Response by Pupillographical Study in the Chemically Sensitive Patient." *Clinical Ecology* 7 (2) (1990): vol. 7, no 2. as in Biblio.

TABLE 13.3
Sources of Hydrocarbons

Coal and petroleum products, including solids, liquids and gases

Solids: a whole array of plastics, synthetic fabrics, roof tar, asphalt, wax coatings (used to coat some fruit and vegetables)

Liquids: gasoline, diesel, and oil. (Industry uses a huge number of related petrochemicals.)

Gases: natural and bottled gas; fumes from any of the hydrocarbon solids or liquids; odor from cleaning compounds, polishes, paints, insecticides; evaporating oil from an electric motor

Auto and bus exhaust

Chemicals used in copying and duplicating machines

Art and decorating supplies

Treated papers and adhesives

Pine wood and turpentine (can affect people sensitive to hydrocarbons since coal, oil, and gas all developed from organic material)

Disinfectant cleaning solutions

---

cally we are all exposed to the vapors or fumes, but at times these chemicals enter our bodies with food or water, or from contact with our skin. These can be toxic to many body organs, especially our nervous system, liver, bone marrow, kidneys, or heart. They can cause the arms and legs to tingle or feel numb or weak. Because these chemicals are fat soluble they are stored in our fat, including the fatty tissue in our brains. The spectrum of illness caused by these chemicals range from minor irritation of the skin or eyes to cancer. Examples of aromatic hydrocarbons are benzene, toluene, xylene, styrene, and trimethyl- or ethylbenzene. You must ask if your child or family are ill in some way from an excessive exposure of any of the following.

There are three major categories of hydrocarbons. They can be called aliphatic, aromatic, and halogenated, both chlorinated and brominated.

Aliphatic Hydrocarbon

Pentane, hexane, and heptane are the most common examples of aliphatic hydrocarbons. These include solvents used in glues, cements, and adhesives for footwear. Some are combined with other hydrocarbons to form paint thinners and as solvents for graphic art colors.

Aromatic Hydrocarbons

The aromatic hydrocarbon compounds include benzene, toluene, xylene, styrene, ethylbenzene and trimethylbenzenes.

Benzene

Low levels of benzene, another common industrial pollutant and component in gasoline, for example, is known to increase the risk of leukemia in humans. Newborn infants of mothers who smoke have more benzene in their blood at birth than babies from nonsmoking mothers. The benzene comes from the cigarettes. In 1979 the surgeon general admitted that some of our so-called pure water supplies were contaminated with benzene, and the pesticides chlordane, aldrin, and dieldrin.

Toluene

Toluene is used as a paint thinner, stripping agent, in lacquers and varnishes, and as an additive in fuel. It is also used extensively in print shops. Solvents containing toluene can cause depression and brain malfunction, and with prolonged exposure, permanent neurological damage.

Xylene

This is used in gums, resins, inks, rubber paints, photographic solutions, plastics, gasoline, synthetic fibers, degreasing agents, insecticides, and to clean microscope lenses. Health effects are similar to those caused by toluene but less severe.

Styrene

This is used in making plastics and synthetic rubber products. Prolonged exposure can cause leukemia and chromosomal changes. Styrofoam cups and dishes contain styrene. Hot liquids dissolve the styrene into the beverage in the styrofoam cup.

Ethylbenzene

It is used as a paint or lacquer thinner and as an antiknock ingredient in motor fuels.

Trimethylbenzene

Trimethylbenzene is used in solvents, for paint thinners, perfume, motor fuel, and dyes.

Halogenated Hydrocarbons

The chlorinated hydrocarbons include chloroform, dichloromethane, methyl chloroform, trichloroethylene, tetrachlorethylene, and dichlorbenzenes. These are used as solvents in dyes and drugs, in paint stripper, deodorants, disinfectants, fumigants, metal polishes, mothproofing, and dry cleaning, as well as in fluorocarbons used in refrigerants, plastics, and propellants. These chemicals can cause skin and respiratory illness, liver and kidney damage, and heart and blood irregularities.

Brominated hydrocarbons, including bromoform and methyl bromide also cause symptoms. These tend to be found in drinking water, disinfectants, and degreasers and fumigants.

Trichloroethylene

Trichloroethylene (TCE) is a carcinogen emitted from some copy machines, correcting fluid, dry cleaning fluids, floor polish, rug shampoos, and the glue used in furniture. It is used as a solvent or degreaser in machines and oils. It is used as a fumigant. Most children are not directly or massively exposed to these items. Sometimes, however, it can be a factor related to a child's illness. In Dr. Sherry Rogers's book, *Tired or Toxic?*, she states that a dozen children in Woburn, Massachusetts, died of leukemia after the town's water was accidentally contaminated with TCE.[8] Others who were exposed developed abnormalities in their protective immune system, excessive infections, or problems with their skin, heart, and nervous system.

Dioxin, Chlorine Bleach, and Paper

Even paper can be needlessly dangerous in today's world. Toilet and facial tissue, milk cartons, coffee filters, disposable diapers, and tam-

8. Sherry Rogers, M.D., *Tired or Toxic?*, 1990. Box 3161, 3502 Brewerton Road, Syracuse, N.Y., 13220.

pons are bleached white with chlorine, which contains dioxin plus, at times, many other organic chlorines that are hazardous to our health.[9] Dioxin is a toxic chemical that causes cancer and birth defects, and weakens our immune defense system. It is not considered safe in any amount. Dioxin can seep from the cartons into our milk, from the coffee filters into our coffee, and eventually into our streams so our fish and water ways are also contaminated. Chlorine bleaching of paper pulp releases up to 700 million pounds of organochlorides into our air and waterways each year.

Other countries such as Sweden, Germany, and Austria use safer, oxygen-based systems to bleach paper. Why don't we? In the meantime, we should all refuse to buy chlorine-bleached paper.[10]

Phenols

Phenols are one type of organic hydrocarbon compound derived from coal tar or petroleum. They are used in oral dentifrices and extensively in household products. The phenols as a class include pentachlorophenol (PCP). Pure phenol (carbolic acid) is a potent disinfectant and antiseptic (see Table 13.4).

There are two types of phenolic compounds. Nonchlorinated phenols are found, for example, in the common disinfectant aerosols that you use in your bathroom or kitchen.

The other group are chlorinated phenols. Chlorinated phenols such as Dowicide are used as wood preservatives, defoliants, and as antimicrobial preparations.

Formaldehyde[11]

Formaldehyde is found in many commonly used substances (see Table 13.5). It is most often in resin glues, plastics, and foams.

The second most common use of formaldehyde is in preservatives, fungicides, and chemical stabilizers.

The third most common use is in fabrics. It is an agent used to make permanent press clothing, draperies, fireproof material, and other fabrics.

9. Contact: Greenpeace, 1436 U Street N.W., P.O. Box 3720, Washington, D.C. 20009. (202-462-1177).

10. This book is printed on nonchlorinated paper.

11. List of sources of formaldehyde and phenol from: Debra Dadd and Allan Levin, *A Consumer Guide for the Chemically Sensitive*, 1982, Nontoxic Lifestyles, Inc. Used with permission. Available through Debra Dadd, P.O. Box 279, Forest Knolls, Los Angeles, Calif. 94933.

TABLE 13.4
Sources of Phenol

Acne medications

Adhesives, glue

Aerosols used as disinfectants for odor or mold control

Allergy extract preservative in traditional allergy extract treatments

Aspirin

Bakelite

Baking powders

Caulking agents

Detergents

Disinfectants (pine)

Dyes

Epoxy and phenolic resins

Explosives

Fiberglass

Flame-retardant finishes

Food additives

Inks: fountain pen, printers, stamp pads

Insulation: thermal and accoustical

Jute or hemp fiber preservative: carpet backing, area rugs, rope, twine

Laundry starches

Matches

Metal polishes

Mildew, mildew-proofing

Molded-plastic articles, such as telephones and toys

Mouthwashes

Nylon

Paints: enamel paint, tempera paint, watercolor paints

Perfume

Pesticides and herbicides

Pharmaceuticals

Phenolic plastics, such as hard saucepan handles

Photographic chemicals

Plastics

Plywood

Polyurethane

Preservatives in cosmetics: mascara, liquid eye liner, cream rouges, and eyeshadows

Preservatives in hair care products: hair spray, setting lotion, shampoo, hair color

Preservatives in medication: nose and throat sprays, bronchial mists, cough syrups, eye drops, antihistamines, cold capsules, decongestants, first-aid ointments

Shaving cream and lotions

Shoe polishes

Spandex: girdles, support hose, etc.

Synthetic detergents

Synthetic fabrics

Tin cans (inner lining)

Tobacco smoke

Wood preservatives, sealants, solvents

Formaldehyde is produced by combustion in poorly tuned engines or from burning cigarettes or wood. Generally the amount of formaldehyde produced by incinerators is proportional to the amount of smoke.

Formaldehyde test kits are available to check any item for formaldehyde. The test is positive if a drop of a test solution turns purple when placed on the item in question.[12]

Heavy Metals

The major toxic heavy metals are lead, arsenic, mercury, cadmium, zinc, and nickel. Some water fountains or pipes continue to release lead and certain workers in industry are exposed to excessive lead.

12. Northeast Center for Environmental Medicine, 2800 W. Genesee Street, Syracuse, N.Y. 13219 (315-488-2856).

TABLE 13.5
Sources of Formaldehyde

Adhesives

Air pollution, i.e., industry

Antifreezes

Beverages, beer, wine

Burning of gas, oil, wood, coal, kerosene, diesel fuel

Carpets, carpet pads

Cleaning solutions, detergents, laundry starches

Clothing: polyester, artificial silk

Construction adhesives

Cosmetics, mouthwash, toothpaste, deodorants, nail polish, nail hardeners, shampoos

Disinfectants, bactericides, fungicides, germicides, deodorizers (room or air)

Dry-cleaning compounds

Embalming fluids

Explosives

Exterior plywood, fabric dyes

Fabrics: wrinkleproof, water-resistant, dye-fast, flame-resistant, moth-resistant, shrinkproof, elastic

Fertilizers

Furniture cabinets

Gas appliances

Gelatin capsules

Hair-growing products, hair-setting lotions

Household waxes, oils

Inks

Insect repellents, pesticides, rodent poison

Jute or hemp fiber preservative (carpet backing, burlap, area rugs, rope, twine)

Laminating materials

Leather tanning agents

Maple syrup (some varieties)

Newsprint

Paints, finger paints, enamels, tempera paints, lacquers, varnish removers, wood preservatives, wood stains, wood veneers

Particleboard, chipboard, interior plywood, wood paneling

Perfume

Pharmaceuticals

Phenol formaldehyde resin

Photographic chemicals and film

Plaster, stucco, wallboard, concrete, Bakelite, cellophane

Plastics, plastic cleaners

Shoe polish

Tissues (facial), toilet paper

Tobacco smoke, tobacco

Upholstery fabrics and finishes (permanent press, water-repellent, dye-fast, flame-resistant, water-resistant, shrinkproof, mothproof, mildewproof)

Upholstery foam

Urea formaldehyde foam insulation (UFFI), glass-fiber insulation

Vitamin E and A preparations

Wallpaper

Wines

Industrial traffic can cause cadmium pollution. Arsenic is found in some seafood. Blood, urine, and hair examinations can verify this form of body contamination.

How to Confirm a Chemical Sensitivity

You can suspect a sensitivity when the same form of illness is noted repeatedly after exposure to a particular chemical odor. Various examinations of your blood or urine may help to detect the levels of chemicals in your body.

If you are suspicious of formaldehyde, for example, there are a number of ways to confirm the sensitivity:

1. You can measure the indoor level of some chemicals, such as formaldehyde. For a list of approved agencies, contact your local health department or a branch of the EPA. They should be able to tell you if the contamination level in your home or in a particular school is beyond the normal range.[13]

2. You can have your doctor send your child's blood to a lab for examination. Such studies can detect and identify a wide range of chemicals. For example, to check for an excessive formaldehyde exposure, a doctor measures the formic-acid level. If it is too high, this suggests an excessive exposure to formaldehyde. If you know the name of the product thought to cause difficulty, it is often possible to call and find out the major specific chemical that is in that commercial product.

   If you believe you may be ill because of some chemical, contact Accu-Chem Laboratories, 990 North Bowser, Suite 800, Richardson, Tex. 75081 (214-234-5577), *as soon as possible* after the exposure. They can tell you how to have your blood, urine, or, if you are a lactating mother, your breast milk measured to see if an abnormal chemical is present. They can monitor the levels of chemicals in your body during the subsequent few months to determine how well the drug is being excreted or stored.

   By checking where a possible offending chemical is found, measures can be taken to reduce a child's future exposure to that item. If a child's symptoms subside when there is no further exposure and at the same time tests show there is no longer an excessive blood level, this would suggest that the cause of that person's problem had been found and eliminated. By the same token, if someone's body cannot excrete or detoxify some chemical in a normal manner, the blood level of that offending chemical or its breakdown product might remain abnormally increased for too prolonged a period of time, which could indicate a health problem if an individual's illness occurred shortly after some chemical exposure. If the chemical exposure is too great, some may have to be stored in the fatty tissues of the body.

3. Some specialists in environmental medicine have special chemical testing booths to ascertain and document whether a chemical is a problem or not. They can expose a patient to a single

---

13. Contact: the Environmental Protection Agency, 230 South Dearborn Street, Chicago, Ill. 60604 (312-353-2205).

chemical if it is thought to cause symptoms. If a provocation test for a chemical reproduces a patient's symptoms, it would indicate there may be a relationship between that exposure and the patient's illness.[14]

Purposeful exposure to the chemical odor that seems to cause mild symptoms can be helpful, but this should be closely monitored by a physician. If you were well before you smelled an odor and worse a few minutes later, you may have found an answer. To document chemical sensitivities, it is best if the tests are conducted when a person is not masked or adapted. *In other words, the challenge with the suspected item, similar to a food challenge, should occur after it has been totally avoided for at least four days. This method will enhance the tendency of the next contact to unmask or reveal a sensitivity so that it will be obvious.* Caution again: Don't you do this. If your response to chemicals is alarming or extreme in any way, talk to your physician first.

4. Some doctors can use provocation allergy testing. Symptoms or other changes that typify an individual's chemical sensitivity can be provoked by means of an allergy skin test. To decrease bias, this can be done single-blindly so that the patient is unaware of the actual chemical being tested. A weaker dilution of a problem chemical will sometimes stop, or neutralize, such reactions.

    Even if the exact chemical that is in an indoor or outdoor area has a characteristic odor that has not been identified, it is still possible to do P/N testing. An air pump can be used to prepare an allergy extract of the air that contains the chemical. One merely bubbles the contaminated air through a bottle of normal saline solution. Commercial kits are available for this.[15] The pump to make the extract works according to the same principle as an aerator in a fish tank. After such an air extract has been appropriately filtered and checked for sterility, it can be used for P/N allergy testing and treatment. Using this type of extract, it is often possible to reproduce and then eliminate some patients' exact symptoms. The neutralization dilution of extract will often enable children to remain in a particular school, for example, without developing headaches or hyperactivity. (See Chapter 11 for good examples of this.)

    If possible, however, it is far better to try to decrease chem-

14. William Rea, M. D., has such a testing booth. Contact: Environmental Health Center, 8345 Walnut Hill Lane, Suite 200, Dallas, Tex. 75231 (214-361-9515).
15. Contact: Larry Ward, P. O. Box 413, Silverado Canyon, Calif. 92676 (714-770-9616).

ical contamination within a school or home, to change schools, or to move. Our major aim should be to eliminate the cause of illness, not treat an illness by increasing the tolerance to a chemical with an allergy extract. We should be concerned about all the children in a school, not just the one who initially manifests illness from an accidental exposure or extreme sensitivity.

5. Many chemicals are stored in our body fat. Although it is helpful to measure the level of certain toxins or chemicals in fat, this test is extremely expensive. Once again, certain levels are considered normal, whereas others are excessive.

How Can Chemical Sensitivities Be Prevented or Diminished?

In general the thrust must be fourfold:

1. You must attempt to avoid or at least to limit any continued chemical exposure in your food, water, air, clothing, home, workplace, or school. Urge that all car and bus motors be turned off unless the vehicles are moving. Buy organically grown, less-contaminated food as much as possible. Grow your own vegetables.

2. You must try to eliminate some of the chemicals that are already stored within the fat in your body and brain. This essentially means that you must take steps to excrete unwanted chemicals through your urine, bowel movements, perspiration, expired air, and saliva. If mothers are exposed to some chemicals, the chemicals can be excreted in the breast milk.

3. After you find out which chemicals affect your family, you must try to learn about the nutrients that are required by your body to help excrete or alter those chemicals.[16]

4. Lastly you should encourage your entire family to drink more *glass*-bottled or purified water. Try to drink six to eight glasses of liquid a day to enhance excretion of all types of waste products in your perspiration, urine, and bowel movements. Liquids help excrete body impurities and soften bowel movements.

16. Sherry Rogers, M.D., *Tired or Toxic?* (see Bibliography); L. Ron Hubbard, *Clear Body, Clear Mind.* 1990. Bridge Publications, Inc., 4751 Fountain Avenue, Los Angeles, Calif. 90029.

Urge your children to drink more water or fresh, pure, un-sweetened, less-contaminated, organic fruit or vegetable juice between meals. You can create a nutritious soda pop by diluting pure organic fruit juice with a large amount of pure carbonated water. Many children drink only sweetened juices or soda pop, which may appeal more to their taste, but for many reasons these are not as beneficial for the body as pure, clean water.

How to Enhance Excretion of Chemicals From the Body: Detoxification Units

Some children and adults have been so polluted with chemicals that they require detoxification. The aim of this procedure is gently and naturally to help the body excrete the chemicals stored in body fat. Such programs entail some or all of the following:

- Nicotinic aid (Vitamin B_3), which helps to mobilize the chemicals in fat so that they can pass into the blood. The use of B_3 must be carefully monitored and the dosage individually adjusted.

- Exercise, which increases the blood flow to all the body tissues so that chemicals that were released from the fat or tissues can be moved to the skin and excreted in the perspiration or through other body channels, such as the intestines or bladder for eventual elimination.

- Carefully controlled low-temperature saunas, which induce increased perspiration to help remove chemicals from the body. The sauna must be well ventilated.

- The use of cold-pressed polyunsaturated oils, vitamins, and other nutrients, which help the liver bind chemicals so that they can be excreted via the intestines in the bowel movement.

- Massage therapy, to stimulate circulation and mobilize body fat.

- The use of substances to bind chemicals that are in the intestines so that they can be excreted more readily.

While this is done, the loss of water, potassium, and various other salts through perspiration must be judiciously monitored and replaced. It is essential to keep vitamin and mineral supplements maintained in a normal balance during this procedure.

During detoxification it is not unusual for the odors of anesthetics, even those received years ago, suddenly to be noted in the air as they are excreted from the body. A beautician might excrete the chemicals she routinely breathed for years. If a patient used large amounts of perfume years ago, those odors might be evident in the sauna air. A painter might excrete solvents. On occasion a patient's perspiration will become green or discolored because of the color of the chemical

TABLE 13.6
Major Detoxification Units*

G. Megan Shields, M.D., HealthMed Clinic, 314 N. Harper, Los Angeles, Calif. 90048 (213-655-5928) (Hubbard expert)

William Rea, M.D., American Environmental Health Foundation, 8345 Walnut Hill Lane, Suite 200, Dallas, Tex. 75231 (214-361-9515)

Allan Lieberman, M.D., Center for Environmental Medicine, 7510 North Forest Drive, North Charleston, S.C. 29420 (803-572-1600)

Jeffrey White, M.D., Enviro-Med Clinic, 3715 Azeele Street, Tampa, Fla. 33609 (813-876-5442)

David Buscher, M.D., Environmental Detoxification Unit, 1370 116 Avenue NE, Suite 102, Bellevue, Wash. 98004-0288 (206-453-0288)

In Europe

H. P. Fredricksen, M.D., Veramed Allergie-Klinik Inzell, Zwieselstr 2, 8221 Inzell, West Germany (011-49-08665-671-0)

Jonathan Maberly, M.D., Airedale Allergy Centre, High Hall, Steeton, Nr. Keighley, W. Yorkshire BD20-6SB, England (0535) 56013

Jean Munro, M.D., Breakspear Hospital, High Street, Abbots Langley, Harts, WD5 OPU, England (011-44-923-261333)

Klaus-Dietrich Runow, M.D., Director, Institute for Environmental Diseases, Tm. Kurpark 1, D-3501 Emstal, West Germany (011-49-5624-8601)

---

*These practitioners are listed in order of number of years of experience.

that is being expelled through the pores of the skin.[17] Sauna areas can present a smorgasbord of unpleasant aromas, depending upon the previous exposures of the persons undergoing detoxification.

Some detoxification centers monitor the decrease of chemicals in the fat and note if this decrease correlates with a patient's physical and emotional improvement. If it does, it would suggest a possible cause-and-effect relationship.

There are a variety of methods used to rid the body of pollutants, chemicals, and toxins. One is called the Hubbard Method.[18] This method has been proven to be safe and effective to help remove some of the three hundred foreign chemicals found in fat, among which are: polybrominated biphenols (PBBs), polychlorinated biphenols (PCBs), polychlorinated dibenzofurons (PCDFs), heptachlor, dieldrin, and DDT. This program requires about twenty-eight days to complete. There are few centers in the country where medical management has the specialized expertise to attempt to detoxify children safely. (See Table 13.6). Unfortunately most are reluctant to see infants or young children under the age of four.[19]

These methods remove a wide variety of toxic chemicals that can interfere with the functioning of many areas of the body, especially the nervous system. They can help relieve the following symptoms in some patients: weakness, tingling, burning, numb arms or legs, and problems remembering. In responsive patients these symptoms can be partially or totally reversed. Children are especially resilient if they are detoxified shortly after exposure.

A Typical Day of Chemical Exposures[20]

Many of the following chemicals are found in the products you are exposed to or eat each day.

Bedroom:
Regular clothing and nightclothes: polyester with formaldehyde
Bedsheets: Polyester with formaldehyde

17. David Root, M.D., Ph. D., et al., "Excretion of a Lipophilic Toxicant Through the Sebaceous Glands: A Case Report," *Journal of Toxicology* 6(1)(1987), pp. 13–17.
18. Contact: G. Megan Shields, M.D., HealthMed Clinic, 314 N. Harper, Los Angeles, Calif. 90048 (213–655–5928).
19. Contact: William J. Rea, M.D., Environmental Health Center, 8345 Walnut Hill Lane, Suite 200, Dallas, Tex. 75231 (214–361–9515); William J. Rea, M.D., *Chemical Sensitivity.* 1991. Lewis Publishers, Inc., 121 S. Main Street, Chelsea, Mich. 48118.
20. Patricia Moore, "Clinical Ecology: Medicine for the Chemical-Sensitive," *Coming Clean at Home—Garbage—The Practical Journal for the Environment* (1990), pp. 30–35.

Mattress with flame-retardant chemicals: polyurethane foam, tolune diisocyanate gas

Pillow: polyester, polyurethane foam

Acrylic, nylon, polyester blankets: dyes, pesticides (mothproofing), plastics

Dry-cleaned clothing: Tetra- and trichloroethylene

Starched clothing: formaldehyde, pentachlorophenol, phenol

Mattress pad: polyester with formaldehyde, plastic

Gas, oil, or kerosene heat: hydrocarbon fuel

Cat or dog flea collar: Carbamates, organophosphates

Mothballs: paradichlorobenzene, naphthalene

Bathroom:

Tap water: chlorine, flourine, heavy metals (lead or copper), chlorobenzene, ethylphenols, chloroform, asbestos, nitrates/nitrosamines, toluene, trichloroethane, trichloroethylene, xylene, pesticides, plastic (vinyl chloride), and possibly other factory chemicals

Soap: halogenated salicylanilides or carbanilides, ammonia, butylated hydroxyanisol (BHA)/Butylated hydroxytoluene (BHT), artificial food color, formaldehyde, fragrance, glycols

Dandruff shampoo: Selenium sulfide, resorcinol

Regular shampoo: ammonia, cresol, detergent, EDTA, ethanol, formaldehyde, fragrance, nitrates/nitrosamines, plastic (PVP), sulfur compounds

Plastic shower curtain: Polyvinyl chloride gas, phthalates

Toothpaste: saccharin, ammonia, benzyl alcohol, sodium benzoate, fluoride, formaldehyde, polyvinylpyrrolidone (PVP plastic)

Antiperspirant spray: aluminum chlorohydrate, ammonia, ethanol, formaldehyde, fragrance, glycerin

Cosmetics: formaldehyde, artificial coloring, artificial flavor, ammonia, BHA/BHT, glycerin, paraffin, plastics (nylon, PVP), saccharin, talc, nitrosamines

Lipstick: glycerol, hydrocarbons, artificial food dyes

Hair spray or aerosol propellants: chlorofluorocarbons, ethanol, formaldehyde, plastic polyvinyl

Chlorinated scouring powder: chlorine fumes, artificial colors, detergent, talc

Air freshener: paradichlorobenzene, naphthalene, phenol, cresol, ethanol, xylene, formaldehyde

Shoe polish: methyl chloride, nitrobenzene, perchlorethylene, tricholoethylene, xylene

Breakfast:

Orange juice: artificial food dyes, fungicides, pesticides (methidathion, chlorpyrifos, ethion, parathion, carabaryl)

Cereal: food dyes, BHA/BHT, pesticide residues, sucrose

Milk: BHT/BHA, formaldehyde, pesticides, plastic residues, paraffin residues, glycols, possibly some antibiotics

Strawberries: pesticide residues, including captan and methylparathion

Bananas: ripened with petroleum-derived gas called ethtylene which causes brown streaks, not small speckled spots as in naturally ripened bananas, pesticides (i.e., diazinon, thiabendazole, carbaryl)

Prunes: treated with sulfur dioxide and methyl bromide

Refined sugar: chlorine, BHA/BHT, pesticide residues, sucrose

Aspartame: (NutraSweet and Equal) made of phenylalanine and aspartic acid. Large doses said to be toxic to the brain.

Bacon: sodium nitrite

Eggs: Some can be dipped in penicillin or injected with formaldehyde or contain pesticide residues, hormones, fumigants, and petrochemicals.

Bread: pesticide residue, talc, chlorine, formaldehyde, BHA/BHT, monosodium glutamate (MSG)

Butter: BHA/BHT, food dyes, pesticide residues

Jelly: artificial food color, pesticides, saccharin

Coffee: hexane, methylene chloride, pesticide residues, trichloroethylene, hydrocarbons if roasted over a gas flame.

Kitchen:

Disinfectant aerosol: phenol, fluorohydrocarbons

Detergent dish cleaner: phenol, ethanol, fragrance, artificial food color

Car

polyvinyl chloride gas, toluene, diisocyanate from polyurethane in seats

Gasoline: benzene, toluene, butane

Auto exhaust: dioxin, hydrocarbons

Heavy smog: chlorinated hydrocarbon compounds, butane, pentane, formaldehyde, benzene

Lawns:

Sprayed with chloropyrifos, propoxur, diazinon, benomyl, prometon, organophosphates, herbicides 2,4-D and banvel, and the fungicides benomyl and daconil, among other pesticides

Rose bushes:
   sprayed with propoxur, chlorpyrifos, and methoxychlor, among other pesticides

School or Work:
   Plastic and pressed wood furniture: dioxin, formaldehyde, PVC and toluene diisocyanate gases
   Permanent ink markers: benzene, toluene, xylene, ethanol
   Crayons: petrochemicals
   Rubber cement: petroleum distillates
   Correction fluid: trichloroethylene, cresol, ethanol, naphthalene
   Cigarette smoke: benzene, carbon monoxide, carbonyl sulfide, formaldehyde, hydrogen cyanide, plus a host of others
   Swimming pool: muriatic acid, chlorine, fungicides
   Plastics: butylbenzyl, phthalate
   Disinfectants: phenols, diethylene or methylene glycol, sodium hypochlorite
   Foam Cushions: formaldehyde
   Vinyl-covered furniture, plastic notebooks: vinyl chloride
   New carpets: Formaldehyde, toluene, xylene, benzene, tetra-chloroethylene, methylacrylates
   Carpet backing: styrene
   Commercial cleaning solutions: toluene, phenol, formaldehyde, xylene, butane, and methylene chloride
   Paper products: formaldehyde
   Floor polish: trichloroethylene
   Copy machine: trichloroethylene
   Wet paint: aliphatic hydrocarbons, ethylene, mineral spirits, and other solvents
   Stains and finishes: mineral spirits glycol ethers, ketones, halo-genated hydrocarbons, naphthal

Snack:
   Juices: artificial flavors and/or colors, petrochemicals, BHA/BHT, glycols, pesticide residues
   Styrofoam cups: polystrene foam
   Potato chips: pesticide residues, BHA/BHT, MSG

Lunch:
   Tomatoes: ripened with ethylene gas; pesticides on tomatoes include methamidaphor, chlorpyrifos, chlorothalonil, permethrin, di-methoate
   Lettuce: pesticides include mevinphos, endosulfan, dimethoate, permethrin, methomyl

Cucumbers: coated with petrochemical wax or mineral oil, pesticides (methamidophos, endosulfan, dieldrin, chlorpyrifos, dimethoate)

Onions: pesticides (DCPA, DDT, ethion, diazinon, malathion)

Mayonnaise: ethylene diamine, tetracetic acid (EDTA), hydrogenated oil

Luncheon meat: sodium nitrite, nitrosamines, pesticide residues

Frozen french fries: bisulfites, sodium acid pyrophosphate, and sodium EDTA (ethylene diamine tetraacetic acid). Pesticides in potatoes: DDT, chlorpropham dieldrin, aldicarb, chlordane

Apple: Ripened with ethylene gas, sprayed fifteen times with insecticides. Pesticides on apples: diphenylamine, captan, endosulfan, phosmet, azinphosmethyl

Cookies: With dates or nuts fumigated with methyl bromide. Fruit-filled cookies have artificial food colors, hydrogenated cottonseed and/or palm oils, modified food starch, sodium

Ice cream: glycerol, artificial food colors, carrageenan, modified food starch

Diet beverage: sodium saccharin, food dyes, artificial flavors

Coffee: hexane, methylene chloride, pesticide residues, decaffeinated with trichloroethylene

Dinner:

Shrimp cocktail: bisulfites

Carrots: numerous pesticides (DDT, trifluralin, parathion, diazinon, dieldrin)

Cucumbers and green peppers: methamidophos, chlorpyrifos, dimethoate, acephate, endosulfar, wax composed of shellacs, paraffins, palm oil derivatives, or synthetic resins. These are ingredients that are also found in some floor and car waxes.

Chicken: fed antibiotics, hormones (diethyl stilbesterol), and various chemicals, even possible arsenic from chicken feed

Sweet potatoes: colored with artificial dyes, pesticides (dichloran, phosmet, DDT, dieldrin, BHC)

Pears: ripened with ethylene gas, pesticides such as azinphosmethyl, cyhexatin, phosmet, endosulfar, ethion

Bread: pesticide residue, talc, chlorine, formaldehyde, BHA/BHT, MSG

Butter: BHA/BHT, food dyes, pesticide residues

Woodburning fireplace: phenol from creasote-treated wood, formaldehyde

This list is very incomplete.

Many of the chemicals mentioned are stored in our fatty tissues. Some are known to cause cancer.

Should our bodies become toxic-waste dump sites?

How Can Additional Chemical Exposures Be Avoided?

Avoid Specific Exposures

If you are accidentally exposed to a chemical for a short period of time, such as from a parked car that has the engine running, hold your breath and look in the other direction. Breathe only when you have to, and quickly distance yourself from the odor.

If a room has an offending odor, do not enter the room, or leave it as soon as possible. If you must remain, try to sit near a door or an open window.

Use an Air-Purifying Machine

It helps to use special air-purifying machines, which remove airborne chemicals, as well as dust, mite feces, molds, pollen, and smoke. A built-in fan circulates air through these machines so that the chemicals in the air are trapped in charcoal and other filters. The result is cleaner air with less or no odor. These units can be used in homes, schools, business offices, and cars.[21]

There are pros and cons to the wide variety of air-purifying machines presently available. The few that we have personally used are listed in Appendix B. Others may be equally effective. Only a few claim to remove chemical odors, bacteria, viruses, and odors such as formaldehyde.[22]

There are two major varieties of air-purifying cleaners. One is called the HEPA, or High Efficiency Particle Air filter; the other an electrostatic precipitation unit. Always try to use a unit before you purchase it to be certain it is well tolerated. Remember, each child is different.

21. Contact: E.L. Foust Co. Inc., P. O. Box 105, Elmhurst, Ill. 60126 (708-834-4952 or 800-225-9549).

22. Contact: AllerMed Co., Martinaire VH–300, 31 Steel Road, Wylie, Tex. 75098 (214–442–4898).

Use a Charcoal Mask to Absorb Odors

Charcoal absorbs odors, so it helps protect an individual from breathing polluted air. If a charcoal mask is carried in your pocket, purse, or car, it can be quickly placed over your child's nose whenever an offending odor is noted. For example, it can be held over the nose during takeoff or landing when airplanes routinely become flooded with noxious exhaust fumes. It can be used in traffic jams or in backed-up traffic lines in heavily polluted toll booth areas.

Some people, however, are sensitive to the specific sources of the charcoal. To resolve this problem, various masks can be purchased that are filled with charcoal derived from either bituminous coal, wood, or coconut shell.[23] Most ecologists can check to determine which type of charcoal is the least offensive for a particular individual.

Buy Organic Food

Attempt to decrease your total allergy load by eating food that is organic or less chemically contaminated whenever possible. The fat in red meat, such as beef, for example, often contains many of the stored pesticides used when the grain was grown or from the chemically sprayed grass the cow ate.

In addition, some meats contain antibiotics and hormones, which are added to animal feed. These make the meat and poultry industry more cost-effective. In Puerto Rico, from 1978 to 1981, there was a striking increase in precocious puberty in both girls and boys aged six months to eight years: Store-bought chicken contained so much female sex hormone that some girls had menses and breast development long before they started school.

Fruits and vegetables are often similarly sprayed, coated, or contaminated *throughout* with various pesticides, herbicides, or other chemical substances. Peeling or scrubbing will only help a little because chemicals typically permeate the entire food, not just the outside.

Live in the Cleanest Part of Your City

You can move to a cleaner, less polluted, or more elevated section of your city. Your home location should be in an area that has the least industrial or environmental pollution. Note the prevailing

23. Contact: The Living Source, 3500 MacArthur Drive, Waco, Tex. 76708.

winds. Does fresh air blow toward your home most of the time or is it contaminated? Check with your local health department about air pollution and toxic dump sites in your area. Ask for a detailed map. If the entire area is too heavily polluted, you may have to move to a less industrial locale.

If you live in a high-rise apartment house, or vacation in a hotel, request the highest floor. The air nearest the street level is usually the most contaminated.

Be wary of condominiums or apartment houses because there is no way of protecting your unit from the pesticides or chemicals used by neighbors. Pesticides can pass through walls, ceilings, and floors.

Find a Locale Where It Is Safe to Live

Many people ask what is the safest, most chemically free area in the United States in which to live. This is not easy to answer. Pilots will tell you that there is a progressively larger and larger haze of smog and pollution around most large cities at the present time. Cities such as Los Angeles or New York are so polluted that a growing number of people cannot go outside or downtown in those areas. Foreign metropolitan areas such as London and Mexico City are equally bad. Rural farming areas are often not better at times because of extensive crop or aerial spraying.

In general, pollution is less in the more elevated areas, such as in the mountains. Another possibility is to live near water *if* the prevailing winds blow clean air toward your home. If odors bother you, try to live in a city that has little or no industry. Cheyenne, Wyoming, for example, is said to have very little pollution.

If you live in a home that is highly contaminated due to construction materials (formaldehyde), furnishings (synthetic carpets), and pesticides or termiticides, and so on, you may not only have to move, you may have to buy all new furnishings and furniture as well. Some chemicals penetrate and contaminate the fabric and fiber of home furnishings to such a degree that they cannot safely be used anymore.

Purchase Products Made From Natural Materials

Whenever possible, buy the least chemically contaminated clothing and home furnishings. Wear 100 percent natural fabrics, such as wool, cotton, silk, linen, and ramie. Buy solid wood, metal, glass, or cotton furnishings.

You can determine if some home item or piece of clothing will be a problem by checking your pulse. Hold a large piece of carpet, for example, directly against your skin for a half hour. Note whether your pulse increases 20 points or your ability to breathe decreases (see Chapter 10).

In addition, a few very sensitive people seem to be able to feel a fabric, floor covering, or wall, for example, and know that it will be a problem for them because they sense "a creepy, crawly feeling" in their hand. This enables them to detect exactly which items bother them and to avoid any direct contact.

Remember, if you can lower your total allergenic load or exposure, you might be able to breathe some chemicals with less difficulty.

Insist on Windows That Open

Chemical sensitivities can be diminished by improved ventilation in chemically contaminated areas. For example, simply open the windows and allow fresh air inside, providing the outside air is cleaner than the inside air. Avoid buildings that have windows that can't be opened.

Avoid Airborne Pollution and Toxins

Toxins in the air are another potential source of illness. For example, about 20 to 25 percent of all toxic pollutants of all the Great Lakes come from polluted air. The emissions from industry, power plants, incinerators, and automobiles turn our sky into a giant global toxic-waste dump site. This contamination can kill our trees and contaminate our lakes, rivers, and food supply. The toxins and other chemicals destroy the earth's ozone barrier, which protects us from the sun's harmful rays. In some areas of the United States healthy adults are urged not to exercise outside, and pregnant women are warned to stay indoors on certain days because the ozone levels are too high.

According to the EPA, over 50 percent of people live in cities plagued by excess spray and dangerous levels of carbon monoxide. Over 133 million people live in areas that exceed the smog standard, and about 78 million are overexposed to carbon monoxide. Many major cities have these serious pollution problems in both the summer and the winter.

Smog is mainly a summer problem because of the interaction of intense sunlight with airborne chemicals, such as auto exhaust. Carbon monoxide problems, on the other hand, are more prevalent in the winter due to temperature inversions, which keep pollutants closer to the earth's surface. Smog can be seen when you look toward the horizon. It creates a discolored, foggy appearance in the air that obscures and blurs the outlines of distant buildings or mountains.

Make Sure the Water You Drink Is Clean

Put a water-purifying system on the water-intake source of your home so that all your water taps will provide less-contaminated water. If you have only a single purifying unit on the kitchen sink, you will have to carry water to the bathroom, for example, to brush your teeth.

City tap water is not really purified. The number of bacteria in the water has been significantly decreased but not eliminated. Chemicals are purposely added to our water supplies to accomplish this. Some children and adults, however, are so sensitive to chlorine, for example, that they become ill from drinking tap water. Chlorine can also react with naturally occurring organic material, such as the tannin in leaves. These reactions can form trihalomethanes (THM), such as chloroform and other chemicals, which are known to cause cancer. Alum is a form of aluminum that is used as a flocculant in some water-purifying systems to remove suspended particles during water treatment. Some people are concerned because this aluminum exposure may contribute to aluminum toxicity, which is thought to be a possible causative factor in Alzheimer's disease. There are no EPA standards for aluminum.

Nationwide over 2,100 contaminants have been found in drinking water, and the vast majority of these are organic chemicals. Present drinking-water regulations test for only about 70 of these. Roughly about 50 out of the 79,000 regulated public water systems in the United States have advanced treatment facilities, which utilize activated carbon. Call your health department to check on yours. Carbon is one of the most effective substances for removing unwanted chemicals from water. Without it, the majority of chemical water contaminants will not be removed.

Sometimes you can spot a tap-water problem easily. Merely test each of your family members first thing in the morning before they put anything in their mouths by counting their pulse for a full minute and noticing exactly how each one feels. Does anything ache or hurt? How is their disposition? Is everyone thinking clearly? Then put a half teaspoon of tap water under each person's tongue. Have them try to hold the water there for a full minute without swallowing. In about ten minutes ask the same questions. If the pulse has increased or your children feel or act differently or ill, you may have found one more answer related to their health.

Even bottled water can be a problem. About 75 percent of bottled water comes from the ground water. Most state regulations only require bottlers to test for a minority of the two-thousand known water contaminants. Bottled water is not regulated by the FDA unless it is sold across state borders. Sometimes water is shipped in plastic-lined transport trucks prior to placing it in glass bottles so the buyer is unaware of the chemical contamination that took place during shipment. Test all bottled water in the same manner that you test tap water.

Remember, however, that you can be fooled. Maybe you are algae-sensitive and there are no algae in the water on that day. Maybe some chemical factories contaminate the water only on weekends, when there is less surveillance. Factory residues are of course diluted in lakes, rivers, or underground aquifers, but will they be diluted enough? Chemically sensitive individuals need very little chemical exposure to cause symptoms. The purity of tap water can vary from day to day depending upon the ground water and when and where factory or other direct or indirect contamination is occurring. Lawn chemicals and aerial chemical sprays eventually seep into the ground water and can at some point come out your faucet or into your well water. Your city's health department or private agencies can examine your water to determine exactly what is in it.[24]

In addition to chemicals in our water, some city water systems are contaminated with protozoa such as *Giardia lamblia*. These organisms commonly cause diarrhea or other chronic abdominal or bowel complaints. If many children from a certain neighborhood all seem to have one infection after another, check your water supply for sewage contamination. It is possible for this to be a problem, even in the United States at this time. Call your health department and ask if you live in a pocket problem area. If the answer is yes and your child has bowel problems, have the feces examined for germs and other organisms that cause illness.[25]

How Do Water-Purifying Systems Work?

A series of filters are usually required to purify water. Each has a specific function that enhances both the efficiency and the cost-effectiveness of water purification. The Herro Care Purification System is one example of such a unit. This system meets the standards set by the Food and Drug Administration and surpasses the requirements of the Environmental Protection Agency. However, these units can be very expensive. The price can vary from two hundred to two

24. Contact: Accu-Chem Laboratories, 990 North Bowser, Suite 800, Richardson, Tex. 75081 (214–234–5577).

25. Contact: Great Smokies Medical Laboratory, 18A Regent Park Boulevard, Asheville, N.C. 28806 (800–522–4762).

thousand dollars. Professional assistance is available and is even necessary to help customers select the most efficient and economical unit
to satisfy each family's special needs.

The Herro purification system consists of a series of three cartridges.[26] The first one filters both large particles and microscopic
material. The second cartridge uses activated charcoal to remove
organic material, as well as a wide range of organic chemicals. This
cartridge makes the water look, taste, and smell clean. An optional
resin in this section can also remove heavy metals. The last cartridge
is said to remove the majority of microorganisms that cause disease.

Once again, each individual must investigate any water purifier
prior to purchase. Make phone calls and do some comparative shopping regarding not only price but also the effectiveness of the unit
you select. Be sure to check on the maintenance costs for the system
you install. If possible, ask to have your own tap water pass through
any system you intend to use. The bottom line is, can you drink the
water without developing symptoms? (See Chapter 10.) If the unfil-
tered tap water causes illness and the filtered water does not, you
may have corrected one more factor that can contribute to the ill
health of your family.

Is Distilled Water an Alternative?

Distilled water is one alternative, but it is far from ideal. To distill
water, you merely evaporate it and then recondense the vapor. The
problem is that the chemicals in the water can also become a gas and
can then condense back into the distilled water again. In addition
essential minerals, such as calcium and magnesium, are removed
during this process. If distilled water is stored in plastic, the chemicals
from the plastic tend to enter the water even more rapidly, because
this water now lacks minerals.

Don't Forget the Shower and Bath Water

Consider purchasing a special filter that removes chlorine and iron
while softening the water in the shower. You can fill the tub with
shower water for bathing if you do not have a purifying unit on your
main water line. It has been estimated that 29 to 91 percent of water
contaminants enter the body during baths and showers, because
chemicals are readily absorbed through our skin surface. The force

26. Contact: Herro Care International, 5121 North Central Avenue, Phoenix, Ariz. 85012
(602–274–6563). (See Appendix B.)

of the shower allows gases such as chloroform or other volatile contaminants to escape from the water. The chemicals in water therefore contaminate our bodies through our skin and, in addition, through the air we breathe. Long, leisurely tub or whirlpool baths may not be as healthy as we once imagined.

Is Water Affected by Lead and Polyvinyl Chloride (PVC) Pipes?

Many homes have lead solder connecting their water pipes or have lead water pipes. For this reason, let your faucet run for a few minutes in the morning before you drink the water that was in contact with the pipes all night. Soft water leaches more lead than hard water into the tap water. Lead contamination has no odor or taste. The EPA estimates that over 40 million Americans have excessive lead in their drinking water. Lead poisoning can cause birth defects, mental retardation, high blood pressure, hyperactivity, and a number of other brain and nervous system problems. The lead in drinking water should not exceed 0.020 mg/liter. Lead is also used as a solder, so it can leach from the seams of canned foods into their contents. It is discharged into our air from certain types of fuel, so we may breathe it into our lungs. It is present in the paint used in older homes.

Polyvinyl chloride pipes are also not free of problems. They cause potential difficulty because they can leach tiny amounts of vinyl chloride, a potent possible carcinogen, into the water. Plastic wrapping can contain acrylic acid, toluene, styrene, and vinyl chloride, which can be released into some plastic-covered food products.

Don't Buy Food or Beverages Packaged in Plastic

Do not purchase, drink, or eat foods supplied in plastic bottles or jars. Try to encourage the use of glass for storage. The chemicals in plastic can leach or seep into stored liquids or food. Some plastic bottles also leach minute amounts of methylene chloride, a known carcinogen, into the contents of the container. Store foods in glass and cover with cellophane.

In this regard it seems irresponsible, unwise, and almost incomprehensible that almost all intravenous fluids and blood for transfusions are now supplied in plastic bags. If a mother receives blood from a plastic container just before her infant is delivered, certain chemicals from the plastic can be found in the baby's blood.[27] Is this

27. John Laseter, Elizabeth Dowty, and James Storer, "The Transplacental Migration and Accumulation in Blood of Organic Constituents," *Pediatrics* 10 (1976), pp. 696–701.

any way to begin life? When we are ill, should we be given the drugs plus a bit of plastic intravenously just because it is modern, more convenient, and cost-effective?

Think About What Neighbors and Organizations Spray on Lawns and Into the Air

What anyone puts on their lawn or into the air affects everyone. Lawn and aerial sprays, as well as the chemicals from many factories, eventually find their way into the water supply. Some of these chemicals are known causes of the symptoms listed in Tables 13.1 and 13.2; others potentially cause cancer. *We must discourage the use of these chemicals by everyone.* Look in your phonebook for the name of *natural* lawn maintenance companies. Help educate your neighbors and friends.

Avoid Taking Medicines That Contain Unnecessary Dyes

Urge your doctor to prescribe white medication whenever possible (see Chapter 26). Many children's antibiotics, for example, contain unnecessary dyes, artificial flavors, and sweeteners, which can make some youngsters hyperactive. Purchase home remedies such as cough syrups that contain as few dyes and chemicals as possible.

Children and adults can develop medical problems not only from the dyes but also from the binders or fillers, such as corn, that are used in the preparation of tablets or capsules. Fortunately relatively few people are sensitive to the beef and pork used to create gelatin capsules.

Increase Your Daily Doses of Vitamin C

Listen to Linus Pauling—vitamin C helps. Scientific studies have shown that vitamin C will help the body in many ways. It has been shown to increase the effectiveness of liver enzymes, for example, which help detoxify pesticides and chemicals.[28]

Exercise

Regular exercise is extremely important. This increases the circulation so that noxious substances can be excreted in your perspiration.

28. Linus Pauling, *How to Live Longer and Feel Better* (New York: Avon Books, 1986).

If you choose to jog or walk, however, avoid heavily polluted urban streets. If you can't exercise, get massages.

Get Away From It All

On a regular basis drive to nearby unpolluted areas to hike, camp, and breathe fresh air. Try to stay in clean-air areas for as long as possible.

Practical Tips for Resolving
Chemical Problems in Your Body Quickly

Breathe Oxygen

Usually three or four liters a minute of oxygen for ten minutes, *as soon as possible after an offending chemical exposure,* will provide beneficial relief. If the exposure has been extreme, oxygen may be needed intermittently for ten-minute intervals throughout the day. If chemicals cause serious problems, an oxygen tank should be kept at home for emergency use, with the school nurse, and in the family car. Oxygen must be prescribed by a physician. Your doctor can provide individualized instruction and appropriate precautionary advice if it is necessary.

Look in the yellow pages of the phone book for lists of oxygen suppliers or providers of home health care equipment. The tanks are easily carried, are about 2½ feet high, and hold 660 liters. You rent the first one and for a modest fee have it refilled whenever the oxygen level is low. In areas where retired people live, some rental fees are exorbitant because of questionable charging practices. Pay for the oxygen used, not a rental fee for the equipment.

To moisten oxygen so that it does not dry out delicate lung tissues, bubble it through water in a *glass*, rather than a plastic, pint jar. The tubing should be Tygon, not ordinary plastic, which can cause symptoms in some very sensitive persons. The masks used to inhale oxygen should be ceramic, never odorous soft plastic. This is especially true for chemical-sensitive asthmatics. Even the odor of some plasticized asthma medicine aerosol chambers can cause symptoms.

Also be careful if your child is placed in a plastic humidity tent with oxygen in the hospital. The odor of that tent or the chemicals used to clean and sterilize it can make some children ill. The same is true for some plastic-coated mattresses used in hospitals or plastic mattress covers used at home. Prior to an awareness of possible health problems as a result of the outgassing of chemicals from plastic, mattress covers of this type were routinely recommended for relieving allergies.[29]

Unfortunately many hospital emergency-room physicians are not aware of the benefit of oxygen in treating chemical exposures. Even with a letter from another physician, they are sometimes resistant to providing this beneficial treatment. If there is a communication problem in an emergency room, merely ask to speak to the medical director. There would be few medical contraindications for the use of oxygen to help most children or adults. The immediate benefit of oxygen would usually far outweigh any risk in a well-supervised medical facility. Discuss your thoughts about your child's possible need for oxygen with your physician. A tank of oxygen in your home and car might make a trip to the hospital unnecessary.

Use Neutralization Allergy Extracts

It is often easy to use provocation allergy testing to show exactly which symptoms certain chemicals cause. Neutralization dilutions of extracts made from contaminated air can be used to relieve symptoms. Such neutralization extract and/or oxygen, can sometimes provide varying degrees of relief after unavoidable exposures. It is unfortunately impossible, however, to test or treat for all chemical sensitivities. Much research is *urgently needed* in this particular area of environmental medicine if we are to help the many sensitive children and adults who cannot realistically avoid chemical exposures.

Try Heparin

At times heparin appears to be helpful. This drug is normally used to thin the blood a bit so clots do not form unneccesarily. One or two drops of the concentrated solution under the tongue sometimes appears to enable some children or adults to tolerate exposure in the heavily polluted areas of downtown New York City, for example, or to shop in stores that have a strong chemical odor. The occasional use of this minuscule dose should not thin the blood. We really don't know why it helps, but in this dose, it should not hurt. Heparin must be prescribed by your physician, so discuss this possibility with your doctor.

29. See Appendix B for sources of Tygon tubing, mattress covers, and mattresses.

Use Antioxidant Preparations

Some nutrient preparations, such as Anti-Ox by Stephen Levine, Ph.D.,[30] and Oxy-Gard, sold by Klaire Lab,[31] appear to help the body excrete chemicals. These are antioxidants, which help to neutralize the harmful free radicals or free electrons that can damage our bodies. They help reverse the harmful effects of toxic chemicals, foreign matter, and allergic reactions within our bodies. These preparations basically contain vitamins E, C, B_2, B_6, and A, as well as selenium, L-glutathione, and taurine. Anti-Ox also contains zinc.

How to Tell Whether an Illness Is Due to a Toxin or to a Chemical Sensitivity

Every reaction to an odor or chemical is not a sensitivity reaction, of course. Sometimes it is due to the toxic effect of some exposure.

The first evidence of a toxic exposure is often an allergylike symptom. Rashes, lung problems, and heart problems can occur. These chemicals tend to hurt the nervous system so that tremors, muscle twitching, dizziness, headaches, and difficulty with the arms and legs can be noticed. More prolonged exposure affects the immune system as well as other body areas (see Table 13.2).

We honestly cannot always be entirely certain what to call it, but it is obvious that chemical exposures can cause illness. In general the symptoms of a toxic reaction are known, specific, and well documented. An allergy or chemical sensitivity, however, can cause a variety of complaints, but some symptoms can be identical to those noted during toxic reactions. In other words the toxic and allergic symptoms can overlap so an exact diagnosis is not always possible. One major difference, however, is that a minute exposure may be required to cause an allergic sensitivity or reaction, whereas in general a larger or prolonged lesser exposure might be required for a toxic reaction.

A toxic chemical response can affect almost any individual. For example, if a gas heater is defective, an entire family can develop similar symptoms of toxicity, for example flulike symptoms, headache, nausea, vomiting, diarrhea, weakness, joint aches, and leg aches.

30. Contact: Nutri-cology, Inc./Allergy Research Group, P.O. Box 489, San Leandro, Calif. 94577-0489 (800-545-9960 or 415-639-4572).

31. Contact: Klaire Laboratories, Inc., P.O. Box 618, Carlsbad, Calif. 92008 (619-744-9680).

In contrast a chemical sensitivity is more prone to affect those who have allergies, allergic relatives, or damaged immune systems. One child may develop a headache or another may become nasal whenever an examination is printed on a chemically treated paper. A few office workers might develop muscle aches or irritability shortly after using a copy machine. Some children may become dizzy and unable to concentrate or type well after using a chemical white-out correction solution to correct errors in a typing class. A child might become depressed or asthmatic shortly after a class is held in a recently carpeted room that smells of a new synthetic rug or carpet adhesive. An entire family may become ill after moving into a trailer or building that has formaldehyde in the particleboard subflooring, paneling, prefabricated walls, cabinetry, carpets, or furnishings. Think back to the time when your child or you became ill. Did the medical complaints begin shortly after or within a few weeks after some chemical exposure inside or outside your home or school?

If you are concerned, find a physician who knows about toxins *and* environmental allergies (see Appendix D). Sometimes they may be able to give your problem a label, but more important, they may be able to help you resolve your medical illness by finding the cause of the problem. Because chemicals affect the brain and nervous system, the symptoms they cause may appear to be emotional or psychiatric in nature. Some affected individuals are therefore treated solely for an emotional disturbance, when in reality they have an unrecognized and possibly treatable medical problem.

To add to the complexity, children, as well as adults, can develop serious secondary psychological problems because of long delays in diagnosing the true cause of their illness. Sometimes years elapse before the role of a chemical in someone's illness is recognized. These patients need appropriate medical care followed by psychological counseling. When someone has been ill for years and no one believes that it is anything but a psychological problem, this can lead to anxiety, anger, confusion, resentment, and other emotional problems.

Having said that, one last word of caution must be added. Good judgment and common sense must prevail, or there may be a tendency to blame chemicals for everything.

One Family's Chemical Sensitivity Problem

The Zimm Family

I would like to relate one family's challenging experience with unanticipated chemical exposures. Every physician practicing ecologic medicine has a few desperate families who truly require special help. These families are unfortunately no longer unique.

Both of the Zimm parents had typical allergies. When they decided to move into a trailer, this young couple were totally unaware of the problems that could arise because of the extensive use of formaldehyde in the construction of most trailers

Nancy

Nancy, the oldest girl, was six years old when she came to see us along with her siblings. She was a happy, playful child until the family moved into the trailer. Within a few months she gradually became depressed, refused to go outside, and was totally exhausted all the time. Within a few days after they moved from that trailer, she was energetic and happy again.

Eve

Little Eve was born one month after the move into the trailer. Her mother drank large amounts of cow's milk when Eve was being breast-fed. Allergy diets excluding milk were finally tried when Eve was four years old. At that time it was found that milk was one factor that caused her to scream and to have insomnia.

Her mother was perplexed during Eve's infancy because she seemed to be too quiet and subdued. She continued to be inordinately tired at the age of two to three years. As a toddler she continued to need three-hour naps. She was ready for bed each day by 11:00 A.M. This could have reflected the fatigue portion of the allergic-tension-fatigue syndrome.

At night she would scream, hour after hour. She had many abdominal problems. She tended to whine and yawn frequently. She had dark eye circles. She sneezed often, her nose ran, and she coughed all the time. She tended to have sudden, inexplicable unprovoked episodes when she would bite and attack her older sister.

She had had ten ear infections during the first year of life, each requiring prolonged antibiotic therapy. She needed ear surgery for ventilation tubes by the time she was two years old because fluid kept forming behind her eardrums. In spite of the tubes, she continued to have seven more ear infections between the ages of three and four years.

She was seen in my office at the age of four years. After taking a detailed history I suggested that the family move from the trailer as soon as possible. Within two days after the move, Eve was better. Her attitude improved. She could sleep better at night, was no longer nasal, and she stopped coughing. We did not check the child's blood, but her mother's blood showed an elevated level of formic acid (formaldehyde).

Jimmy

Little Jimmy was born after the family had lived in the trailer for two years. He also seemed to be an exceptionally unhappy infant and toddler. Jimmy was tired and cranky when we saw him for the first time at the age of two years. He had a raspy voice, baggy eyes, scarlet earlobes, and a miserable disposition. He had had six ear infections between the ages of one and two years, as well as two bouts of pneumonia. His mother noticed that if Jimmy bathed in water that had a strong smell of chlorine, his ears became scarlet. This suggested a possible sensitivity to chlorine. Like the other children, he was also better two days after his family moved.

The Zimm Family Finds Answers

Once Mrs. Zimm became aware that chemicals were a problem, she was faced with the almost impossible challenge of constantly protecting her family from future chemical exposures. On one occasion she was forced to come to Buffalo in someone else's van because the family car was malfunctioning. Although the children were happy when they left home, all three children were irritable and exhausted by the time they arrived in Buffalo.

Eve reacted as she typically did to chemical odors: She wet her pants within fifteen minutes after she was in the van and then began to scream. She developed her typical four-day headache. Nancy slept most of the time they rode in the van, but by the time the family was near Buffalo, she was coughing and had a chest rattle, headache, and abdominal pain. She awoke up with a temper tantrum. The van was unfortunately new and smelled of chemicals, as well as automobile exhaust fumes.

Similarly when the family replaced their old car, all the children became ill whenever they went for a drive.[32] They continued to have difficulty until their mother cleaned the upholstery with baking soda

32. William J. Rea, M.D., et al., "Food and Chemical Susceptibility After Environmental Chemical Overexposure: Case Histories," Annals of Allergy 41 (1978), pp. 101–110.

and covered the seats with heavy-duty aluminum foil and then layers of cotton blankets. The children could then go on long drives in that car without feeling ill or misbehaving.

If Eve went into grocery stores, malls, or hospitals that smelled of chemicals, her chest would quickly fill up with mucus, her ears and cheeks would become brilliant red, her throat would feel tight, and her head would begin to pound. As was typical for her, the headache would not subside for four or five days. If she drank water stored in a plastic container, she had diarrhea six to nine times that day. If water is stored in glass, she has no bowel disturbance.

On one occasion, Eve was fine when she accompanied her brother to the pediatrician's office for a routine immunization. The doctor had just remodeled his office and installed some new paneling that smelled of formaldehyde. Within fifteen minutes her eyes were glassy, her ears were red, her throat hurt, and she began to race about, flipped her body in the air, kicked, and could not sit still. She cried in pain for three days and nights because of the headache caused by this particular exposure.

After the move from the trailer to an apartment, the children did well. Their home was austere but environmentally safer. Then, unexpectedly, the landlord sprayed for ants. The children's behavior quickly changed. Nancy began to hit and scream. Eve was coughing, irritable, whining, hitting, and wetting the bed. Her headaches returned. She again began to tell her parents, "I hate you and I want to leave home."

On one occasion the children were all feeling well when they went to visit their grandmother. However, she had just installed a new carpet, and the entire family became ill within fifteen minutes and had to leave very quickly to return home. Eve's eyes became glassy and she began to scream, cry, and hit. Her nose became congested and her typical four-day headache began. She had to be physically removed from the house. Jimmy began to wheeze. Nancy whined, cried, and complained of abdominal pain and muscle aches. She remained ill for three days.

The children all became sick or misbehaved when the family shopped in a store selling polyester clothing. Eve routinely ran through the clothing racks and suddenly acted like a "monster." She had to be physically carried from the store. Once again she began to say she wanted to die and asked her parents what they would do if she died.

The children's blood was examined about a year after they initially came to our office because of the accidental ant-spray exposure. There was evidence of high levels of benzene, xylene, trichloroethylene, and tetrachlorethylene in each child's blood. This entire family needs detoxification, but the units that do this are too far away, too expensive, and most do not care for children as young as Jimmy. We were faced with a difficult problem: How could we remove some of the chemical pollution in their bodies? They need to regain enough tolerance to chemicals so that future everyday unavoidable exposures will not make them so ill.

Parents Can Find Answers on Their Own

One of the most encouraging aspects about this family's problems is that the children's parents learned to determine exactly what caused their children to become ill. In the past they had felt forlorn, perplexed, and helpless. They needed others to resolve their children's health problems, and many times they had to depend upon drug, hospital, or surgical treatment. Repeated medical efforts to detect and eliminate the cause of the children's recurrent ear problems or Eve's incapacitating prolonged headaches had been totally unsuccessful.

By noting when the children developed red ears, red cheeks, bloated abdomens, or sudden changes in their affect or behavior, the parents now have little difficulty determining exactly what is causing each symptom to develop in each child. In addition, they know that when the children's pulses are about 80, they are fine, but whenever their pulses increase above 100, something is wrong. For the first time, efforts can be made to pinpoint, diminish, and possibly eliminate specific exposures that make their children ill. Once parents know why, they can better protect their youngsters and prevent future flare-ups of illness.

Why Are Allergic Families Prone to Chemical Problems?

We must ask why chemically sensitive children appear to have so many allergies. In part it appears to be genetic. Children inherit their immune systems and their tendency to develop allergies along with their eye and hair color. This tendency passes along from one generation to the next, so that affected children often have many relatives who have similar medical problems. But remember that chemical exposures also weaken the immune system and diminish the ability of the body to detoxify chemicals.[33] Chemically sensitive children often have not only the typical allergies but the less frequently recognized allergies as well. You can easily see why some families with these sensitivities cannot begin to cope with the insurmountable physical, emotional, and economic problems that face them.

Recognize the Characteristic Patterns, Then Figure Out Why

Before the true cause of the Zimm children's illnesses were recognized, one medical problem led to another. The allergically swollen tissues made them prone to one infection after another. The antibiotics used to treat the infections led, in turn, to yeast problems. The recurrent infections led to tonsil, adenoid, or eardrum surgery. Many secondary emotional and family problems arose because the children never felt well.

The chemical sensitivity caused by a prolonged low-level chemical exposure such as living in a trailer is not totally resolved by moving. Once a person has been sensitized, every slight odor, from automobile exhaust to a freshly waxed floor in a neighbor's kitchen, can cause symptoms. An increasing number of chemically sensitive children are unable to attend schools because of the chemical contamination, e.g. synthetic carpets, inside the classrooms and buildings. The scenario of an ecologically ill family can be tragic unless it is recognized. Parents usually have no choice but to become knowledgeable about how chemicals can affect their family's well-being.

Related Medical and Social Problems

The parents of affected children typically have the same sensitivities and often feel as sick, both physically and emotionally, as their youngsters. Because the children are so ill, they need their mother, so she can't work outside the home. The father often has to work two jobs to pay the bills. This leaves him exhausted and tired when he finally returns home, only to find an equally weary, ill wife trying to manage several sick, screaming unhappy children.

Because there are simply not enough physicians trained to meet

---

33. William, J. Rea, M.D., "Toxic Volatile Organic Hydrocarbons in Chemically Sensitive Patients," *Clinical Ecology 2* (1987), p. 70.

the needs of the public at the present time, many parents are faced with the need to travel long distances to have their children tested for their allergies and ecologic illness. Even after parents know what to do and why the children are ill, they are often too busy, exhausted, discouraged, ill, and financially drained to cope with day-to-day medical challenges. They find it difficult or impossible to maintain a rotation diet or even find a "safe" home in which to live. To add to their stress and overload, their insurance company often balks at paying their medical bills, even when the children improve quickly and dramatically after ecologic care. If such a family can survive as a unit, it is truly a miracle of love, perseverance, and determination.

There are answers for the Zimm family and for others who have chemical sensitivities. The answers, however, are neither fast nor inexpensive. Antioxidant nutrients that contain vitamins, trace metals, minerals, and essential fatty acids help to strengthen the immune system and aid in the excretion of body chemicals. Some children, however, are so sensitive they can't tolerate even the less allergenic brands of vitamins. Some families who have extreme chemical sensitivities may need detoxification so that they can tolerate more unavoidable pollution exposures associated with day-to-day living. If they can eat a rotation diet of the more expensive organic foods, if these are available, their food allergies should diminish. If their home is relatively ecologically safe, they should have fewer flare-ups of illness and behavior problems. If they receive allergy extract therapy for the major substances causing them to be ill, they should improve. This combined comprehensive allergy approach should diminish health problems in many families, but it can be difficult to do without help. They need the support of loved ones, and a source of private funds or an insurance company that faces its responsibility.

There is genuine hope and encouragement for chemically ill children. Many parents meet their challenges day by day and gradually accomplish what needs to be done. Unfortunately, they have few positive alternatives. Most loving parents will make every sacrifice possible and necessary to help their children. Once chemically related illness is recognized and children are treated, the reward should be an improved level of health and happiness for *every* family member. One must pray that such families have the inner strength and faith to face each new challenge. As they overcome one obstacle after another, they find encouragement and satisfaction. Each success adds to their storehouse of knowledge so that parents can prevent future illnesses in their little ones. The Zimm family certainly improved remarkably and responded favorably to treatment for one and a half years. However, they must continue to retest the children's allergy extracts approximately every two to three months, avoid chemicals, and follow a comprehensive allergy-treatment program to keep their children well.

What Can You Do If Your Child or Family Is Suddenly Exposed to a Chemical?

For example, if:

- The school sprays with insecticides while school is in session.
- A certain factory is polluting a city and making a large number of individuals ill.
- Some chemical at work or school makes you or your child unable to perform competently.
- Aerial spraying with a potentially harmful chemical is planned in the area of your home or in your child's school.
- If the landlord uses a termiticide or pesticide.

Contact the following:

- Environmental Health Network, c/o Linda King, P.O. Box 1628, Harvey, La. 70058 (504-340-2321)
- National Pesticide Telecommunications Network (800-858-7378)
- Environmental Protection Agency, 230 South Dearborn St., Chicago, Ill. 60604, (312-353-2205)
- J. Laseter, Ph.D., Accu-Chem Laboratories, 990 North Bowser, Suite 800, Richardson, Tex. 75081 (214-234-5577)
- Citizens Commission on Human Rights, 5265 Fountain Avenue, Suite 2, Los Angeles, Calif. 90029 (800-522-0247)

For the nearest specialist in environmental medicine, see Appendix D.

PART FOUR

SPECIFIC PROBLEMS OFTEN NOT RECOGNIZED AS ALLERGY

CHAPTER 14

Is Your Child Always Sick?

Many parents complain that their child has one infection after another and never seems well. Sometimes this is related to a child's allergies, which can cause the nose and lung tissues to swell so that germs can invade more easily. Many of the children in this book have a history of one ear infection after another from early infancy on. The average normal child develops about four infections a year, but it is not uncommon for some allergic children to have one to two infections each month. They will be ill for about one to two weeks, well for a few days, and then another infection begins. One way of breaking the cycle is to recognize the basic allergic tendency, give these children appropriate allergy treatment, and improve their nutrition. This combined approach appears to diminish the repetitive need for newer and better antibiotics.

RECURRENT EAR INFECTIONS

Emily

Little Emily was only three years old when we initially saw her. Her major problem was repeated ear infections. In time, we determined that if she drank milk, a specific sequential pattern always occurred. Within an hour she would have a typical temper tantrum and become hyperactive and very difficult; her total disposition would change, and she would become impossible to console; she would throw her favorite toy on the floor and jump up and down on it; she tipped over furniture, cried, whined, stamped her feet, kicked things, and pounded the walls. A few hours later she would complain and cry because her legs ached. That night she would wet the bed, and the next day she would start with another ear infection. She would be treated with an antibiotic for about ten days, be fine for a few days, and then the entire pattern would begin again.

In time, her mother realized that popcorn or corn chips caused Emily to develop a headache and become irritable. In addition, her mother found that in spite of treatment for sugar, Emily had to limit sugar for a long time because it continued to cause her to become hyperactive, cranky, and irritable. Emily's mother now knows that she must continue to watch carefully to be certain that milk does not cause new or different symptoms as time passes. This is especially true if she notices any physical or emotional complaints during a period when Emily craves dairy products.

Emily's Early History

Once again, Emily's allergy history did not begin shortly before she came to see us. Her mother had many allergies, and her grandmother could not drink milk without becoming sick. Milk formula caused Emily to vomit. She had three formula changes in nine months and vomited every milk and soy milk formula that was tried. By the age of two years Emily began to have hay fever whenever she was near cats. Approximately every other day she complained of tummy aches, muscle aches, and headaches. At times she acted excessively tired.

Milk—One Cause of Her Ear Problems

Emily's major problem, however, was recurrent ear infections. Her tonsils and adenoids were removed when she was two and a half years old. Her ear specialist was knowledgeable about milk allergy and wisely suggested that Emily be placed on a milk-free diet. She improved for the next few months. Her mother then became ill and could not monitor Emily's diet. Shortly after Emily began to eat dairy products and drink milk, her ear infections recurred and she complained about leg and muscle aches, abdominal pain, fatigue, and coughed, and had temper tantrums. She also became irritable and started to wet the bed again every night.

By observing her response to different foods, her mother determined that soy caused intestinal symptoms and dark eye circles. Her headaches were due to excessive orange juice.

Emily's Treatment

We initially treated her only with her neutralization allergy extract for milk, soy, and orange under her tongue. She responded very well.

At first her mother had to limit the quantity of milk she could drink. After five months of milk treatment, however, she could ingest ice cream and yogurt every four days without difficulty, provided she was also given lactose. Part of her milk problem appeared to be an inability to digest milk sugar, or lactose. Because milk caused symptoms that were not exclusively intestinal, and because we could reproduce her personality changes with provocation allergy testing, it was obvious that at least part of her milk problem was due to a milk allergy. The excessive abdominal gas and diarrhea that Emily had at times were typical of a lactose intolerance, but that could not account for her leg aches, temper outbursts, and ear problems. These complaints are classic for many youngsters who have common and unusual forms of allergy.

After comprehensive allergy treatment, which included the P/N allergy testing and treatment, plus a rotation diet and changes in her bedroom, Emily improved dramatically. Five years later her mother continued to report that her earaches, leg aches, muscle aches, and headaches were no longer a problem.

AN UNHAPPY TODDLER WHO HAD EXCESSIVE INFECTIONS THAT STARTED IN INFANCY AND CONTINUED UNTIL ALLERGY TREATMENT

Mark

Mark was seen for the first time in our office when he was thirteen months old. He had many allergic relatives. He had one infection after another, starting at the age of two weeks old. In spite of repeated antibiotics for two weeks out of every month, his ear infections became progressively worse each month. A series of physicians made his mother feel that she was not taking proper care of Mark and accused her of not giving him his medication properly.

Mark was breast-fed for four months, then he was started on a milk formula. From then on, three or four times a week, he began to scream for as long as four hours at a stretch. He was extremely irritable, disliked cuddling, and refused to smile or eat. Whole milk was tried at nine months, but he continued to be unhappy, could not sleep, and was sick all the time.

Milk Allergy Diagnosed and Treated

At eleven months an allergist and a pediatrician referred him for surgery to place ventilation tubes through his eardrums. His parents, however, refused. They chose instead to investigate the possible role of allergies. At thirteen months he was placed on a soy milk formula, instead of cow's milk, and to everyone's surprise he stopped screaming and crying. However, he still could not sleep at night. Sometimes he slept less than two hours after he was put in bed.

When Mark was about fourteen months old, his mother began to observe other cause-and-effect relationships. She noticed that he became irritable and would cry all night mainly after he played outside. After playing in grass, he wheezed, sneezed in bouts, and rubbed his nose upward, indicating that he had typical asthma and hay fever.

With P/N allergy testing we found that we could produce both irritability and screaming during the grass allergy tests. These complaints were relieved when he was given a weaker dilution of grass allergy extract.

One day we were surprised in our office because after we allergy-tested him for dust, mites, and molds, he smiled for the first time! In addition, after three months of allergy treatment for these items and a number of foods, he began to show a genuine interest in eating solid foods for the first time. Prior to that he had existed mainly on a soy formula and apple juice, but routinely spit out table foods. Before allergy treatment, on a "good" day he never swallowed more than two tablespoons of solid food a day.

His Response to Treatment

By the age of seventeen months his mother was delighted. He stopped hitting and slapping. Mark began to sleep all night and he awoke in the morning with a smile instead of a frown. He seemed happy and he giggled, laughed, and smiled like other toddlers.

Over time his mother has observed that chemical odors, such as tobacco, chlorine, lawn chemicals, household paint, and finger paints make him depressed. She tries to limit these exposures as much as possible. Food colors in soda pop, bubble gum, or suckers continue to cause a marked change in his personality. For example, at the age of three years, when someone gave him a glass of red soda pop, he became totally uncontrollable, tore off his clothing, and tried to jump out of a moving car. He was hanging halfway out of the car window before his mother could pull the car to the side of the road. His mother thought she'd need the help of the police to take Mark home safely.

For the past five years, since we began to treat him, he has continued to remain 95 percent improved. His disposition and sleep problems are gone. His ear problems are no longer evident, and the need for surgery was eliminated. Whenever he has an occasional flare-up of symptoms or stops smiling, his mother usually recognizes exactly what has caused the recurrence. He is retested for suspected allergenic substances and his treatment is adjusted. He usually improves dramatically while he is still in the office, on the way home, or within twenty-four hours.

This boy is now rarely ill. He averages one cold a year. His mother is extremely cooperative and is delighted to have a healthy son who smiles. She no longer fears calling her doctors as she did before. She no longer feels it's her fault when Mark is sick. His mother continues to try to maintain a rotation diet, keep their home allergy-free, avoid chemicals, provide adequate nutrients, and give him allergy extract treatment under his tongue. It is reassuring that since treatment he has changed from a sickly, unhappy toddler to an unusually healthy, happy child.

What Can Parents Do to Decrease Family Infections?

Children who have allergies and recurrent infections are thought to have a deficient or weak immune system. In part this is genetic, because most allergic children have at least one parent who has known typical or atypical forms of allergy. In addition to the genetic factor, environmentally oriented physicians believe that the immense number of indoor and outdoor chemicals and pollution to which we are all exposed can damage the immune system. Long-term studies by the Russians on rats, for example, show that their immune systems are weakened if they are exposed to microwave energy. There is some evidence to suggest that these machines can also adversely affect some humans.[1]

1. Robert Becker, M.D., *Cross Currents* (Los Angeles: Jeremy P. Tarcher, Inc., 1990).

Parents often ask how they can strengthen their child's immune system. Our bodies must be supplied with essential building blocks. You cannot build a brick house without mortar. Each body has in-dividual and specific needs, which change according to age, diet, life-style, and stresses. In order for the body to resist infection and feel optimally well, each cell must contain the proper nutrients. Vitamins, enzymes, trace metals, minerals, essential fatty acids, and amino acids are the mortar needed to build healthier bodies and immune systems. These, combined with fewer ingested and inhaled pollutants and toxins, should enable our bodies to function at a higher level and help us to feel truly well.

Physicians and nutrition specialists such as Linus Pauling, Ph.D.; Alan Gaby, M.D.; Jonathan Wright, M.D.; Leo Galland, M.D.; Abram Hoffer, M.D., Ph.D.; and Jeffrey Bland, Ph.D., are only a few who have written and taught many about how to improve their nutrition. Some of their publications are listed in the Bibliography.

CHAPTER 15

Hyperactivity Is
a Mixed Bag

Many parents are justifiably frightened about their children's futures in school. Some young mothers of hyperactive children are continually apprehensive that there may be a call from the kindergarten teacher telling them to come and take their child home. Many mothers truly live in daily fear that when the phone rings, it is because their child is being sent home again because of disruptive behavior. According to Lendon Smith, M.D., in 1950 there was one hyperactive child in every classroom. Today there are five or six. The problem is increasing, and the answer is not more Ritalin but more attempts to find out why this is happening. Some of these children merely have undetected allergies affecting their brain.

Specialists in environmental medicine and allergists see many children who also have typical allergies and hyperactivity. These youngsters usually have many of the other characteristics associated with allergic tension fatigue syndrome (ATFS), such as headaches, muscle aches, clumsiness, irritability, aggression, and "impossible" behavior. Some have periods of extreme fatigue alternating with their uncontrollable overactivity. Most of them also have classical nose and eye allergies (see Table 15.1).

Children with ATFS have behavior and activity problems in school and at home. They are often thought to have attention deficit disorder (ADD), or if they have hyperactivity, attention deficit hyperactivity disorder (ADHD). Both ATFS and ADD youngsters are so impulsive that they can't sit still, can't concentrate, and are easily

Table 15.1
Allergic Tension Fatigue Syndrome (ATFS)

Possible Nervous System Symptoms:

Hyperactive, uncontrollably wild, unrestrained
Fatigued, weak, weary, exhausted, listless
Nonstop talk, repetition, loud talk, stuttering
Inattentive, disruptive, impulsive
Short attention span, unable to concentrate
Restless legs, finger tapping
Clumsy, poor coordination, tremor
Insomnia, nightmares, inability to fall asleep and wake up
Nervous, irritable, upset, short-tempered, moody
High-strung, excitable, agitated
Depressed, easily moved to tears, temperamental
Oversensitive to odor, light, sound, pain, and cold

Other Possible Medical Symptoms:

Nose: hay fever
Aches: head, back, neck, muscle, or joint; "growing pains," or aches unrelated to exercise
Intestinal complaints: bellyaches, nausea, upset stomach, bloating, bad breath, gassy stomach, belching, vomiting, diarrhea, constipation
Bladder problems: wet pants in daytime or in bed, frequent need to rush to urinate, burning or pain with urination
Face: dark eye circles, puffiness below eyes, red earlobes, red cheeks
Glands: swollen neck glands
Ear problems: fluid behind eardrums, ringing ears, dizziness
Excessive perspiration
Low-grade fever

distracted. When they are not racing wildly about, they tend to be fidgety, irritable, and wiggly. They exhibit a variety of learning problems.

Ecologists have found such a definite overlap between ADHD and ATFS that they often appear to be in the same mixed bag (see Table 16.1). Many children labeled with these diagnoses have the same typical cluster of characteristics. Studies have shown that 25 percent to 50 percent of ADHD children have learning disabilities. About 30 percent bed-wet or soil their underpants. These characteristics are certainly seen in youngsters who have ATFS or unusual forms of allergy. When ADD or ADHD youngsters have allergic relatives, an allergic appearance, and an obvious allergy to pollen, molds, dust, foods, and/or chemical sensitivities, they usually have ATFS and many respond favorably to appropriate allergy care.

In both groups of children, regardless of the original medical label, many appear to respond remarkably well and quickly in a week or less to the Multiple Food Elimination Diet. Many mothers have successfully tried this diet on their own prior to the time they are seen in our office. In fortunate children continued improvement has been noted merely by excluding one or two favorite foods from their diet.

Other children, however, are more complex and challenging. These children often require the expertise of a specialist in environmental medicine or/and an allergist who can implement a comprehensive diagnostic evaluation and allergy treatment program. Many need counseling or a psychologist. Others have problems that are totally unrelated to allergy. They require the expertise of various other medical or psychology specialists who treat specific emotional or learning problems, as well as medical complaints related to the ears, bladder, intestines, nervous system, and so on.[1]

Hyperactivity can be caused by a wide range of nervous system disorders, by genetic problems, birth injuries, previous infections, accidents, stresses, emotional problems, endocrine abnormalities, biochemical disturbances, toxins, and even enzyme defects. Dr. Jonathan Brostoff's book, *Food Allergy and Intolerance,* discusses one theory of why Dr. Feingold's diet to control hyperactivity helped so many children.[2] The Feingold diet did not allow the children to eat food coloring, artificial flavoring, salicylates, or additives. Additives must be

1. B. J. Kaplan, et al., "Dietary Replacement in Preschool-Aged Hyperactive Boys," *Pediatrics* 83 (1989) pp. 7–17.
2. Jonathan Brostoff, M.D., and Linda Gamlin, *Food Allergy and Intolerance.* 1989. Bloomsbury Publishing Limited, 2 Soho Square, London, W1V 5DE, England.

detoxified by body enzymes. Dr. Brostoff states that some hyperactive children appear to lack phenolsulphotransferase-P, an enzyme needed to detoxify certain intestinal bacteria. Food dyes inhibit this enzyme so that it does not function properly. The result can be hyperactivity, which can be due to the presence of certain intestinal bacteria that were not detoxified. These sorts of problems, however, can occur with or without allergies to foods. We need to have a better understanding of such relationships and their relevance to specific children's problems.

Evaluation of hyperactive children often includes some combination or all of the following:

- An extensive, detailed review of the child's past and present history. The details of the prenatal period, birth records, immunizations, and any major infections or injuries can be very significant.

- A discussion of classical, as well as less obvious allergies in closest family members. Many parents are unaware that their own chronic medical complaints could be an allergy.

- Any evidence in the hyperactive child of either typical or unusual allergies from infancy on. This must be discussed in great detail.

- Each child's school history and the results of evaluations by educators, psychologists, or counselors must be considered.

When indicated, detailed *individual* instruction must be given to the parents concerning the following:

- How to conduct environmental and allergy changes within a youngster's home and/or school.

- The value of a long-term rotation diet if foods appear to be significant factors in a child's problem. Dietary and nutritional consultation may be required to assure proper growth and development of children.

- Practical advice concerning chemical and pollution avoidance and treatment.

- Allergy extract therapy, especially if the above has not sufficiently eliminated a child's symptoms.

- Nutrient supplementation to enhance the total body's immunity and help restore normal digestion and natural detoxification mechanisms. These may help to diminish allergies and the propensity to other medical problems.

A number of additional studies are often required to help confirm whether an allergy is present and to rule out other common causes of hyperactivity and learning problems. These studies must be highly individualized and could include, for example, attempts to determine if hypoglycemia, lead poisoning, yeast, or parasites are a problem. Sometimes selected amino acid therapy is needed.

The following is a rather typical history of a child whose mother figured out some answers by doing the Multiple Food Allergy Test.

AN AGGRESSIVE TEN-YEAR-OLD BOY WHO HAD UNCONTROLLABLE TANTRUMS AND INCREASED ACTIVITY

Donald

Donald first saw us when he was ten years old. He had many allergic relatives and obvious typical allergies. His parents were particularly concerned because he had episodes when he spit and bit himself and other people. He had temper tantrums as often as five times a day. He could not sit through a meal, a television show, or a game. His teachers noted that he could sit still in the morning, but that after lunch his school performance and behavior deteriorated.

Four months before we saw Donald, his mother tried the Multiple Food Elimination Diet. Within a week he was 75 percent better, and during the second week his parents found that wheat, chocolate, and sugar made him hyperactive and disagreeable. After avoiding these foods for three months his mother called to tell us he was "a joy." Friends could not believe he was the same child. His teachers were delighted and very pleased. His Conner's Hyperactivity Score decreased from an abnormal high of 23 to a normal 13 within one week. Shortly after treatment he went to a state fair with his family and they said that it was the first time in Donald's entire life that they had ever had a good time with him.

When given provocation allergy tests for mold in our office, he suddenly became extremely violent. He kicked and was ready to hit anyone who came within range. He was negative, uncooperative, and inordinately angry. After a tiny drop of the correct dilution of mold allergy extract was placed in his arm, he returned to the pleasant child he had been during the many previous hours of allergy testing. Most children act normal in the office until they are tested for some item to which they are exceedingly sensitive. Then the change becomes obvious to anyone.

Typical of many families with an allergic child, his parents soon became expert in the detection of the major foods that caused him difficulty. After they learned how to watch for early clues of allergy, they noted that ten minutes after he ate a bowl of cereal, he would become bouncy, unable to concentrate, irritable, and hyperactive.

His most remarkable response occurred when we used P/N to test him for wheat. He scribbled when asked to write. Then he tore the paper up after attacking it vigorously with the pencil. He crumpled what was left of the paper and began to cry. Then, in exasperation, he pounded the table with his fist. He was so angry at one point that he even punched the air. As the reaction to the test subsided, he held his head with his hands and complained of a headache. A few minutes after the correct wheat neutralization extract was given, he acted perfectly calm and entirely normal. He said he'd felt "mad" when he was being tested for wheat.

Two months after his treatment his mother wrote to tell us that their lives had changed. Donald was responding very well to his allergy extract therapy and they could "live" with their son again. His muscle aches, joint pains, headaches, and leg aches had subsided. His intestinal symptoms and associated red earlobes made it very easy for them to tell that he was reacting to a food or some other allergenic substance. His dark eye circles and sleep problems disappeared. They were all delighted that his previous physicians' diagnoses had been wrong. His problems were not emotional.

Five years later this boy continues to be 95 percent better. On one occasion he stopped all his treatments for several months because he had been so well for several years. His original symptoms slowly recurred. He resumed his allergy therapy and quickly and dramatically improved again.

The following patient represents the classic allergic child, one who had hyperactivity, obvious food allergies, plus elusive chemical sensitivities. He vividly illustrates how challenging it can be initially to differentiate the role of multiple factors in a child's illness. Specialists in environmental medicine attempt effectively to ferret out each of the various pieces of the allergic puzzle. Once they have completed their evaluation, the total picture should be more clearly evident.

HYPERACTIVITY WAS PART OF RYAN'S MIXED CHEMICAL BAG

Ryan

Ryan's mother brought him to see us when he was four years old. His mother had noticed that the yellow antihistamine, which he had used every day for one year, helped his nose allergies but always made him hyperactive. He had had similar problems in the past with an orange antihistamine. His teachers said they thought Ryan had neurological problems because at times he had poor muscle coordination, acted clumsy, twitched his face, and hit his head. He had a poor memory and attention span.

Ryan's Early Infant and Toddler History

Similar to many allergic children, both parents had typical allergies. Ryan kicked and hiccupped more than his sister when he was in the uterus. From about five to six months on, his mother's abdomen bulged in different areas. He punched and poked so vigorously that her stomach muscles hurt.

After he was born, she described him as too active. He preferred to be held with a swinging motion as his parents walked and did not tolerate quiet cuddling. He occasionally had diarrhea but he had no colic or feeding problems. He slept poorly; the slightest sound awakened him.

When he was fourteen months old, his family moved into a brand-new home. Four months later, when the weather became cold, the windows were closed and the heat was turned on. At about that time, he began to have classical nose and eye allergies. This type of history suggests a possible dust or chemical sensitivity.

From the age of eighteen months to three years he had a constant series of monthly ear infections. This suggested a milk sensitivity. Later on he had flulike symptoms every two to three weeks. These problems were diminished when he began to take daily antihistamines.

As time passed, his year-round hay fever seemed to become more evident during the warm seasons, when pollen and mold spores were in the air. This is a typical pattern for many allergic youngsters. However, Ryan's pediatrician assured his mother that he was too young to be tested for allergies.

By the age of two years on, his parents also noticed that he was always tired when he arose in the morning and again, on occasion, shortly after he ate. He had daily nausea, bloating, and loose bowel movements. He wet his pants from April to October. In the winter these problems occurred once or twice a week, *but almost always on school days*. He had ten temper tantrums a day and daily headaches in the summer, but again, these were evident in the winter mainly on the two days he attended school.

Why did he have so many problems in the warm months and why was he worse in the winter, but only on school days? Pollen and mold allergy could explain his hay fever, but what about his summer intestinal complaints and wet pants? There must be a sensible reason, and if it could be found, this child might be helped. A more detailed history revealed an abundance of helpful clues, which provided a plausible explanation.

Clues to Ryan's Symptoms

When Ryan was about eighteen months old, he had the classic ATFS (Allergic Tension Fatigue Syndrome) symptoms. He had periods when he was "hyperactive and out of control," and this could be quickly followed by extreme fatigue. His mother said he would become "a lump on the floor and act totally exhausted." This tended to occur again during the summer months whenever he was outside. He acted similarly whenever he was exposed to tobacco smoke or went to a circus.

If he was near a wood-burning fireplace, he acted bizarre. He would walk in a strange, stiff manner, hit his head, become hyper, and then suddenly become limp and be unable to stand. Shortly after he was removed from the odor of the fireplace, he returned to his normal self. His mother noticed similar personality changes when he went into certain clothing stores in the nearby mall. He would suddenly become very antsy and fidgety for no apparent reason. This suggested that chemical odors could be a problem.

His preschool teachers complained that at times he acted too hyper, too tired, or walked or acted in a strange manner. He tended to be shy, and he had strange periods when he did not want to be touched or to be near anyone. His mother decided to check his schoolroom. She learned that his napping cot and the tabletops in the kindergarten class were sprayed six times a day with a commonly used disinfectant aerosol. This suggested that some chemical in the aerosol might be affecting Ryan adversely. This proved to be an extremely important clue.

From the age of three years on, he had growing pains and leg aches that were unrelated to exercise. In time his mother realized that every time he drank pure orange juice or ate a whole orange, he became so tired that he was unable to walk up the stairs "because his legs ached." Without treatment this lasted about one half to two hours. Then he could bound up and down stairs easily.

Ryan could never stay very long at birthday parties. After he ate, he became so bouncy and antsy that he always had to be taken home before the entertainment began.

Ryan's Traditional Allergy Treatment

Finally, because of his hay fever and inappropriate behavior, his mother took Ryan to a well-trained board-certified pediatric allergist. He tested Ryan and found strong pollen and mold sensitivities by prick allergy tests. Stronger intradermal tests revealed he had a slight sensitivity to dust and pets but no reaction to five foods. The doctor said that the problems in his temperament and activity were unrelated to his outdoor allergies. He assured Ryan's mother that his behavioral problems were not associated with foods or the food coloring in antihistamines. He said that neither her son's history nor his food-allergy skin tests indicated a food allergy. The doctor gave Ryan's mother a printed sheet that recommended a plastic mattress cover and an air conditioner. He prepared an allergy extract for her son.

After Ryan began to receive his allergy extract treatments for pollen, molds, and dust, however, *every treatment appeared to precipitate a repetitive pattern of illness*. He received his injection every Tuesday at noon. Within one to three hours his arm would swell and became very red and tender. Then he developed a headache and became markedly overactive. He became progressively more sick throughout Tuesday, and by Wednesday his nose and eye symptoms were much worse than usual. He would lie on the couch all day complaining of a headache, leg aches, and nausea. He acted extremely fatigued, whined, laid around, and even developed a low-grade fever. By Thursday he could return to school but he remained fussy, tired, and irritable until late that day or early Friday. From Tuesday night to Thursday night he wet his bed, and then he would be dry until he received his next weekly allergy injection.

This type of complaint is certainly rare. Ryan's allergist assured his mother that her son's symptoms after each injection were *not* due to the allergy extract. Again we must ask, if it was unrelated, why did all these symptoms consistently happen *only* after he received his allergy extract?

Specialists in environmental medicine, however, often hear this type of complaint from patients who are sensitive to chemicals. Phenol is routinely used as a preservative in most allergy extracts. This part of the history again suggested that chemicals might be one part of this child's problems. Phenol and hydrocarbons are also two ingredients commonly found in aerosol disinfectants, as well as in the vapors produced when wood is burned. Now the clues were beginning to fit together.

Ryan's Attempt at Following an Allergy Diet

A friend suggested that Ryan's mother try our Multiple Food Elimination Diet. There was no change after the first week. During the second week, however, when he ate each potentially problematic food one at a time, his mother saw distinct changes. Sugar, yellow and orange antihistamines, and *orange drink* definitely caused him to become hyperactive. This was a surprise because by history pure *orange juice or oranges* had repeatedly caused fatigue and difficulty climbing stairs. This suggested that some ingredient other than orange in the orange drink was causing that problem. Orange drinks often contain sugar, corn syrup, and artificial coloring or flavors. All these items are common causes of hyperactivity in some children. Later on we ascertained that yellow, red, or orange food coloring appeared to make Ryan hyperactive.

In time, Ryan's mother read more books about allergy and she found that his eyes and nose were better if she closed the air vent in his bedroom so that the dust from the furnace did not circulate in that area. This change also seemed to make him less active in the morning, and he awoke happier. A year later, shortly after she had the ductwork cleaned and then opened his bedroom vents, his previous symptoms recurred. This often happens in dust-sensitive individuals. When furnaces are professionally vacuumed, this temporarily loosens dust in the ductwork so that it is circulated through the house for a short while as soon as the furnace is turned on again. This type of transient, dust-related flare-up of symptoms usually subsides within a few days after furnace cleaning.

When sugar and yellow, red, or orange food coloring were removed from Ryan's diet, he definitely was less active and behaved better. The odors of perfume, paint, stain, incense, potpourri, tobacco, lawn spray, and smoke, however, repeatedly continued to cause extreme hyperactivity and/or fatigue.

How Do the Pieces Fit Together?

Now let's try to put all the pieces of Ryan's history together. Ecologic-allergy histories often fall into surprisingly tidy packages that sensibly explain the majority of a child's complaints. Ryan's overactivity in the uterus might be explained by the fact that his mother drank an excessive amount of orange juice or ate much more chocolate and pasta than usual at that time. His sensitivity to orange juice later on might be related to the amount his mother drank when she was pregnant.

They also lived in a heavily polluted section of town at that time. Almost every day a tire factory and oil storage area contaminated the air near the vicinity of their original home. In retrospect, this might also have been a factor related to his future sensitivity to chemicals.

Ryan's family moved to a new location and new house when he was fourteen months old, and a number of medical problems began four months later, shortly after the heat was turned on. New homes are not usually dusty or moldy, so that was an unlikely explanation for his winter complaints. Most new homes, however, smell of many chemicals, especially hydrocarbons, formaldehyde, and phenol. These odors often become more evident when a new house is suddenly closed during the colder months. The outgassing of chemicals from construction materials and furnishings found in new homes frequently causes the types of symptoms that Ryan had.

Phenol is a chemical commonly found in disinfectants. The disinfectant spray used repeatedly at school could explain why he was worse in so many ways during the winter but only on school days. That same chemical, phenol, is used as a preservative in allergy extract, and this could easily explain why he was worse after each allergy treatment. It is also found in some treated wood, so it could account for his problem related to burning wood.

Ryan's seasonal summer history was still perplexing. When he was three or four years old, he seemed worse shortly after he went outside in the summer. He was better within a few minutes after he went inside or was in an air-conditioned area. This can happen with a typical pollen and mold allergy. Hay fever often improves in a home that has an air cleaner or air conditioner. Personality and activity changes, although frequently not recognized, also can be due to mold and pollen allergies. It is even possible for intestinal complaints and wet pants to be caused by a pollen and mold sensitivity, but these would be less frequent causes of these particular problems. The next summer, however, when Ryan's mold allergy extract treatment needed adjustment, his mother noticed that on rainy or damp days he again developed abdominal pains and temper tantrums and wet his pants. After the mold treatment in his allergy extract was corrected, these problems stopped.

In addition, we considered that his outdoor summer symptoms might be due to a sensitivity to outdoor pollution. With more questioning, we ascertained that the family had moved from a factory- and oil-polluted area of the city to a locale that was heavily infested with mosquitoes. The city used mosquito-control sprays every two weeks all summer. In addition, the neighbors and Ryan's father had to spray their yards whenever they wanted to eat outside during that summer. Half of their nearby neighbors also routinely used lawn chemicals. Maybe these chemicals were factors contributing to his problem.

In time, Ryan's teachers complained that he had to be bodily removed within three minutes after he entered his gym class. When his mother checked, she found that they used a hydrocarbon or petrochemical type of oil that had a strong odor on the gym floor. This smell caused the same type of symptoms that he had after exposure to burning wood, another source of hydrocarbons.

In addition to Ryan's proven classical pollen, mold, and dust allergies, this child's history strongly suggested that he had both unrecognized chemical and food sensitivities. His repeated symptoms related to diverse chemical exposures were difficult to ignore.

Proof of His Chemical Sensitivities

To confirm these suspicions, we videotaped his responses to a skin test for phenol, hydrocarbons, and formaldehyde, as well as exposure to a popular home disinfectant aerosol. This disinfectant contains 0.1 percent phenol, 79 percent ethanol, and 20.9 percent "inert" ingredients.

Prior to his test for the disinfectant aerosol, Ryan acted normal except for an occasional grimace. About twenty minutes after being exposed to the spray on a paper towel, he began to whine, lay on his mother, became clingy, cried, and repeated the same phrase over and over again. Within one hour all these symptoms intensified, and eventually he lost total control and refused to write. His mother said his limp posture and total personality change were typical of what tends to happen on school days or after exposure to burning wood.

Figures 15.1–15.3 show how his drawing changed after he breathed the odor of the disinfectant spray. At the peak of the reaction, he could not even pick up a pencil. His symptoms subsided

Before test   During test   After treatment
                                          with oxygen

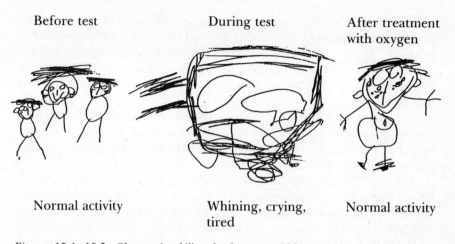

Normal activity   Whining, crying,   Normal activity
                     tired

Figures 15.1–15.3. Changes in ability of a four-year-old boy to draw due to exposure to disinfectant aerosol

nicely after he received oxygen for a few minutes.

We allergy tested Ryan to determine if he was sensitive to the phenol contained in the diluting fluid used by most allergists to prepare allergy extracts. He developed wiggly legs, whined, made faces, talked like a baby, pouted, developed a runny nose, and became tired. These symptoms are similar to what happened when he received his allergy extract. During the test his pulse rose from 68 to 88, and after we found what appeared to be the right treatment dilution, it decreased to 64. His writing deteriorated during the test and returned to normal after we found his treatment dosage. He seemed fine that evening, *but the next morning he had a large red area at the site of his phenol test.* This indicates a delayed allergic reaction to the phenol skin test, similar to the type his allergy treatments had repeatedly caused in the past. This delayed reaction also indicates that his neutralization treatment dilution, which we determined the day before, was *not* correct. Such delayed reactions to allergy tests or treatments can be difficult to treat.

Similar again to his response to all his previous traditional allergy extract treatments, the day after the phenol skin test, he awoke with eye and nose allergies, said he was exhausted, cried, whined, and lay on the couch. His leg aches and nausea recurred. He was irritable and aggressive. He continued to be temperamental and was tired for two more days. His response certainly mimicked the repeated reactions he had had after each of his previous traditional allergy extract treatments.

His mother has since noticed that phenol exposures, in particular, cause facial twitching, hyperactivity, and changes in his speech. For example, on one occasion she tried to use nose drops to treat his stuffiness. He became very temperamental, irritable, and hyperactive. His mother told the doctor that they must contain phenol and she was correct.

During P/N testing for hydrocarbons he acted tired, became whiny, impatient, temperamental, and developed a runny nose. His mother now recognizes that when he is exposed to hydrocarbons, his major symptom is fatigue.

During P/N testing for formaldehyde he pouted, acted tired, talked like a baby, developed glassy eyes, acted fidgety, and became aggressive. His mother has noticed that this chemical seems to cause symptoms similar to either hydrocarbons or phenol. He can act tired or tense in particular.

After five months of sublingual allergy extract therapy, a rotation diet, and changes in his home, he was 75 percent improved. He rarely makes strange faces or grimaces unless he is exposed to chemicals. His school replaced the previous disinfectant aerosol spray with aqueous Zephiran,[3] and he has fewer behavioral problems on school days in that classroom. His mother urged the school officials to use a different substance on the gym floor. He can now participate in gym for almost a full half hour without any change in his behavior, but if he remains in the gym area too long, his behavior again deteriorates, probably because of the new waxes they continue to use on the floor.

At Halloween his mother found that the odor of a "suede" cowboy suit that contained formaldehyde and the plastic chemical smell of masks made him act inappropriately. His mother must be wary of every odor at this time because this youngster is one more example of how the spreading phenomenon becomes obvious after a child has developed a chemical sensitivity. (See Chapter 13.)

Summary

In summary, Ryan seemed to be too active, before birth, as an infant, toddler, and child. In addition, he developed classical infant forms of allergy including nose and eye symptoms and the typical associated ear infections. In time, his traditional allergies were overshadowed by his chemical sensitivities. These were clearly and repeatedly evident in many ways and they interfered with his schoolwork and nor-

3. Available at drugstores.

mal play activities. Routine allergy treatment had to be discontinued, probably because of reactions to the phenol in his allergy extract. In contrast, he appears to be helped by the P/N form of allergy extracts that are devoid of the preservative phenol. Comprehensive environmental allergy treatment has unquestionably helped. Most gratifying, however, is the fact that his mother now recognizes *why* her son is not feeling right, or is too active or too tired. She knows what to do to help eliminate his symptoms. She now recognizes delightful aspects of his personality that simply were never evident before.

Most hyperactive youngsters are not nearly as complex or challenging as Ryan. Merely watch your child and when the red ears, dark eye circles, and inappropriate activity and behavior changes occur, ask: What did my child eat, smell, or touch? The answers are often only a thought away.

CHAPTER 16

Tourette's Syndrome Overlaps With ATFS and ADD

Tourette's Syndrome (TS) was first described in 1885 by a physician named Gilles de la Tourette. Articles did not appear in the medical literature until the sixties and seventies. It is not a common problem, so the correct diagnosis is easily missed.

At a medical conference about environmental illness Marshall Mandell, M.D., from Norwalk, Connecticut, presented some patients who had TS.[1] He discussed his study of children who had a combination of both TS and classical allergy. He found that some of these youngsters responded well to allergy treatment. These children are often seen by allergists because they complain about throat clearing, sniffling, and coughing as well as the typical signs and symptoms of Tourette's Syndrome (see Table 16.1).

It must be clearly stated, however, that most physicians do not believe that allergy is in any way related to TS. It appears, however, that when some children's allergic symptoms respond favorably to allergy treatment, their manifestations of TS are also simultaneously relieved (see Table 16.2).

TS symptoms are usually initially recognized between the ages of three and ten years. In retrospect, however, clues sometimes date back to early infancy. Various aspects of TS are sometimes evident in several relatives, suggesting a possible genetic or hereditary factor.

1. Marshall Mandell, M.D., *"Unsuspected Allergies Play a Major Role in Tourette's Syndrome."* Presented to the Society for Clinical Ecology, November 1984.

Table 16.1
Symptoms of Tourette's Syndrome (TS)

1. Twitchy face
2. Making faces
3. Facial tic
4. Eye rolling
5. Eye blinking
6. Neck snapping
7. Shoulder shrugging
8. Trunk arching
9. Arm twisting
10. Finger tapping
11. Leg swinging
12. Leg jerking
13. Jumping
14. Skipping
15. Touching
16. Kissing
17. Biting
18. Inappropriate laughter
19. Sniffling
20. Snorting
21. Throat clearing
22. Hissing
23. Blowing
24. Grunting (with eating)
25. Barking
26. Chicken sounds
27. Other strange sounds
28. Hearing problems
29. Hurting self
30. Poor concentration
31. Licking lips
32. Repetitive actions
33. Repeating own words (palilalia)
34. Repeating others' words (echolalia)
35. Vulgar speech

Symptoms of Allergic Tension Fatigue Syndrome (ATFS)

1. Excessive fatigue
2. Muscle aches
3. Headaches
4. Nose allergy
5. Eye allergy
6. Asthma
7. Allergic cough
8. Irritability
9. Destructiveness

10. Easy crying
11. Red earlobes
12. Dark eye circles
13. Glassy, glazed eyes
14. Red cheek patches
15. Excessive perspiration
16. Perspiration odor

Symptoms of Attention Deficit Hyperactivity Disorder (ADHD)

1. Hyperactivity
2. Short attention span
3. Restlessness
4. Poor concentration
5. Poor impulse control

Children who have TS usually have at least half of the medical complaints listed in Table 16.1.

The characteristics of TS are quite easy to miss unless the children have extreme bilateral eye blinking, make peculiar sounds, such as barking, or manifest unusual vulgarity. The diagnosis, however, can be made at times when these particular complaints are not evident.

There are similarities in the symptoms of children who have the Tourette's Syndrome (TS), allergic tension fatigue syndrome (ATFS), and attention deficit hyperactivity disorder (ADHD) (see Table 16.1). About 25 percent of children who have TS have been given stimulant medicine such as Ritalin because they were originally diagnosed as having ADHD.

However, if a child looks and acts allergic and has allergic relatives, plus the characteristics of either ADHD or TS, it is possible that the child has allergic tension fatigue syndrome (ATFS). It is possible to help relieve many of the combined TS and/or ADHD symptoms in some of these allergic children by using the newer, more comprehensive ecological methods of allergy treatment. This is true even though medically they may be classified as three distinct entities.

If parents become lax with their child's allergy diet, control of common allergy-causing home factors, or neglect to retest for known allergenic substances when indicated, any combination of the symptoms related to these three entities can recur. Fortunately, reinstitution of appropriate allergy care usually diminishes or eliminates the varied complaints quickly (see Table 16.2).

CHILD WITH TOURETTE'S SYNDROME AND ALLERGY

Edward

Edward was a clever, attractive, mischievous six-year-old when he was first seen in our office. Most of his relatives had allergies. Three close relatives had symptoms typical of Tourette's Syndrome.

His allergies began during infancy. He cried excessively every day from the age of two days until he was two years old. His mother sometimes had to put him in his room, go into her own room, shut the door, and put a pillow over her head because she needed to drown out his screaming.

Edward as an Infant

During infancy he had colic for nine full months. Milk caused diarrhea and screaming during the first three months of life, and after a switch to soy milk, although his diarrhea stopped, he continued to cry. He had dark eye circles, perspired excessively, and was overactive. He never crawled; instead he walked by the age of nine months. He had one ear infection after another from early infancy to the age of five years. Removing milk from everyone's diet proved that it had been a family problem. It appeared to have made his sister do reckless and dangerous things. It had caused his mother to develop a postnasal drip, fatigue, watery eyes, itchy skin, and difficulty thinking. Subsequent to the milk-free diet again as an infant, his diarrhea stopped. Subsequent to the milk-free diet again at age five, Edward no longer had ear infections.

Edward as a Toddler

As a toddler Eddie refused to wear clothes. As soon as his mother dressed him, he took his clothes off. His mother called him a "holy

TABLE 16.2
Edward's Response to Allergy Treatment
(Each fraction represents the number of
characteristic symptoms Edward had that were typical
of each of the medical problems listed in Table 16.1.)

| | Complaints Typical of: | | |
	TS	ATFS	ADHD
8/82 *Before* any allergy treatment (Retrospective score at time of diagnosis)	21/35	10/16	5/5
10/83 Scores *14 months after* TS diagnosis and allergy treatment	4/35	1/16	2/5
10/85 Scores *3 years after* TS diagnosis and allergy treatment	2/35	0/16	0/5
8/89 Scores *6 years after* TS diagnosis and allergy treatment	0/35	2/16	0/5

terror" because he was so active. He moved furniture faster than she could replace it. He would throw pillows and move chairs and coffee tables from the living room to the kitchen. He emptied the cupboards in much less time than it took his mother to replace the contents.

Edward as a Child

In kindergarten, however, his teacher complained because he made siren noises. By the first grade he barked, and the teacher joked that she wanted to give him a dog biscuit. His mother could hear him when he was a block away from their home because of the strange loud noises he made on the street.

As a child he had headaches and abdominal pain every night at bedtime. He had difficulty playing with his sister or the neighborhood children. By the age of seven or eight years he was always touching and kissing everybody. The other children at school harassed and intimidated him because he acted "different." By the age of nine he had typical hay fever plus the classical symptoms of the TS and ATFS.

He was such a distressing activity and behavior problem that his grammar school principal confided to me that it really didn't matter how he did on his exams. He was going to be passed so that he would attend a different school in the fall.

During his episodes of inappropriate Dr. Jekyll/Mr. Hyde behavior he often had glassy eyes and red ears. On one occasion when we were allergy testing for molds (because he tended to be worse on damp days), he threatened to urinate down his mother's leg. His behavior changes during allergy testing were often vulgar, most unusual, and at times spectacular. As soon as we found his treatment dosage, however, he would act in a subdued, appropriate manner, and his vulgarity totally disappeared.

Typical of TS, he tended to touch everything, twitch his face, flap his arms, blink, throw his head backward, bang objects, hide under the furniture, and bark, grunt, or make other strange noises. His mother said that he sometimes beat himself with the washcloth and pounded himself until he was bruised. He had episodes of extreme vulgarity in action, speech, and drawings. He had received the drug Haldol to treat his TS, but it did not help. While taking the drug, he was forced to stay indoors because ordinary sunlight hurt his eyes.

His TS behavior tended to be particularly evident in one certain school. Surprisingly his TS symptoms could be provoked repeatedly when he was skin-tested with a tiny drop of a special allergy extract prepared from the air in that school. Figures 16.1–16.3 show how this boy's writing became vulgar during an allergy skin test for his school air. He refused to draw at the peak of his reaction.

His TS symptoms routinely seemed worse after he had been in the school cafeteria. This was noted especially the day after the previous night's Bingo games had permeated that area with cigarette smoke and when he visited his grandfather's home, which also smelled strongly of tobacco.

On one occasion when he was seven years old, his personality suddenly changed after he ate an egg salad sandwich while he was attending a Baptist school. His mother was called to come to school immediately because he was in the midst of an especially vulgar episode. She brought him directly to our office, and when they arrived, he was very agitated. His ears were bright red and he was giddy and smiling as he inappropriately blurted out obscene phrases. We began

Drawing before allergy test	Writing during allergy test	Drawing after allergy test

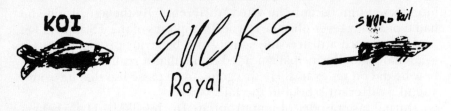

Pleasant and cooperative	Vulgar, overactive and aggressive; refused to draw	Pleasant and cooperative

Figures 16.1–16.3 Vulgarity in the writing of an eleven-year-old boy during testing with school air extract

to allergy-test for egg. He proceeded to spit, crawl under the furniture, bounce all over, hit the testing nurse, and continue to use foul language. During this reaction his mother struggled unsuccessfully to keep him from unzipping his pants as he bounced up and down on a sofa. As soon as he received his neutralization dose of egg allergy extract, he was quiet, polite, pleasant, and engrossed in reading about rockets in a *National Geographic* magazine.

His mother found that he improved about 50 percent after the Multiple Food Elimination Diet. When milk was put back into his diet at the age of six, he developed glassy eyes, hyperactivity, aggression, and irritability.

During the next few years all of his allergy and Tourette's symptoms were approximately 85 percent better if his room was kept allergy-free, he followed his diet, and he was treated with allergy extract. His mother always knew when he needed to have his allergy treatment adjusted because he would again begin to bark like a puppy, blink, make blowing noises, and move in a jerky manner. Initially, even with his milk allergy extract treatment, he could not drink milk because his undesirable symptoms reappeared. At the present time, however, milk does not cause difficulty, providing he continues to receive his milk allergy extract treatment.

On one occasion when he was disturbed after a change in schools, he began to jerk his head back and bang it on the furniture. His mother became distraught and didn't know what to do. She said he was "driving her nuts." She was surprised and pleased when ten minutes after his allergy treatment made from the air in that school, he was normal again. This episode could easily have been attributed solely to an emotional upset. The rapid favorable and complete change that repeatedly occurred after his allergy extract treatment, however, suggests that he probably was manifesting an unusual and undesirable allergic reaction to something in the air in that school.

When his mother related his improvement with allergy treatment to the local Tourette Society, they did not believe her. She said the doctor and other mothers seemed disinterested. Amazingly they did not want to hear why or how her son's TS symptoms had improved.

Table 16.1 shows the typical characteristics associated with Tourette's Syndrome (TS), allergic tension fatigue syndrome (ATFS), and attention deficit disorder (ADD). Table 16.2 clearly illustrates how his symptoms in each category changed from the time he initially saw us at the age of seven years until the present time at the age of sixteen years.

Eddie's school grades improved remarkably after treatment. He was naturally an unusually bright youngster, but prior to treatment his scholastic achievement was never on a par with his ability. Before treatment he simply could not sit still long enough to concentrate or learn.

Edward as an Adolescent

When Eddie was sixteen, he returned to our office because he was fatigued and had difficulty reading. He had not had any form of allergy treatment for two years.

While we were retesting for his mold allergy, he tried to do his homework. During the testing he was surprised because he said he could read with less difficulty and for longer periods of time.

This type of observation obviously needs more validation, but if molds affect our vision, could this mean that visits for eye examinations for certain sensitive individuals should not take place on damp days or in moldy, chemically contaminated offices? (See Chapter 3.) Could textbooks that smell moldy or dusty create visually related learning problems for some allergic children? There is much we do not know.

In Summary

Edward initially had only the ATFS, but as time passed, he developed classical TS as well as ADD symptoms. Allergy treatment repeatedly relieved many of the symptoms characteristic of each category. One cannot generalize about how many other TS patients might respond similarly, but it certainly appears that some TS children might benefit from comprehensive environmental and allergy treatment.

We also cannot predict Edward's future. He is at a critical age and we must hope that he does not falter as others have done as he exerts his adolescent independence. We believe he must maintain his diet, keep his room environmentally sound, and keep his allergy extract updated because his past history indicates that he has so many typical and unusual forms of allergy.

CHAPTER 17

Is Ritalin Necessary?

Ritalin (methylphenidate) is a drug that is used mainly to quiet hyperactive children, who are impulsive, inattentive, easily distracted, and unable to concentrate. It is usually prescribed for children who have attention deficit disorder (ADD), which is called ADHD if it is associated with hyperactivity. There are almost one million children receiving Ritalin (or similar activity-modifying drugs such as Cylert) in this country. Twenty-five percent or more of students in special classes are placed on Ritalin in certain areas of this country. The use of this drug has increased by 25 percent in the past five years.

There is no doubt that Ritalin quiets innumerable children in many classrooms and homes. The question is not so much whether Ritalin helps, but rather is it necessary? What are the problems and potential dangers associated with its use? Do parents have other alternatives that might help as much and be safer? Parents and educators must be aware that Ritalin is _not_ the only or the best way to quiet some unruly, inattentive children.

One study that I did in 1978 indicated that about 65 percent of hyperactive children on Ritalin can be helped by appropriate diets and allergy extract therapy without the use of any pills or drugs.[1] Others can be helped with substances that naturally quiet the brain when individuals are agitated or distressed. If the kitchen faucet

1. Doris Rapp, M.D., "Does Diet Affect Hyperactivity?" _Journal of Learning Disabilities_ 11 (1978), pp. 56–62.

leaks, we don't call for a demolition crew. If pills must be tried, milder and safer ones should be considered first. Medications might not be necessary if the cause of the hyperactivity can be found and eliminated.

What Are the Indications for
Prescribing Ritalin for a Child?

Physicians make the diagnosis of ADD after a thorough history and physical examination. Then they frequently prescribe Ritalin if certain medical criteria are met. The criteria listed below should have been noted before the age of seven years and *should be evident considerably more frequently* than in most children of the same mental age. Of course, many children normally manifest these characteristics at times.

According to the *Diagnostic Manual of Mental Disorders* (DSM-III-R), children who have attention deficit hyperactivity disorder (ADHD) should have manifested at least eight of the following symptoms for at least six months:

- fidgety hands and feet;
- difficulty staying in their seat;
- easily distracted by things around them;
- difficulty waiting for their turn in games or activities;
- blurting out answers before questions are completed;
- inability to stick with a task or play activity;
- difficulty playing quietly;
- frequent excessive talking;
- interrupting or intruding in the activity of others;
- switching from one uncompleted activity to another;
- inability to follow through with simple instructions or chores;
- not listening when spoken to;
- losing or misplacing toys, books, assignments, and so on;
- doing physically dangerous things, such as running into the street without looking.

According to the *Physicians' Desk Reference* (PDR), used to inform doctors about exactly how and when to use most drugs, Ritalin is *"not intended for use in the child who exhibits symptoms secondary to environmental factors."* I wonder how many general practitioners, psychiatrists, pediatricians, neurologists, psychologists, teachers, or parents are aware that foods, pollen, molds, dust, mites, pets, and chemical pollution are all clearly environmental factors. Any of these can cause some children to become hyperactive, inattentive, and impulsive. If each of these factors is not considered, many children can be needlessly placed on this drug.

According to the *Physicians' Desk Reference,* Ritalin should not be prescribed for any child under the age of six years, or children who have epilepsy, nervous tics, psychoses, normal fatigue, or in families in which members have Tourette's Syndrome. It should be used with caution if there is a history of seizures or if the drug causes visual disturbances.

What's Good About Ritalin?

Ritalin is said to calm many, but certainly not all, learning-disabled ADHD children so that they can sit still, concentrate, and behave better in school. There is no proof that it improves academic performance or reading.[2] In one study, educational intervention alone was found to be as successful as or superior to any program using Ritalin. When this drug is helpful, busy parents who work and teachers who have overcrowded classrooms are grateful. Ritalin is easy to administer to a child and requires little or no change in a family's life-style.

What's Bad About Ritalin?

Most drugs have side effects, and some of the major problems noted in some children who use Ritalin are as listed below. For a detailed list of hazardous side effects with multiple references, see Dr. Richard Scarnati's article.[3]

- Loss of normal appetite with a subsequent decrease in normal growth.
- Better behavior in school, but when the drug wears off, parents

2. Gerald Coles, *The Learning Mystique* (see Bibliography).
3. Richard Scarnati, D.O., An "Outline of Hazardous Side Effects of Ritalin (Methylphenidate)," *The International Journal of the Addictions* 21(7) (1986), pp. 837–841.

often notice their child can become much more active and difficult to control than usual; this is often noted after school.

- Intestinal complaints.
- Drowsiness, loss of personality (a few become zombies).

Less common complaints include:

- rapid heartbeat;
- depression, mood changes; anxiety, tension or agitation;
- hyperactivity (caused by the dye on the tablets—the generic form, which is not colored, is called Goldline Methylphenidate.

The long-term effects of this drug in children are, surprisingly, not well established. This should be of concern because almost a million children are presently taking Ritalin.

Ritalin is a Class-2 controlled substance, listed in the same category as cocaine, codeine, morphine, and amphetamines. Class 2 drugs can cause some children to develop a tolerance. This means that 5 or 10 milligrams might be enough to quiet your child now, but as time passes, your child may need larger and larger doses to produce the same quieting effect. I saw one teenager who needed 120 milligrams a day to control his activity. He was finally able to discontinue his Ritalin medication entirely after he simply eliminated dyes and sugar from his diet.

A campaign of radio and television public education, led mainly by Dennis Clarke of CCHR (Citizens Commission on Human Rights), has repeatedly informed the public about the multiple potential dangers of this drug. Their research, for example, shared little-known information about the present major street drug problem in certain Canadian cities, in which abusers are combining Ritalin and a commonly used pain-killer drug.

Ritalin is addictive, according to the criteria in the DMS-III-R used by the American Psychiatric Association. This means that, similar to a drug addict on heroin or a cigarette smoker, it is not easy to stop. The manufacturer of Ritalin, Ciba-Geigy, claims it is not addictive if used as directed. The *Physicians' Desk Reference,* however, used by most doctors to explain more about drugs, definitely states that it is addictive. Addictive drugs cause withdrawal symptoms when they are not taken on a regular basis. If Ritalin is stopped too quickly, or sometimes even if it is gradually decreased and stopped, it is possible that this drug can cause fatigue, disturbed sleep, depression, Tourette's Syndrome, psychosis, or suicide.

In our office we often see children whose parents do not want their children given a narcoticlike drug. We also see some who were not helped when the drug was given, or who cannot tolerate Ritalin because of some undesirable side effects. The following patient clearly demonstrates how dangerous this drug can be for some youngsters. (See Charles in Appendix E.)

Severe Depression in a Child Using Ritalin

Paul

Paul's mother had been advised to see a doctor for his hyperactivity within three days after he started kindergarten. He was already "too much" for his frantic teacher. His mother was not surprised. Paul had exhausted his entire family for years. He never slept. He would grab an umbrella and jump off the staircase with it. He was known to roller-skate through the living room at 3:00 A.M. He was so out of control that he drove his mother "crazy." When she complained to the doctor, she was told that "she would have to accept Paul the way he was."

A neurologist saw Paul and started him on Ritalin even though he was only five years of age. He remained on the drug for about fifteen months. His parents said they were told "not to read about the drug or believe anything about side effects because it was not true." They were reluctant to start the drug, but more than one doctor had suggested that Paul really needed Ritalin.

The first dose of Ritalin made him act very quiet and a little depressed, but his parents were assured that he would be all right in a little while. The school psychologist saw him three times a week for a year. She was concerned because Paul would go out onto the playground and just stare at the other children. She suggested that the drug be stopped, but the doctor told his parents to continue it. His mother repeatedly noticed that fifteen minutes after he took the pill, he became silly and active. Then he acted very withdrawn and quiet, and this was followed by overwhelming sadness.

By the time he was in the first grade, his teacher noticed that Paul was different from the other children who were on Ritalin. His teacher was concerned because he became very withdrawn, acted like a zombie, and *never* smiled anymore. Before Paul started Ritalin, he was a happy, spirited, but uncontrollably exuberant boy.

It did not seem possible to his parents, but he seemed to be worse on Ritalin. It relieved his overactivity and enabled him to sleep, but at times he refused to eat or drink. The school nurse said she could barely get him to drink enough water to swallow his Ritalin tablet. He gradually became more and more moody, nasty, and very depressed. In contrast to the jovial, playful boy he was before, he had developed a totally different personality. Now when he came home from school, he angrily went directly to his room. He slammed his door and told everyone to leave him alone. He stopped laughing, smiling, and playing. Every day he complained that no one liked him and repeatedly said, "Everyone hates me." He had no friends. He had to be forced to get on the school bus every morning because the other children pushed him in the aisle, refused to let him sit next to them, and made fun of him.

He repeatedly told his mother he wished he could go to heaven because he'd be happy up there. Each week he asked his parents, if people killed themselves, could they go to heaven? At night when he said his prayers, he would beg God to please let him die before morning so that he could go to heaven and be happy. He routinely cried himself to sleep each night. His mother admitted she also had a nightly cry because she was so worried about what might happen to him. She felt she was such a poor mother that on one occasion she was ready to "give him up because she felt she wasn't good enough to raise him." When she informed her pediatrician about Paul's depression, she was told to continue the drug.

On two occasions he tried to kill himself. The first time he took the screen off the bedroom window and tried to jump out. The second time it was shortly after his mother decided to stop the Ritalin because Paul's problems might be an allergy.

His mother reported that she had checked with Paul's neurologist and was assured that an instant, complete withdrawal of the drug could not harm Paul because Ritalin "was not addictive." After all, he was only receiving 10 milligrams of Ritalin a day. Two weeks after stopping Ritalin, however, he became hysterical. He was crying and kicking his feet. When his mother checked his room, he was holding a pillow over his head as tightly as he could. As he tried to suffocate himself, he kept repeating, "I wish I was dead, I wish I was dead."

Paul in the Uterus

Similar to many other allergic children, Paul's problems did not suddenly begin the day he started kindergarten. He was hyperactive in the uterus, hiccupping all day and kicking so hard and so early that even the obstetrician was surprised. His mother's ribs were bruised, and she said it hurt to breathe. His father could not sleep next to his mother because Paul's kicking in the uterus woke him up. During the pregnancy, his mother said, she ate an excessive amount of dairy products. Unfortunately Paul was six years old before his sensitivity to milk was discovered. Could the milk Paul's mother drank have caused her unborn baby's distress? This is certainly a possibility.

Paul as an Infant

As an infant Paul continued to be hyperactive and at times acted like a "maniac." He walked at nine months, ran by ten months. He never slept more than an hour at a stretch. When he was awake, he cried and screamed constantly. He rocked his crib in excess. He had extreme colic, which lasted the entire first year of life. He spit up excessively and vomited so much and so hard that surgery was considered. He vomited his milk, soy, and baby formulas that contained corn. He needed to be rocked, walked, and bounced. He often had raw, bleeding buttocks. He had bags under his eyes and extremely dark eye circles.

By ten months his behavior became impossible. This happened shortly after he began to drink cow's milk. Paul's mother begged her pediatrician unsuccessfully for help. Paul was so active that she had to restrain him in a harness. By the age of one year he was aggressive and kicking everything. His infancy was not what a mother would fantasize. It was a most difficult, unpleasant period in both Paul's and his mother's life.

At two months he had his first ear infection. By the age of six years he had had surgery for ear tubes four times, and his tonsils and adenoids had been removed. This history is typical of certain milk-sensitive children. In retrospect we must wonder if any of these surgeries could have been prevented if his milk sensitivity had been recognized earlier.

Paul as a Toddler

As a toddler Paul was destructive. He spilled the contents of jars and bottles on the floor, put holes through walls, ruined furniture, ran into walls, jumped off banisters, smeared his bowel movements on the walls, and kicked the dog. By the age of three years he had year-round hay fever, and contact with grass caused a rash. No one, not even his grandparents, wanted to baby-sit with him.

Paul as a Young Child

When Paul was about the age of four, his mother was told by a psychologist that Paul was intelligent and *not* hyperactive. She was told that his behavior problems were *her* fault because he was not disciplined correctly and she let Paul manipulate her.

As a small child he hit, kicked, and punched not only his sister but also his father. Paul frequently had red earlobes, red cheeks, puffy eyes, and wiggly legs. He complained about frequent bellyaches, nausea, and sometimes had diarrhea. Peanut butter in particular caused this problem. He ate fish on one occasion and his eyes swelled shut and he could hardly breathe.

By the age of six he "leaked" urine in his pants everyday and at times created an embarrassingly large wet area on his pants in school or a large puddle on the floor because he could not wait to get to the bathroom. He wet his bed about two to three times a week. Shortly after he began his allergy treatment, these urinary problems subsided completely. Later on we found that he seemed to have allergic spasm of his bladder rather than his lungs. His mother repeatedly noticed that whenever he ate sugar, he would wet his pants and wet his bed that night.

Prior to his allergy treatment he perspired excessively during the day and at night, and it was not unusual for his bedclothes and sheets to be totally wet in the morning.

He never slept through the night until he was almost five years old, and he was always up before dawn. His headaches were so frequent that he needed Tylenol daily for a year.

His family felt like prisoners. Paul's behavior was so bad that they could not take him anyplace. They were fearful of leaving him with a baby-sitter, if they could find one who would tolerate his behavior. One teacher confided to his parents that he was "hated by every child in the class." Paul laughed uncontrollably in school, could never sit still, and either did not play at all or "drove the other children crazy." His mother noticed that dyed antihistamines and the odors in science class made him wild.

Even though Paul was very young, he was well aware that children did not want to be with him. He never let his father or siblings hug or kiss him. He destroyed his and their toys and could not play nicely with anything or anybody.

There was no doubt that this little boy had many allergies and a wide range of emotional problems. Few would realize that these could be secondary to his allergies and not vice versa. He had suffered for years because his classical and unusual forms of allergy were not recognized and appropriately treated. His mother had asked her pediatrician about allergies at one time and was told not to waste her money. In spite of that advice, she took him to a board-certified allergist when he was six years old but was assured that diets were not helpful in treating hyperactivity. The doctor said his behavior was unrelated to allergy or foods. He also told Paul's mother, "He'll have to be put away someday," and "He'll never have any friends." One pediatrician and one school psychologist said that he was learning-disabled. His kindergarten teacher said that in spite of his innate superior intelligence, he was unable to learn or perform at a level comparable to his ability.

Paul's Life Changes

The turning point in this six-and-a-half-year-old child's life occurred after his parents saw the 1987 *Donahue* show. They cried tears of joy and relief as they saw the program that showed a hyperactive child "just like Paul." They immediately began the Multiple Food Elimination Diet, and within two days he was 80 percent better. Within a week he was suddenly transformed back to a happy but normally quiet child. They knew they had found the right answers when his teacher commented that she was pleased because she saw Paul smile. That teacher had never seen him smile before!

When his allergies were detected and he no longer needed Ritalin, he repeatedly asked, "Am I a good boy now?" The final confirmation of his improvement was dramatic and heartrending. He came home and rang his own doorbell. His mother opened the door and there was Paul, all smiles, tightly clutching a little boy's hand. Bursting with happiness he said, "Mommy, I have a friend."

After P/N testing and two days of allergy extract therapy for foods and other common allergens, he was 80 percent better, and after two years of allergy extract treatment he is 95 percent better. He is happy, affectionate, lovable, polite, and has friends. He now acts like other children. He no longer has headaches, abdominal complaints, problems urinating, insomnia, aggression, or destructive tendencies. He can sit still, carry on a conversation, and go places with his family without difficulty. He is even so considerate and cooperative that he asks if he can help with simple chores about the house.

Yes, he occasionally regresses, but his parents know exactly why. When he goes into a store that smells of polyester clothing, he lies on the floor, cries, and fusses like a two-year-old. His parents recognize that the cause is most likely the chemical odor of formaldehyde in the polyester clothing. They know that he will be fine when he is no longer near that smell.

He no longer has difficulty concentrating and has been doing very well scholastically and socially in school. His present teachers are totally unaware that he was ever a problem in the classroom. His parents are grateful that their child, who was previously ill and truly impossible, is presently a simply wonderful friendly, healthy youngster.

We videotaped Paul while we monitored his brain waves and blood both before and during allergy testing for a sensitivity to grass. Changes occurred in his brain waves and blood during his reaction to the grass test that were not evident before the test or during the placebo test period.

His brain waves during his reaction to grass appeared to reflect what was seen clinically during the grass test. There were significant changes, mainly in the forehead and temple areas. These changes occurred at the same time that he became fidgety, cried, fussed, wiggled, and complained that his head hurt. After his grass-allergy extract neutralization treatment, the brain waves changed again, returning toward the levels noted during the baseline and placebo periods. His pulse also increased when he reacted to the grass and then returned to normal.

During this pilot study his blood showed changes in certain critical amino acids needed for the transmission of nerve impulses through the brain. In particular, the levels of critical amino acids that produce acetylcholine, a major neurotransmitter, were altered.[4]

Should Schools Insist That Children Receive Ritalin?

Schools certainly have the right to say that a student cannot remain in a certain school setting because of that pupil's inappropriate behavior or activity. It seems incomprehensible and wholly inappropriate, however, for any school personnel to state that any child cannot return to school unless Ritalin is taken by the child. This drug can be dangerous, and as Paul's case clearly demonstrates, in spite of repeated evidence that this drug was harmful to his health, his parents were told to continue it. Educators and parents must be aware of alternative methods for helping hyperactive children.

4. The above study was done in conjunction with David Cantor, Ph.D., a psychologist associated with the University of Maryland School of Medicine. J. Alexander Bralley, Ph.D., at Metametrix Laboratory, in Norcross, Ga., kindly interpreted the amino acid data.

What Alternatives to Ritalin Are Available?

As indicated in this chapter, some hyperactive children can be helped by diets and appropriate allergy treatment. Studies done in 1978[5] and 1985[6] indicate that about two-thirds of hyperactive children respond to the diet. Shouldn't a simple two-week diet be tried first, before a narcoticlike drug?

Leo Galland, M.D., in New York City, and David Horriben in Nova Scotia, believe that some hyperactive children can gradually stop Ritalin after their diet is enriched with essential fatty acids.[7]

Mary Coleman, M.D., Ph.D., found serotonin, a brain chemical, to be abnormally low in hyperactive children. She found that vitamin B_6 could raise serotonin levels. This increase was associated with less hyperactivity in some children.[8]

Natural Products for Hyperactivity, Anxiety, and Sugar Craving

Billie Sahley, Ph.D., is a psychotherapist and orthomolecular nutritional specialist. She is the director of the Pain and Stress Center located in San Antonio, Texas. She has written educational material to help parents of children who are unable to cope normally at home or at school because they are too tense, nervous, passive, or overactive.[9]

Dr. Sahley helped design a number of preparations to quiet children and enable them to learn more effectively. They do not contain common allergenic components such as corn, yeast, dyes, sugar, soy, wheat, or caffeine. Some of her preparations can be tried as an alternative for the strong addictive drugs Ritalin or Cylert. See Table 17.1 for a number of natural preparations that Dr. Sahley has suggested to help reduce pain, stress, hyperactivity, depression, and the consumption of sugar.

5. Doris J. Rapp, M.D., "Does Diet Affect Hyperactivity?" (see Bibliography).
6. Joseph Egger, M.D., et al., "Controlled Trial of Oligoantigenic Treatment in the Hyperkinetic Syndrome," *Lancet* 1: (1985); pp. 540–545.
7. Leo Galland, M.D., and Diane Buchman, Ph.D., *Superimmunity for Kids* (New York: E. P. Dutton, 1989).
8. Mary Coleman, Ph.D. "Physiology and the Neurosciences," editorial, *Biological Psychiatry* 14 (1979): 1–2.
9. See Bibliography.

TABLE 17.1
"Natural" Aids Recommended by Dr. Sahley*

Name of Nutrient	Content of Nutrient		Use
For hyperactivity—instead of Ritalin, try:			
Calms Kids—6 capsules contain:	GABA	800 mg	To help hyperactive children by restoring their biochemical balance or homeostasis.
	Tryptophan extract	800 mg	
	Glycine	500 mg	
	Vitamin B$_6$	50 mg	
	L-Taurine	500 mg	
	Calcium	100 mg	
	Magnesium	50 mg	
	Ester C (long-acting vitamin)	60 mg	
For anxiety or headache:			
SAF—4 capsules contain:	GABA	650 mg	Helps balance the body's own chemistry to aid with relief of stress and anxiety.
	L-Tyrosine	650 mg	
	Siberian ginseng	100 mg	
	Inositol	100 mg	
	Vitamin C	100 mg	
	Vitamin B$_1$	3 mg	
	Vitamin B$_2$	3.1 mg	
	Niacin	50 mg	
	Vitamin B$_6$	4 mg	
	Magnesium	100 mg	
For pain: DLPA	750 mg of a 50/50 mixture of a D- and L-phenylalanine		Helps acute and chronic pain.

For anxiety:

GABA 750	750 mg of GABA, an amino acid	Beneficial for anxiety or muscle tension. Most effective if the capsule is opened and the contents are mixed with 1/2 cup water before drinking.

For sugar craving:

1. Gymnema sylvestre	Gymnema sylvestre, an ancient Indian herb (known to the Hindus as Guramal, or "sugar killer")	Impedes the absorption of a certain amount of the sugar or carbohydrates you eat, allowing only some to pass through the body unused.
2. Glycine	500 mg glycine, the simplest nonessential amino acid, so called because it resembles the sweet taste of glucose and glucogen	Open the capsule and put a small amount on the tongue. It is said to decrease sugar craving.
3. L-Glutamine	500 mg of L-Glutamine, an amino acid	Also used in the past for craving of sweets.

*All "Natural" Sahley Aids are available through: The Pain and Stress Therapy Center, 5282 Medical Drive, San Antonio, Tex. 78229 (512–696–1870).

As Dr. Sahley has frequently stated, these children's brains are not malfunctioning because they have a Ritalin deficiency. She states that certain amino acids can help to restore a normal biochemical balance within the brain. Amino acids literally are brain food. These are essential to make neurotransmitters, which allow the brain cells to communicate with one another and the rest of the body. There are a number of amino acids that tend to quiet the brain. Most individuals normally increase their production of calming types of amino acids during periods of stress or anxiety. Certain amino acids such as tryptophan, taurine, GABA (gamma amino butyric acid), and glycine slow or inhibit excessively excitatory brain impulses and help to reestablish a normal, balanced state within the brain. All these ingredients are found in Calms Kids, which appeared to be helpful for some hyperactive children.

This nutrient preparation has helped some hyperactive children aged four to fifteen years who cannot learn or who cannot behave appropriately. Sometimes it helps within seventy-two hours. The usual dose is the contents of one to two capsules three times a day. Let's look at each component separately.

Tryptophan

To date, unfortunately, no comprehensive published scientific studies have been conducted in relation to the effectiveness of tryptophan to treat hyperactivity. In 1990, this substance was temporarily removed from the market because one shipment of the drug was accidentally contaminated by a toxic substance. Tryptophan was subsequently released again for sale when it was proven that it was not the cause of a well-publicized toxin-related illness. (See Chapter 27.)

Tryptophan is an essential amino acid that helps maintain the protein balance within the body. It is known to promote sleep and decrease depression. Tryptophan is needed to produce serotonin, a neurotransmitter that helps control our moods or disposition. To help convert tryptophan into serotonin, the body also needs vitamin B_6, or pyridoxine. Ritalin also raises the serotonin level, but tryptophan is thought to do it more gently, slowly, and naturally. Sources of tryptophan include dairy products, wheat germ, and avocado. Unfortunately many hyperactive or allergic children seem to be sensitive to milk and dairy products, so this source of natural tryptophan can be limited in some allergic children's diets.

GABA

The second amino acid in Calms Kids is GABA, which tends to slow down the excitatory or stimulating chemical messages sent from cell to cell within the brain. GABA is thought to fill the receptor sites in the brain so that anxiety and stress-related messages do not overwhelm the thinking portion of the brain. GABA acts like a natural tranquilizer but does not cause the user to become too sleepy or tired. In essence it reduces anxiety. It is thought to help hyperactive children, as well as those who are too tired and passive.

Taurine

Taurine is another neurotransmitter needed for normal brain function. This amino acid also inhibits or quiets the brain in such a way that it appears to act as another natural tranquilizer and sedative. It supposedly helps to control hyperactivity and excessive body movements. This amino acid requires a supply of both zinc and manganese.

Glycine

Glycine is thought to help balance and soften dramatic mood swings, which can vary from unusual highs to extreme lows. It can act as a sedative. Combined with inositol, a substance found in some vitamins, glycine is thought to decrease aggression.

Vitamin C

This vitamin is also said to have a calming effect on children.

Magnesium and Calcium

Magnesium and calcium are two minerals that are included in Calms Kids because they are both thought to quiet the brain and central nervous system. Magnesium deficiencies can be associated with twitching, tremors, apprehension, irritability, noise sensitivity, confusion, and disorientation. Calcium deficiencies are known to cause irritability, sleep problems, anger, inattentive behavior, stomach upsets, cramps, and tingling in the legs and arms. In general, it is urged that these minerals be taken at least four hours before or after vitamins so that there is less competition for absorption.

What Does Paul's Medical History Illustrate?

Paul's basic allergy history is similar in many ways to that of innumerable other hyperactive children. He had an abundance of evidence indicating that he had typical, as well as many of the less frequently recognized forms of allergy, from infancy throughout early childhood. Unlike many other children, however, he was placed on Ritalin in an effort to control his hyperactivity, behavior, and learning problems. While he was on this drug, and shortly after it was withdrawn, he became depressed and suicidal. His many physical, emotional, social, and learning problems persisted until his allergies were detected and appropriately treated at the age of six and a half years. Brain-wave and blood tests all confirmed that changes did occur during single-blinded grass allergy tests that were not present before the test or during a placebo challenge period. These results suggest that provocation/neutralization allergy testing with a grass pollen allergy extract can alter Paul's brain function and cause immunological changes in his blood. He illustrates what we have seen so often. Children who become hyperactive after exposure to grass sometimes have an allergy affecting their brain. Paul's entire family suffered greatly for a long time because his brain allergy and other forms of allergies were neither recognized nor acknowledged earlier.

CHAPTER 18

Aggression in Children
Due to Allergy

MOTHER BATTERING

Kari

Some youngsters appear to be amazingly aggressive at a very early age. Kari was almost four years old when her distressed parents came to see us. Every morning started with a fight. She always woke up unhappy and unpleasant. The first words of the day were "I hate you." She would start her day by trying to kick her mother in the stomach. She would bite or scratch her until she drew blood. She used two hands to slap, batter, dig into, and bruise her mother. She punched, hit, kicked, and slammed doors. She routinely refused to put on her clothing, and by the time her mother had her left sock on, the right was already removed. Every day both Kari and her mother were in tears by the time Kari left for day care.

At times Kari would crawl into a dark corner, become very negative, act withdrawn, and absolutely refuse to be touched. Sometimes she would scream at the top of her lungs for as long as ninety minutes. She would growl, snarl, grind her teeth, claw, and throw herself at doors. She would attack her mother with such explosive violence that her mother was truly frightened. One parent alone could not contain this child. It was not unusual for two people to hold her down when she was having a tantrum so that she would not hurt herself or others. These episodes could occur five or six times a day, and some lasted for several days. She did inexplicable things, such as urinating in her sneaker. Her mother felt guilty and ashamed because she justifiably dreaded the time when Kari would awaken each morning and again when she would return from day care.

Kari's mother had no idea what was causing her attractive little girl to be so challenging to raise until her physician grandfather suggested the possibility of allergy. He had seen a movie at a medical conference during my presentation of a hyperactive child who seemed strikingly similar to Kari. Kari's mother knew there were many relatives who had typical allergies, but only a few family members were hyperactive. Some had depression or wide mood swings, but none had the vast range and degree of personality and physical problems that were so frequently and painfully evident in Kari.

Kari's Response to P/N Allergy Treatment

When we first saw four-year-old Kari, her favorite words were "Nobody likes me." Within two weeks after her initial P/N allergy testing and treatment for yeast, grass, and a number of foods, it was obvious that she had improved significantly. She even awoke smiling and dressed herself without getting angry. She increasingly displayed intermittent periods of unbelievably pleasant and calm behavior. Her mother was very encouraged. Shortly after treatment she even slept one night for twelve hours without awakening.

After two and a half years of our comprehensive approach to allergies and P/N treatment, she continued to be approximately 85 percent better.

Most children probably will not have as many problems as Kari had, but some of the challenges related to raising Kari may have been similarly experienced by other desperate parents. This child's history is typical of many aggressive children. Her history is discussed in some detail so that you can possibly recognize if unsuspected clues relating to allergies could be a part of your child's special behavior problem.

Kari as an Infant

When she was only a day old, Kari did not sleep well. As an infant she was fussy, active, and moving. Her grandfather first suspected that she was hyperactive at the age of three months. She could not be cuddled; she had to be bounced. She was rocking her crib all over the room at eight months of age. Once when she was nine months old, she kicked her mother so hard during a diaper change that her mother could barely breathe. Kari's buttocks frequently looked as if they had been scalded in hot water. At ten months she had to be restrained or physically held down or she bounced all over the car.

At fourteen months she climbed so well that she crawled out of her crib, opened a locked window, knocked out the screen, and was hanging precariously out of the window when her mother rescued her.

Kari as a Young Child

Starting at the age of three years, she had a headache once or twice a week. Her mother had already noted the characteristic red earlobes, red cheeks, glassy look in the eyes, and wiggly legs. At that time she did not realize that these were typical clues of unrecognized allergies which might also indicate that her daughter's brain was being affected.

By the age of three and a half years she had classical nose allergies. She had a runny nose and frequent throat clearing. She sneezed not once, but several times in a row, and tended to pick her nose.

Kari's Life Changes

The turning point in Kari's life occurred when she was almost four years old. Her grandfather suggested that Kari be placed on our Multiple Food Elimination Diet. She improved tremendously within one week. Her Conner's Hyperactivity Score (see Glossary) fell from an extremely abnormal high of 27 before the diet to a normal 9 within one week. Her crying significantly decreased. She no longer raced wildly from room to room. She offered to help her mother set the table. She sat through an entire meal and even used a knife, fork, and napkin without fighting. She allowed her mother to brush and comb her lovely red hair. She spoke more clearly and colored neatly in her picture book. She sat still and enjoyed listening when her mother read her a book. For the first time she was attentive and seemed to hear and understand what was being said.

During the second week of the diet, when she was purposely given milk for the first time in seven days, it definitely made her hyperactive. This reaction lasted for four full days! It is no wonder that she never felt or acted well. Chocolate made her nasty, violent, and extremely unhappy. Food coloring caused insomnia. Eggs caused her to cry and become argumentative. Later on it was obvious that potatoes caused a total personality change so that she hid in a corner and could not be held, touched, or consoled. Mold testing caused dramatic changes in her disposition and behavior.

After three months of treatment Kari was not perfect. She still had periods when she was demanding, crying, arguing, and unable to sleep. Her parents, however, were beginning to recognize an increasing number of specific items that were related to certain radical changes in her mood and behavior. More and more often she had precious periods when she would be demonstrably affectionate. She stopped arguing about every *no*. She woke up in the morning without a fuss. She left her clothes on for longer periods of time. Her attention span was much longer. She would eat from her own plate. She helped to keep her room neater. She would, surprisingly, get in and out of the car without creating a family crisis. She minded her parents. She could even entertain herself. She stopped her extreme clinging and whining. For the first time, and for longer periods of time, she seemed happy and content to be with her mother.

Hypoglycemia Was Also a Problem

In addition to the typical complaints of allergic children, Kari's mother related clues that suggested that Kari had possible hypoglycemia or low blood sugar. When she was hungry, which was almost constantly, she did not ask for food, she demanded it. Her blood sugar was definitely too low—56 mg/dl—on one occasion when she acted very hungry, irritable, and whiny in our office. Hypoglycemic symptoms indicated that her brain needed glucose or sugar. These types of complaints were particularly evident at about 11:00 A.M. and again between 3:00 and 4:00 P.M., when the blood sugar tends to drop because no foods have been eaten for several hours. Kari's personality routinely improved quickly and dramatically as soon as she was fed.

Her glucose tolerance test, however, failed to confirm that this was a problem for her. We see this frequently, for some perplexing reason, in our office, (see Chapter 3). If such children are fed every two hours, however, their disposition sometimes improves significantly. The answer, of course, is to continue to feed them nonsweet foods at frequent intervals. As time passed, Kari's inordinate craving for food stopped after she responded to our allergy treatment. After children who demand constant food respond favorably to a total ecologic-allergy approach of treatment, we often find that both their excessive need for food and their hypoglycemia tend to disappear.

Odors Affect Kari

On one occasion her mother found that the odor of a scented aerosol used in a commercial airplane caused Kari to suddenly scream violently and develop a red body rash. Kari crawled under a seat and screamed constantly for thirty minutes. Her behavior was extremely upsetting for everyone. Only her mother understood exactly why Kari acted this way. Knowing what caused her daughter's personality change made Kari's outbursts more tolerable. There was no longer any need to blame anyone or to become angry or disappointed with either Kari or herself.

When Kari was five years old, her mother tried a natural, unscented shampoo. It was the first time in her life that Kari allowed her hair to be washed without creating a furor. After some causes of allergies are eliminated or treated, many children can tolerate exposures to known offending items with much less or no difficulty.

Greater understanding sometimes relieves very stressful problems and helps tremendously. Parents have no difficulty being sympathetic and caring when a child has allergies causing wheezing in the lungs. When allergies affect the brain, however, it is quite a different matter. Once her parents understood why Kari acted as she did, it was possible to endure more patiently their child's alarming, exasperating, and frightening responses to allergenic substances or offending odors.

In contrast to most children, Kari initially needed frequent office visits for retesting. However, after two years, she was seen only twice a year. In time we ascertained that she responded well to either sublingual or injection treatment of allergy extract. For obvious reasons, most children and parents prefer sublingual therapy.

Some parents might ask why Kari seemed to hit her mother so much and so often. This is an inordinately frequent complaint in my practice. "Mother battering" is immensely common in allergic families but is not the type of thing most mothers would complain about. Children often feel most secure "letting it all out" in front of their mothers. Mothers tend to tolerate much more inappropriate behavior than fathers. Mothers often have to set limits and decide about disciplinary action while fathers are at work. Kari's father's response to his daughter was to quickly give Kari whatever she wanted so she would not create a family furor.

We suggested behavioral counseling shortly after we initially saw Kari because so many of her responses to normal daily activities such as getting up, dressing, washing, eating, and even taking a ride in a car were so extremely negative and unacceptable. Her parents needed immediate help to cope with her actions until she had time to respond to our allergy treatment. There is no doubt that Kari's parents had to learn better ways to cope with their own feelings and moods, as well as hers. Parents can better tolerate extremely embarrassing or stressful situations after they learn to recognize the cause of their child's Dr. Jekyll/Mr. Hyde behavior. It is most reassuring for parents to realize that they are not inadequate and their child is not bad. To the contrary, many parents of children who have behavioral problems due to allergy are truly mortal saints. The emotional, financial, and interpersonal stresses caused by a child such as Kari can be overwhelming even for the most secure families.

Counseling, however, is much more helpful if the therapist or psychologist is knowledgeable about how allergies can affect behavior and activity. To suggest that some children sit in a corner or go to their room for "time-out" periods during an explosive allergic behavioral response to a food, such as a dyed sugar cereal, for example, would be sheer folly. Some of these children would pick up the nearest chair and throw it at the parent. Many of these children do not reason logically or even hear what is being said during extreme reactions to allergenic substances and some appear not to recall their "impossible" episodes.

At one time Kari was seen by a psychologist who specialized in diagnosing the attention deficit hyperactivity disorder. She confirmed that this was Kari's problem. Her doctor felt that her difficult temperament was aggravated by allergies but that the basic problem was psychological. Many well-trained and excellent psychologists and physicians do not agree that allergy could be the basic cause of some hyperactivity and behavior problems. All aspects of Kari's behavior, however, appeared to respond very quickly and remarkably well to a comprehensive environmental and allergy approach to treatment.

She has remained 85 percent better for approximately three years. She is no longer aggressive and abusive physically, verbally, or emotionally. Her mother can tell when retesting for her allergies is necessary because she begins to become a little touchy, withdrawn, negative, or hyperactive. Her mother, however, must continue to sharply limit chocolate, sugar, and orange, or Kari will become hyperactive or withdrawn and again say, "Nobody likes me."

MORE MOTHER BATTERING

Earl

When Earl was initially seen, he was an adult-sized eleven-year-old. His family had many allergic relatives. His mother stated that he kicked and hiccupped too much when she was pregnant.

Earl as an Infant and Child

As an infant he had trouble sleeping. He cried for hours until he vomited. He rocked his crib excessively and perspired more than normal. He started with hay fever during the pollen season when he was only one year old.

When he was a young child, he had lower-rib-cage pain and leg aches that were called "growing pains." These complaints are typical of a dairy sensitivity. Later on Earl found that the only time he could exercise without leg pain was if he did *not* drink milk.

By the age of ten years he developed headaches twice a day. He tended to become very sleepy on car rides, suggesting a possible chemical sensitivity to automobile exhaust.

Earl Has Allergies

At the age of four years, his parents took him to a well-trained, board-certified allergist who confirmed that he had pollen and dust sensitivities. No food allergies were detected. The allergist placed Earl on routine allergy injection treatments, but his arm swelled up "like a grapefruit," so they discontinued that form of allergy therapy.

Earl's Outbursts

His major problem, however, was always his Dr. Jekyll/Mr. Hyde personality. He had mild moody periods twice a day that were barely tolerable. He tended, however, to have four or five violent episodes each year that were exceptionally aggressive or hostile. These episodes seemed to become more frequent and more severe each year. He would seem normal and then suddenly become belligerent and manifest bizarre behavior. During one episode near a pool, he used a hose to dampen everyone in sight, including an eighty-one-year-old woman. During another episode, at the age of eleven, after he had eaten three omelets for dinner, he stood in the middle of the living room sofa. He sobbed uncontrollably because he was unable to do his homework. Shortly after he was given a form of bicarbonate called Alka-Aid to help stop allergy reactions, he acted appropriately again and found that his math was no longer a problem.

On another occasion at the age of eleven years, Earl took a drug to quiet his activity along with some caffeine-free cola beverage. He grabbed a kitchen knife and threatened to kill his mother. His father could not control him and when they finally managed to bind his feet and hands and take him to the hospital, five hospital attendants could not restrain him. He had been aggressive before, but he had never lost total control to this degree.

Earl's Response to an Allergy Diet

When his mother tried the two-week Multiple Food Elimination Diet, within a week he was much less hyperactive. She felt he had improved 75 percent. During the second week, when foods were added back into his diet one at a time, she found that eggs caused hyperactivity and crying and peanut butter caused hives. Artificial colors caused him to crawl under his bed. He refused to come out and stated he wanted to go to an orphanage.

His mother wisely placed her entire family on the diet. A sibling developed puffy eyes and dark eye circles from milk. Another sibling developed diarrhea from milk, and a disposition change from corn.

Earl's Reactions to P/N Testing

During P/N allergy testing for weeds, we provoked a most unusual reaction. On this one occasion, he made strange noises and suddenly bolted wildly out of our office. We had to chase him down the street to give him another dilution of a weed pollen extract. He was extremely angry and totally uncooperative until he received the correct neutralization allergy treatment of weed extract. Then he calmly returned to our office and sheepishly admitted he felt better.

With a few of his other P/N allergy tests Earl would suddenly change from a quiet, polite youngster to an unpleasant, hostile, and angry boy. During provocation tests for yeast and tree pollen, he tended to become very angry and aggressive toward his mother. After he was given the neutralization dilution for yeast and tree pollen, he again was happy and smiling. His yeast allergy tests also caused muscle aches. When he was tested for wheat, his pulse rose and he acted like a dog. During mold allergy tests he became testy, moody, and irritable.

How Much Did Allergy Treatment Help?

Within one month after Earl began his P/N therapy, and his mother changed their home environment and attempted to comply with the

Practical Rotary Diet, his mother said he was 75 percent improved. His Conner's Hyperactivity Score (see Glossary) diminished from a highly elevated 29 to a normal 10 within three months of treatment. After four months of treatment, he was 95 percent better. Within five months this youngster could sit quietly through a meal and watch television without wiggling.

Although he was not perfect after allergy treatment, he was much improved. His teacher sent a note home that his schoolwork was much better. His grades changed from C's and D's, to A's and B's. The teachers said that he became remarkably cooperative and less disruptive in the classroom.

In time, his mother found that she could usually pinpoint exactly which food or contact caused inappropriate behavior. The family realized that he routinely became violent if he sneaked certain types of caffeine-free soda pop. His mother also recognized whenever his mold treatment needed adjustment because his behavior would routinely deteriorate on damp days.

His parents, however, disagreed about discipline and the dietary restrictions. As a result, Earl continued to sneak offending foods. His father purposely gave him foods that were known to cause the child to become difficult. Family counseling was repeatedly encouraged.

What's Happened to Earl Now?

Five years later, at the age of sixteen, his parents were separated and Earl now lives with his father. All his allergy therapy has been discontinued. His father says that Earl rarely explodes even though he eats whatever he likes. This is difficult to explain. It seems unlikely that this young man no longer has unacceptable episodes or loss of control. There are a number of possibilities. His father could be thinking wishfully or maybe he considers his son's behavior a normal variation, or it is possible that the young man simply no longer has any allergies.

Could Counseling Have Helped Earl and His Family?

In general, parents must take a united stand when their child acts inappropriately. They must agree about how to handle "impossible" behavior. To accomplish this, counseling is often essential. Earl's parents did not agree and gave their son mixed and confusing messages. Time alone will tell which parent was correct. Will Earl have sporadic and inexplicable behavioral outbursts that interfere with his future education, employment, and relationships? We do not know at this time. I am seriously concerned about the future of this youngster.

Father Battering

Bill

Five-year-old Bill had responded well to his allergy extract treatment for seven months when his father brought him back to our office. He was concerned because shortly after he took Bill to an aquarium that smelled strongly of chlorine, Bill suddenly would not listen to his father. He was no longer content to stay with him, refused to mind, and atypically darted off on his own. Because of his strange response, his father wondered if the odor of chlorine could be a problem. We therefore tested him with an allergy extract of chlorine and videotaped his response.

Before we gave Bill his first allergy test for chlorine, he was acting in a normal manner. He is is basically an extremely quiet, shy youngster. After the first test he changed dramatically. His patient and caring father warded off repeated blows from Bill's frantic little arms as he tried to hit his dad over and over again. When Bill wasn't striking his father, he was trying to bite his father's arms. As his reaction intensified, he began to drool an excessive amount of thick, frothy saliva. At times, as he thrashed his entire body about, he was so totally out of control that his dad had to press Bill's small body tightly against his own in an effort to protect his tiny son, as well as himself.

After Bill was given a drop of the right dilution of a chlorine allergy extract, he once again became the tranquil, calm, and polite youngster he had been before we started to test him. Bill's reaction to chlorine was certainly extreme and suggests that his parents will have to watch his response to other odors in the future. More details about this child's history are provided in Chapter 29.

Drawing of a Child During an Allergic Reaction to Orange

The intensity and degree of anger, rage, resentment, and hostility in some allergic children can be illustrated clearly in the pictures that they draw during reactions caused by a routine provocation allergy skin test (see Figures 18.1–18.4). These pictures clearly show how this ten-year-old child felt during an allergy skin test for orange.

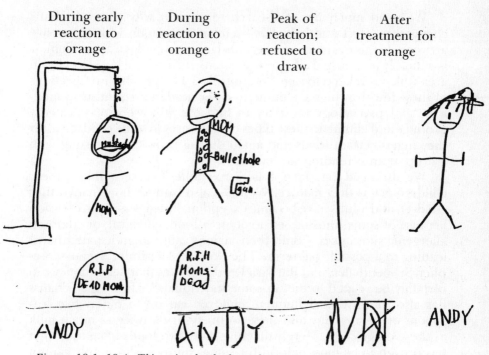

Figures 18.1–18.4. This series clearly shows the emotional changes that the child undergoes during allergy testing. In this case, the child is reacting to orange.

Normally, when he was being treated for his allergy to orange, he could drink a little orange juice every four days without having symptoms. He could not, however, drink larger amounts at more frequent intervals without developing negative behavior. This type of history often indicates a major sensitivity to an item.

For a few weeks prior to this test in our office, he no longer was able to tolerate a drink of orange juice as he had previously. If he took half a glass, he became obnoxious, disobedient, destructive, and both physically and verbally abusive. His mother recognized that this indicated his allergy treatment for orange needed to be adjusted.

Prior to the first drawing he played nicely with the other children. He became aggressive at the same time that he drew the first picture. He pinched his mother, broke his pencils, and acted very upset and angry. After he was given one drop of the correct dilution of an allergy extract for orange, he was again playful and happy within a very few minutes. His writing also illustrates obvious changes associated with his responses to different dilutions of an allergy extract for orange (Figures 18.1–18.4).

We need much more research to explain why these dramatic changes in affect and behavior occur in association with aggressive artwork. Is this evidence of a serious latent psychological problem or is it merely an unusual allergenic response to a critical but select brain area which is related to rage and hostility? The possible ramifications of these few drawings are immense. The academic scientists in medicine and psychology must try to find out why we can repeatedly produce and eliminate these types of responses in some children after they ingest certain foods and again during provocation testing with a drop of an offending substance.

We also need long-term follow-up studies to ascertain how these children act as they mature. We must also wonder how many other children and adults have become exceptionally aggressive on occasion because of some unusual sensitivity to a food, chemical, or common allergenic substances. Could their actions cause unanticipated harm leading to a possible jail term? The work of Alexander Schauss, Stephen Schoenthaler, and Barbara Reed indicates that delinquency can certainly be related to diet in some individuals.[1] Alexander Schauss has also found that delinquent children eat up to ninety-five teaspoons of sugar a day and they routinely drink twice as much milk as the average child. Merely deleting these two foods from their diet has proven to be most helpful for some children who simply cannot adhere to the rules and regulations of a civilized society.

One Caution in Relation to All Aggressive Children

Parents of children who are aggressive must be very careful not to do things that will enable their child to become more effective in that regard. Do not send an assertive, hostile child to a judo, wrestling, or boxing school. Beware of contact sports such as football, hockey, or wrestling. Rather, encourage swimming and tennis. These would diminish the opportunity of aggressive children to hurt others while being praised for their skills. Some people might argue that any vigorous contact sport would enable spirited children to work off their excess energy; to the contrary, under certain circumstances it might enhance their ability to hurt or maim.

1. Alexander Schauss, *Diet, Crime, and Delinquency* (Berkeley, Calif.: Parker House, 1981); Stephen Schoenthaler, "The Effect of Sugar on the Treatment and Control of Antisocial Behavior: A Double-Blind Study of an Incarcerated Juvenile Population," *International Journal of Biosocial Research* 3 (1982), pp. 1–19; Barbara Reed, *Food, Teens, and Behavior*, 1983. Natural Press, P.O. Box 2107, Manitowoc, Wis. 54220.

If siblings are repeatedly hurt by an aggressive child in your family, consider sending the child who is attacked, rather than the aggressor, for lessons in defense or judo.

Remember, if the cause of the aggression is not found and eliminated or appropriately treated, these children could become the batterers of wives (husbands) or their own youngsters in the future.

CHAPTER 19

Is Your Child Really Slow,
or Could It Be Due to
Allergy?

Why are some children so bright one day and so dull the next?[1] Some parents realize that their child is slow, but they are perplexed because the ability to learn simple things seems to be erratic. Some youngsters can comprehend certain complex concepts easily but fail to grasp seemingly simple ideas. They write and draw well one day; the next day they can only scribble or refuse to even hold their pencil. Many parents know their child is bright, and they wonder why he or she cannot learn in a manner that is comparable to the child's obvious intellect and potential.

Parents should ask themselves, could my child have an unrecognized form of allergy affecting her or his ability to learn? Could allergy be part or all of my child's problem? If your child looks or acts allergic or if you have allergic relatives, allergy might be one important missing link that needs to be considered.

COULD HIS SPEECH AND BEHAVIOR INTERFERE WITH HIS EDUCATION?

Robert

Robert was four and a half years old when his mother brought him to see us. His well-educated, cultured, but distraught mother had

---

1. Daniel O'Banion, B. Armstrong, et al., "Disruptive Behavior: A Dietary Approach," *Journal of Autism and Childhood Schizophrenia* 8(1978), pp. 325–337.

asked for years why her son had such unbelievable spells of uncontrollable behavior. She worried that his education might present a serious challenge because his actions were so unpredictable. He simply never could sit still long enough to learn.

As a toddler he was disturbingly hyperactive and aggressive. On a daily basis he kicked, spit, hit, bit, punched, and refused to wear clothing. He had sudden, alarming mood changes, which were accompanied by a spacey look, dark eye circles, and bags under his eyes. At other times he seemed to become easily frustrated and he would suddenly burst into tears. He tended to have recurrent ear infections in spite of the best possible medical treatment. He drooled excessively, and had bad breath and a bloated abdomen. He was clumsy and had difficulty using crayons and scissors. He tended to fall frequently when he tried to run.

His mother fortuitously saw the 1987 *Donahue* show. She recognized that some of her son's behavior patterns were surprisingly identical to those of one hyperactive boy on that program. For the first time she had some insight as to why her son's behavior switched from Dr. Jekyll to Mr. Hyde. She had repeatedly observed that Robert was always calm and loving in the morning, but that by mid-morning his behavior would begin to deteriorate. As the day wore on, he routinely became progressively more and more difficult. For the first time, she wondered if the foods he ate during the day could possibly be the cause of his problems or if some inexplicable changes in the clarity of his speech could possibly be related to his diet.

Robert's Response to an Allergy Diet

His mother started the first week of the Multiple Food Elimination Diet with immense skepticism. She was truly surprised and comforted by his dramatic, rapid response. Within three days after the diet was begun, his behavior was unbelievably calm and consistent throughout the day. By the end of the first week he could sit still and cut with scissors. He could write and draw better and could even speak in sentences. He stopped racing impulsively down the street. He was cooperative, pleasant, happy, and less easily frustrated. He no longer attacked his mother. His parents found the change incredible.

During the second week of the Multiple Food Elimination Diet, when foods were added back again into his diet, one at a time, his mother found specific answers. Within twenty minutes after he ate a slice of wheat bread, his total personality changed. Eating wheat was associated with attacking his dog, babbling, spitting, laughing uncontrollably, and even trying to eat a plate. He was completely out of control. When milk was reintroduced into his diet, the reaction was so violent that he put his head through a glass window. At that time his intestinal symptoms, bloating, and bad breath also recurred. Subsequent P/N allergy testing reproduced similar dramatic personality changes, especially from wheat and milk.

Robert's Response to Allergy Extract Treatment

Within nine days after his initial allergy extract therapy, he improved about 50 percent. Within six weeks he was 95 percent improved. By then he could eat and tolerate all foods, except for wheat products, at a four-day interval. His sensitivity to wheat was so intense that despite months of allergy extract treatment for wheat, he could not eat a slice of bread for approximately one year. At that time wheat was finally tolerated, but only if it was eaten in small amounts. Since then he has been able to eat gradually increasing amounts of wheat products every four days. Presently, after five years of treatment, he is even able to tolerate large amounts of wheat products, every four days, without any difficulty.

Within six months after allergy treatment his IQ, which was initially gauged to be near 81, had increased to 125. Likewise, his previous medical complaints and behavioral problems were no longer evident. Imagine how his school performance would have been if he ate toast or wheat cereal for breakfast and had not been treated.

It was truly imperative that his allergy to wheat and other allergenic items be recognized and appropriately treated *before* he started school. Based upon extensive testing at ages three to five conducted by the public school system, Robert, at the age of five years, could have been labeled mildly retarded, emotionally disturbed, and limited because of a number of motor handicaps. A preschool teacher told his mother that he could never be placed in a regular classroom.

Early and appropriate recognition of his unusual allergies with a diet, provocation testing, and neutralization allergy extract therapy have resolved the baffling enigma that Robert initially presented. Figures 19.1, 19.2, and 19.3 show the differences in his writing and drawings before and after P/N treatment for wheat.

Robert After Six Years of P/N Treatment

At the present time ten-year-old Robert attends a prominent private school for gifted children. Recent academic testing with the Iowa

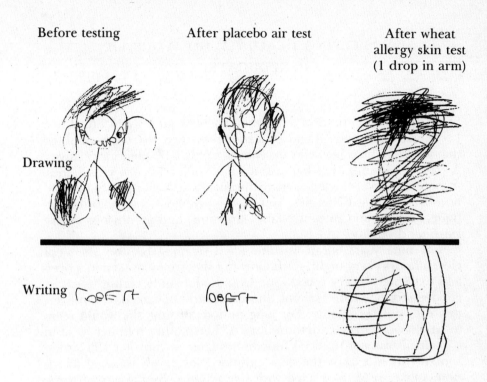

Figures 19.1–19.3. Changes in drawing and handwriting during a wheat allergy skin test in a five-and-a-half-year-old boy

Basic Skills Test showed that although he is only in the fourth grade, he scored at a seventh-grade level. His social studies were at a tenth-grade level. Some of his scores were so high that they exceeded the maximum for that test. He has extraordinarily high skill levels in the areas of engineering and architecture, and his motor skills are excellent. He has been described by his school's cofounder and headmaster as "an encyclopedic young man" with an immense thirst for knowledge.

All children do not demonstrate such an outstanding improvement, but it is not unusual for allergic children to find their C's and D's become A's and B's after their allergies are recognized and appropriately treated.

A SLEEPING BEAUTY WHO WOKE UP
UNEDUCATED

Sarah

Sarah saw us for the first time when she was nine years old. When I looked at her medical and educational history, I strongly doubted that we could help her. Her parents had only a few allergic relatives. A paternal grandfather had asthma and milk and corn sensitivities. A maternal great-uncle has many incapacitating allergies. Sarah had no obvious typical allergies. Her major problems were extreme fatigue, sudden and uncontrollable tantrums, and an obvious severe learning disability.

For nine years Sarah was literally a sleeping beauty: She slept eleven hours every night. Each morning she would awaken in a tired and extremely angry mood. She would adamantly refuse to eat or get dressed. She hated school. She spent most of each day, however, in a dull state of apathy. For long periods of time she would seem to be oblivious of her surroundings. If her mother told her to sit in a chair, it was not unusual four hours later to find her still sitting contentedly in exactly the same position. She rarely watched television, spoke, read, or played with her siblings. By the age of three years her prolonged periods of lethargy became spotted with violent, frightening, and inexplicable outbursts. She was a drowsy angel most of the time, but five to six times a week she had screaming tantrums that were almost unbelievable. These episodes could last a very long forty minutes or a seemingly endless two hours. On one such occasion, she stood on the furniture, pulled at her mother's clothing, hit her, and grabbed at her throat. She repeatedly said the same sentence over and over again.

Her childhood pattern of lethargic periods was evident very early in infancy. At that time she slept twenty hours out of twenty-four. Her mother was repeatedly reassured by their physician that Sarah was all right. In the brief intervals when Sarah was awake, she would scream and seem inordinately irritable. Her parents thought that in time that would change, but mornings became worse, not better. As an infant Sarah was never happy when she woke up in the morning.

Sarah Is Tried on an Allergy Diet

When Sarah was nine years old, her grandmother read an article in a ladies' magazine that discussed how allergies could affect some children's ability to learn. Her mother, who was a nurse, subsequently read about allergies and decided to see if foods could be part of Sarah's problems. After the first week of our Multiple Food Elimination Diet, Sarah's energy level increased "100 percent." She was a "new" child. She could easily stay awake until 11:00 P.M. She awoke happy and by 6:00 A.M., amazingly, not only bounced out of bed on her own but was already dressed for school and anxious to eat breakfast. She actually danced and sang. She had never done this before. She played with the other children in her family. She showed interest in television. Her speech was clearer and she even engaged in normal conversation. Her memory and concentration improved. She seemed anxious to learn. Her dark eye circles disappeared.

During the second week of the diet her mother found that when Sarah ate wheat, dairy products, or chocolate, she became tired, fatigued, irritable, and moody. Milk caused her dark eye circles. Later on her mother recognized that when she ate popcorn at the movies, she screamed and became so extremely irritable and upset that the family was forced to leave the movie. She simply would not quiet down and repeatedly disrupted the entire theater.

Sarah's Response to Allergy Treatment

After five months of allergy extract therapy she could print her name, recall things that happened months ago, follow directions, play simple games, discuss her school day with her mother, count ten objects, remember people's names, and use words more correctly. She had friends for the first time in her life.

After one year of allergy environmental control, a rotation diet, avoidance of chemicals, and nutritional and amino acid supplementation, Sarah was definitely better. Sarah's behavior and activity continue to be markedly improved. Her energy level continues to be much greater than ever before. When she has an occasional emotional outburst, her mother can usually determine the specific cause. Her schoolwork, however, remains far below grade level, although her interest to learn is now intense. Her mother said that at times she has to be "pulled from" the computer after sitting there from 6:00 to 11:00 P.M.

Sarah's Educational Problems

In spite of many educational programs, Sarah has truly fallen between the cracks in our school system. Although not autistic, at one time she was placed in an autistic children's class. Her mother was told Sarah was supposed to "set an example for the other children so that they would learn how to sit still." Instead Sarah mimicked the autistic children. In the language-development classes Sarah could not concentrate because there were too many children and too many distractions. In the neurologically impaired class, even though she became alert and improved with allergy treatment, her previous school program was merely continued as it had been in the past. It was not appropriately adjusted to compensate for her newly acquired alertness and evident capabilities. The school system had no time, insufficient special educators, inadequate funds, and few facilities to help her. It took months for them to provide her with a computer to help her catch up after the many years when she had been inordinately subdued, inattentive, and unable to learn.

At the age of eleven years she was placed in a learning skills and language development program. They taught her to speak more clearly. She learned activities related to daily living, such as how to cook, clean, and eat in restaurants. Her parents, however, had to hire a private tutor to help her learn what Sarah was most anxious to do: She wanted to read and write. She is presently progressing in that she appears to be learning to do things that she could never do before. Allergy is obviously not the total answer for Sarah, but with therapy she is presently awake, pleasant, happy, interacting with others, and eager to learn. It is unfortunate that her parents have had to provide for so much of her basic educational needs and catch-up learning. With special tutoring she is only now learning her ABCs and simple arithmetic. In the fall of 1990, however, she finally began to receive a special academic program which was better adapted to her needs. Hopefully this can alleviate the necessity for private tutoring. It is unfortunate that it required over two full years before her academic needs could be individualized and nurtured in a more appropriate manner.

A Child Who Had So Many Food Allergies He Could Not Do a Diet

Gary

The two drawings (Figures 19.4 and 19.5) demonstrate the type of changes that occur when children are properly diagnosed and treated. When Gary was five and a half years old, he still could not write, color, or draw well. Within five months after treatment this same boy could easily color within the lines.

**DRAWING/WRITING OF 5½ YEAR OLD BOY
PRIOR TO ALLERGY TREATMENT
Unable to Write, Color, or Draw**

How will we
unbounce
Tigger?

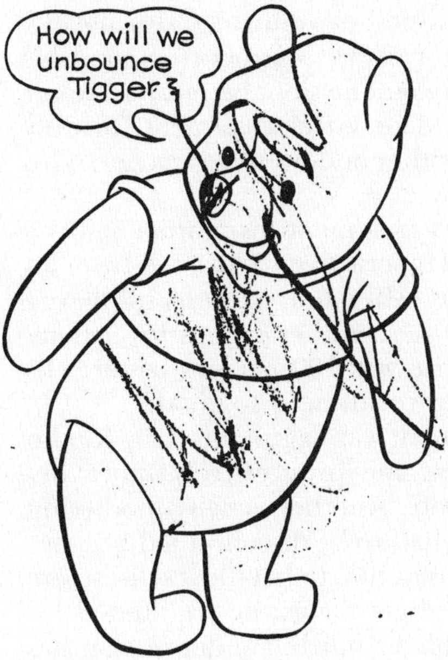

*Figure 19.4. Gary is unable to write,
color, or draw before treatment.*

**DRAWING/WRITING OF A 5 YEAR 11 MONTH
OLD BOY AFTER 5 MONTHS OF
ALLERGY TREATMENT
Able to Write, Color, and Draw**

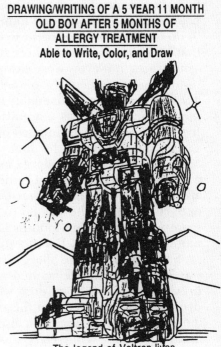

The legend of Voltron lives .

*Figure 19.5. After five months of
treatment, Gary can color within the lines.*

Gary's mother was the principal of a school and she thought that her son was intellectually normal. His IQ was well within the normal range. His school evaluation, however, indicated that he had some mild learning problems. When he was four years old, she was concerned because he still did not speak well and he tended to make animal sounds. He would walk into walls and stare into space. When he was in school, he could not sit still and he was easily distracted. He was thought to have attention deficit hyperactivity disorder (ADHD).

Allergy Testing Reveals Food and Other Sensitivities

His mother came to see us because the Ritalin he was taking did not control his hyperactivity or inability to concentrate. His mother wondered if allergies could be part of her son's problems, because she had allergies. Unlike most of our patients, however, he did not improve on the Multiple Food Elimination Diet. His mother was unable to do the diet correctly because he was so sensitive to so many foods that it was impossible to adhere strictly to the diet. His food and other sensitivities, however, were easily detected or confirmed during P/N testing and treatment. One week after allergy extract treatment his atypical writing and personality improved, he slept better, had fewer mood swings, and was more affectionate. After treatment for only five foods and dust, he hugged his mother and even his teacher. This was extremely atypical for him.

After two weeks of allergy extract treatment his mother said he was 50 percent better. His Conner's Hyperactivity Score fell from an abnormal high of 29 to a normal 11. After four months of allergy extract treatment, he was 80 to 100 percent better and his activity score was only 5. Ten months later he was 100 percent better. His mother said, "I think I'm in a dream world, he is so good."

Six months after his allergy treatment was begun, his daily Ritalin was discontinued. He tended to become progressively more depressed and sad as each dose wore off. Another activity-modifying drug, Cylert, was tried, but this, too, had to be discontinued because it not only did not help, but it also caused him to have low self-esteem and depression. While Gary was on these drugs, he frightened his parents because of his suicidal thoughts. Inordinate depression has not been evident since these drugs were discontinued. These drugs were tried in spite of his obvious improvement on allergy therapy because he continued to have intermittent unexplained spurts of hyperactivity.

After fifteen months of comprehensive allergy therapy, his mother stopped his allergy extract treatment. He continued to do well. Many foods that he repeatedly could not eat before no longer caused symptoms. She found, however, that she had to continue to sharply curtail all food coloring, chocolate, and sugar because these continued to cause impulsive, wild, and "crazy" behavior. Their home was kept relatively allergy-free. He was not as well as when he received his allergy extract, but his mother stated he was 90 percent better than he was before he began allergy treatment four years ago.

Gary's Early Medical History

Similar to other children who have allergies affecting their behavior and ability to learn, his symptoms began early in life. By the age of one year he had year-round hay fever, which in turn made him prone to repeated infections and asthma. His constipation, bad breath, and craving for cheese and ice cream, combined with his preference for water instead of milk, strongly suggested a milk sensitivity.

By the age of one year he had symptoms compatible with allergic tension fatigue syndrome. He was restless, irritable, and in constant motion. He was unhappy, hit both his parents, chewed on things, and had temper tantrums and nightmares. He had sudden, unusual episodes of Dr. Jekyll/Mr. Hyde behavior. He would inexplicably crawl under the furniture and not allow anyone to touch him.

Not Everything Is Due to Allergy

When Gary was seven years old, his personality inexplicably deteriorated again. He was doing very poorly in school. He had nightmares. He ran out of school saying, "I wish I was dead." His mother ascertained that he had had a substitute teacher during the period when he was so distraught. As soon as the former teacher returned, his behavior was again exemplary. This is mentioned only to point out that every recurrence of emotional problems in allergic children is not necessarily related to allergy. All facets of a child's environment and life must be evaluated when a child who has been doing well is suddenly unable to cope with his daily pattern of living. Gary's usual teacher used a copious amount of reinforcement, instead of rejection, with the result that he tried in every way possible to please her and to achieve academically.

Gary is presently continuing to receive some counseling and he is in a special education class. It is anticipated that he will be placed in regular classes next year. His parents are pleased because his schoolwork is better and in many ways his other symptoms have vastly improved since his allergies were originally treated. He no longer has congestion, asthma, intellectual problems, frequent urination, or drastic mood changes. His mother continues to maintain a four-day rotation diet most of the time, and their home is as ecologically sound and as allergy-free as his parents can make it.

This youngster illustrates that the Multiple Food Elimination Diet is of little value if it can't be done correctly. Some parents erroneously assume that foods are unrelated to their child's medical and learning problems because their children did not improve on our diet. Sometimes this is because the parents did not do the diet correctly. The newer P/N allergy testing and treatment methods, however, quickly help to detect and relieve certain food sensitivities, even though diets may not have been helpful for a variety of reasons. Had Gary's mother not followed through with the newer allergy testing methods to detect and treat her son's allergies, Gary would probably have become a greater challenge as time passed because of his physical, emotional, and learning problems.

A Retarded Child With Complex Medical Problems

Kathy

When I first saw eight-year-old Kathy, I really did not believe we could help much more than her obvious nose allergies. She was friendly, but definitely overactive. She was obviously retarded and had typical dark eye circles so characteristic of allergy. She was very small for her age because of a rare medical problem affecting her adrenal glands. Her mother had classical allergies.

Kathy's Infant Period

Kathy had colic for the first eighteen months of her life. She could not tolerate cow's milk because it caused congestion. Goat milk seemed to cause less mucus. She was never a cuddly baby. During infancy she often banged her head. She had recurrent ear infections that began during infancy and she needed tubes placed through her eardrums by the time she was three years old. She had many abdominal complaints and wheezed between the ages of one and three years. All of these complaints suggested a possible sensitivity to cow's and/or goat's milk.

Kathy as a Child

By the time she was eight years old, she was extremely hyperactive. Her mother could not take her to a store or even for a short walk because she was simply uncontrollable. She had periods of exceptional fatigue, hostility, and depression. She had received drugs such as Ritalin to quiet her, but they only caused her to act more depressed and moody. She could not sit still in school. She made clucking throat sounds and craved milk, cheese, and yogurt. This again suggested that the strong dairy sensitivity noted during infancy had not subsided. Her hyperactivity and coughing seemed to be worse during the pollen and mold seasons. Her mother noted that exposure to chalk, crayons, synthetic carpets, and perfumes preceded some of her most unpleasant outbursts. She wondered if there was a relationship. Chemical sensitivities were suggested by this part of her history.

Kathy's Response to an Allergy Diet

Her mother placed her on the Multiple Food Elimination Diet. Within one week she was 75 percent improved. She was calmer, more cooperative, and less cranky. Her speech was easier to understand. She had more energy. Her abdomen was less distended. Her teachers and grandmother commented on her dramatic improvement. During the second week of the diet her mother said that milk and yogurt caused lethargy, irritability, and congestion of her nose, food coloring appeared to cause irritability, corn caused hyperactivity, and eggs caused congestion and a red, itchy nose.

After the Multiple Food Elimination Diet her mother realized how easy it was to recognize cause-and-effect relationships. Within twenty minutes after Kathy ate certain foods, she routinely became ill or acted inappropriately.

Kathy's Response to Allergy Testing

During provocation allergy testing the effect of certain allergenic substances was clearly evident. An allergy test for house dust made her speech unclear, while the dog test made her suddenly become very irritable. She became spaced out, drooled, and was untouchable during the mold tests. The sugar test made her tired and apathetic. All these complaints subsided after her correct neutralization dose of the corresponding allergy extract.

Classroom Carpet and Chemicals Were a Problem

At one point Kathy's schoolroom was recarpeted, and the school was fumigated. Shortly after these changes her teachers noted that Kathy acted moody and irritable and could not concentrate as well as before. We prepared a special allergy extract of the classroom air. When she was tested with it, she became uncooperative and angry. She began to bite, scream, and throw her toys. There was no doubt that treatment with this classroom air extract enabled her to think and act more appropriately in school.

Her teachers' special interest and increased awareness enabled them to detect additional offending items. On one occasion she was given some clay that had an odor. Within ten minutes she was having a tantrum and pulling things off the walls. On another occasion a teacher noted that exposure to a perfumed shampoo caused Kathy to act most inappropriately.

Ways That Kathy Improved

After six weeks of provocation testing and neutralization allergy treatment, her highly abnormal Conner's Hyperactivity Score of 29 dropped to a normal of 14. Her extreme drooling stopped. Her temper, disposition, and behavior improved 70 percent. Her attention span was 50 percent better. After four months of treatment she could string beads and draw a straight line. Because of her improvement her mother could take Kathy places without her creating a scene. Kathy responded so well that her mother decided not to institutionalize her child but to continue to care for her herself.

Can Vitamins Help Children Learn?

Dr. Stephen Schoenthaler, from California State University in Turlock, has almost completed a comprehensive definitive million-dollar study funded by a branch of the British government. His research suggests that vitamin supplementation can raise IQ in approximately 30 percent of randomly selected children by an average of 20 points. This study verifies his previous studies and those of Dr. David Benton in Britain.[2] Part of a comprehensive environmental and allergy treatment program is nutrient supplementation. Some children who have learning problems might benefit by an individualized evaluation of their levels of vitamins, trace metals, and essential fatty acids, as well as blood and urine amino acid analysis.

Allergies Can Affect Any Child

Allergies show no favorites. They can be shared equally by slow, normal, and gifted children. Children similar to Robert can initially

2. Stephen Schoenthaler, Ph.D., Publication of research and book for public due February 1991; David Benton and Gwilym Roberts, "The Effect of Vitamin and Mineral Supplementation on Intelligence, the Sample of School Children" *Lancet* 664(1988) pp. 140–143.

appear to be slow in some ways when in fact they may be gifted. Others, like Gary, need special education, but their ability to learn can take a very positive turn after the role of allergy is recognized. Retarded children such as Sarah and Kathy can learn and act better after the allergy portion of their complex medical and learning problems is treated. We can only hope that educational systems try harder to design individualized instruction programs for children such as Sarah so that their specific needs and capabilities are satisfied more adequately. The educational programs that were indicated prior to allergy treatment may no longer be appropriate after the allergic component of a child's learning and emotional problems is recognized and treated. The instruction of such children must correspond with their increased ability and not be solely dependent upon their past performance.

CHAPTER 20

Fatigue, Headaches, Tics, Seizures—Could They Sometimes Be Due to Allergy?

It has been noted that the brain can be affected by a wide range of common allergenic substances. Observation dating back to the mid-1930s indicated that odors, foods, pollen, molds, and dust could cause a wide range of problems in the nervous system. Entire chapters in texts for physicians written between the thirties and the fifties were devoted to the role of allergy in relation to headaches, fatigue, epilepsy, behavior problems, minimal brain dysfunction, psychological problems, and a wide range of other neurological or learning problems in some children. Unfortunately this valuable information was and is not included in the medical training of many past or present-day physicians specializing in allergy or neurology.

Certainly not all children who have the medical complaints just listed have an allergy causing their illness. It must be stressed, however, that *allergy should at least be considered as one possible cause* of these symptoms, especially when physicians admit they don't know why some child is not feeling or acting appropriately. Once again, the answer is not always more, newer and better drugs to temporarily relieve a child's symptoms. Sometimes it is possible for parents and physicians to ascertain the cause of a youngster's problem so that there is no need for drugs, especially if the child looks or acts allergic and has allergic relatives.

Fatigue—The Tired Child

We have all heard about how allergies to foods such as sugar and red food coloring can cause some children to become hyperactive. Only rarely, however, do we hear or read about the many children who are too tired and unable to function at their full intellectual capacity at school because of allergies. These children cause little disruption compared with an overactive child with a behavior problem. Young children, but more commonly allergic teenagers and women, complain of being tired, irritable, and depressed. These children and adults often have the "fatigue" so vividly described by Drs. Albert Rowe and Theron Randolph in their books and articles written in the thirties and forties. In today's medicine, extreme fatigue is sometimes due to allergic tension fatigue syndrome, a term coined by a pediatric allergist, Dr. Frederick Speer, in the fifties. When I was trained in pediatric allergy in the late fifties, I was told that this syndrome did not exist. Some physicians training to be allergists today are unfortunately still erroneously taught that this medical diagnosis is not a reality. (See Roger, Appendix E.)

A YOUNGSTER WHO SLEPT THROUGH HIS MORNING CLASSES

Kurt

About fifteen years ago I saw a twelve-year-old youngster named Kurt. I vividly recall his history because he was one of the first patients in whom I recognized this problem. He had a long history of typical allergies. His mother was concerned about his school performance because in spite of his intelligence, he simply could not stay awake. He routinely fell asleep each morning in class. The diagnosis was really quite simple. He *always* had peanut butter and milk for breakfast. We ascertained that four tablespoons of peanut butter caused drowsiness and nausea within twenty minutes. We did P/N allergy testing, and within ten minutes after the first skin test for peanut he was extremely sleepy. He was asleep sitting in a chair. When he was given a weaker dilution of that same peanut extract, he suddenly woke up and appeared very alert. We knew we had found the neutralization dose that would relieve his problem. We also found that P/N tests for milk caused extreme drowsiness. After treatment he was able to eat these foods every four days and not fall asleep in school. Three of his teachers wrote us to relate that he was "more alert and less dazed" in school after he began his allergy treatment for peanuts and milk.

Our Study to Document Kurt's Response Fails

We decided to try to document this observation a few weeks later. A local open-minded neurologist agreed to do an EEG-type brain-wave test on Kurt in his clinic. We prepared two solutions. One was ground-up peanuts in water, and the other was a similarly colored mix using ground wheat. We passed a tube from his nose to his stomach so he would not taste the test food. Our "blinded" challenge failed, however, because shortly after we put the peanut mixture into his stomach, he burped and said he tasted the peanut. His EEG showed no significant change. He merely become slightly more tired after the peanut test but he did not fall asleep.

In this regard it should be mentioned that the food that is tasted during a burp often provides a clue to a possible food allergy. It is truly amazing that our bodies seem to be so discriminating that the stomach can hold back a problem food and move other nonoffending foods along their way through the intestines. Although the peanut mix caused Kurt to become tired within a half hour, there was no change in his brain wave.

One challenge facing doctors who try to document that foods cause a certain medical problem is that parents or children often limit or stop eating certain foods as soon as they know that they cause symptoms. If a food is not eaten for several weeks, even if it caused an allergic response before, it may initially no longer cause obvious immediate symptoms when it is eaten again. After that problem food is eaten again, however, for several weeks, the sensitivity often returns. Then if that food is eaten only every four days, i.e., Wednesday and Sunday, the problems caused by that food will again become evident.

We now know that new special types of computerized brain-wave analyses called neurometrics appear to document certain types of reactions in some patients, such as Kurt. Pilot studies in this area certainly suggest that this is sometimes possible. It is only a matter of time until newer research techniques to study specific areas of the brain enable us objectively and unequivocally to validate whether and how foods, chemicals, and other allergenic substances can adversely affect certain parts of the nervous system.

A Mother and Son With Similar Unconscious Episodes

We commonly see children and parents who have similar medical complaints. Let me share the history of one such family. All members had classical allergies. The father and older son both tended to pace back and forth. The daughter tended to cling to her mother so much when she was younger that her mother said she had to be "peeled" off her body. The youngest son, Albert, and his mother each had a similar, severe, and most unusual form of allergy. They collapsed and could not be roused if they ate certain foods or were exposed to certain odors.

Albert—A Collapsed Child Who Could Not Be Awakened

We saw Albert when he was only four years old. His mother had been desperate, alarmed, and frightened for a period of over a year because she repeatedly would find him totally unconscious on the floor. She could not awaken him. Several hours later he would wake up on his own and act perfectly normal. In time his mother noted that this problem seemed to occur after he ate certain foods, especially fresh cherries from a tree in their backyard.

He was the first "tired" child we tested using the newer P/N technique. A tiny drop of cherry allergy extract in his arm caused him suddenly to become limp and unconscious. I must admit I was amazed, startled, and a bit apprehensive at the time because I had never seen a child react in this manner. Ironically his mother reassured me, rather than vice versa. She said this was exactly what always happened about an hour after he ate fresh cherries. We were accustomed to seeing children become hyperactive from P/N testing, not tired. We quickly found his correct neutralization dose for cherry, and he woke up again.

He was treated with an allergy extract that contained a combination of his correct neutralization doses for each allergenic substance to which he was sensitive during testing. This treatment relieved much of Albert's drowsiness, as well as his puffy eyes and dark eye circles.

Albert's Drowsiness Returns, Nine Years Later

Albert did well for the next nine years. His mother maintained a partial Practical Rotary Diet and tried to keep their home allergy-free, ecologically sound, and free of chemicals. When he was thirteen years old, however, he again began to have difficulty staying awake. Although he was innately a bright child and had previously received high grades in school, he now had brain fag or problems remembering. This was noted especially on humid days, when he was in damp places, and after he ate moldy foods, such as grapes or raisins. This suggested a mold or yeast sensitivity. We videotaped him as he became drowsy and fell sound asleep after the provocation skin test for yeast and when he woke up shortly after his neutralization treatment. Once again, after his yeast and mold allergy treatment he stopped falling asleep in school and his grades dramatically improved.

His initial blood study for total IgE failed to show any evidence of allergy, even though he had typical hay fever. Once again we must be careful not to assume that a child does not have an allergy because this type of allergy test is negative.

Albert's Early Childhood

As is typical of many allergic youngsters, this boy's history began long before he was four years old. He was congested shortly after his mother stopped breast-feeding and started cow's milk. Finally Kool-Aid was given to replace milk, and he no longer had nose allergies. In time, however, it was thought that his milk allergy was outgrown, so milk was restarted. In a while he began to complain of excessive abdominal gas, insomnia, dark eye circles, and puffy eyes. Milk was not suspected as the cause of these symptoms because he did not develop congestion as he had during infancy. When all dairy was finally discontinued at the age of four years, his intestinal symptoms finally improved. We frequently note that a specific food will cause one set of symptoms during infancy and that later on, that same food will cause medical problems in a totally different area of the body.

Albert Develops Asthma While on Allergy Treatment

It was disappointing when he developed asthma at the age of eleven years during a pollen season. This, however, responded well and quickly to an updated neutralization allergy treatment for pollen, and he has rarely wheezed since then. Total comprehensive allergy treatment appears to help prevent asthma, but not always. To a large degree, the success will depend upon how well parents follow the suggestions made by the specialist in environmental medicine and how great the child's propensity is to develop allergy in the lungs.

Albert is presently approximately 90 percent better. An occasional episode of extreme drowsiness can usually be attributed to an over-indulgence in a food or contact known to have caused fatigue in the past. If symptoms recur from a food, mold, or during any pollen season, adjustment of his neutralization allergy treatment promptly eliminates his symptoms.

This child has such a long history of serious allergies affecting so many areas of his body that he will have to stringently maintain the principles of dietary, ecological, and nutritional management for a long time. He must also be careful to have his allergy extract therapy updated prior to each pollen and mold season. These measures hopefully will diminish or prevent future flare-ups of allergic symptoms. He has not outgrown his allergies but must remain alert to recognize how they change and which different body areas are affected as he ages.

Karen—A Tired Mother Who Had Spells of Unconsciousness

Albert's mother, Karen, had typical nose, intestinal, and skin allergies. In addition, for years she had perplexed many medical specialists in spite of repeated and extensive neurological evaluations, because of severe muscle aches, extreme fatigue, irritability, depression, and unconscious episodes. She spent much of her married life in bed, too weak and tired to move.

A walk in a typical shopping mall with the usual smorgasbord of chemical odors from stores is always a challenge for her. She routinely becomes weak and collapses unless she shops quickly. This is especially true if she passes a leather-goods store.

If Karen eats in a restaurant, it is always potentially hazardous. She knows that she can become weak and unconscious from sugar, lobster, cherries, coffee, cola, chocolate, or the odor of perfume. These items cause weakness, and in particular, pain in her previously injured right leg and back.

Karen's Response to Rice Allergy Test

In December 1988 she participated in a pilot study to learn more about what happens to patients when they react during provocation allergy skin testing. Her brain waves were constantly monitored during the entire study.[1] In addition, she was videotaped during placebo

1. This above study was done in conjunction with David Cantor, Ph.D., a psychologist associated with the University of Maryland School of Medicine. J. Alexander Bralley, Ph.D., at MetaMetrix Laboratory in Norcross, Ga., kindly interpreted the amino acid data.

and real allergy testing. Certain immunological factors in her blood were measured before, during, and after she was tested with a typical rice allergy extract.

She was her normal, witty self before and after her allergy test with a placebo solution. But after one droplet of rice allergy extract was injected into her arm, she became very quiet and started to act spaced out. Within nineteen minutes her hands and feet were clenched in severe spasm and she was unconscious. As she was given progressively weaker solutions of rice allergy extract, her hands and feet gradually started to relax. In a short while she could open and then blink her eyes in response to questions. However she still *could not talk.* When she was given a drop of allergy extract that approached her neutralization dose, she could smile, but surprisingly she still could not speak. When she finally received a drop of her exact correct neutralization dilution of rice allergy extract, she was able to speak and acted in a normal, jovial manner again.

The constant videotape of her reaction documented her obvious dramatic changes in personality and state of consciousness. These correlated with the exact times that changes were noted in certain immune factors in her blood during her reaction to the rice test. Her level of histamine, a substance released during allergic reactions, progressively dropped during her response to the rice testing. Her blood amino acids showed seven abnormal elevations before, twenty-two elevations during, and twenty-six elevations after the test was completed. The changes indicated she needed to generate energy and that substances related to the function of her sympathetic nervous system were mobilized during the stress of her response. Special neurometric brain-wave recordings, however, which evaluate changes on the *outer* surface of the brain, *failed to show* statistically significant alterations at the time of the test. Her baseline brain wave initially showed some abnormalities and these barely increased during the dramatic reaction period. This was surprising in view of the dramatic differences in her appearance and level of consciousness during testing. We wonder if her obvious reaction was possibly located in the brain stem rather than on the surface of the brain.

With more studies and advanced methods to study brain function we hope that we can eventually determine exactly why both Karen and her son have similar unusual incapacitating reactions to normal substances. Repeated extensive neurological evaluations of Karen in the past have failed to provide answers to explain the "strange episodes" that we can reproduce and relieve, at will, with P/N testing. It is also hoped that the preliminary pilot studies attempting to correlate brain-wave and blood changes with her obvious personality changes during P/N testing will encourage academic research physicians to help us find more answers. The lack of sincere interest of neurologists in Karen's responses during single-blinded P/N allergy testing is almost as astonishing as her remarkable reactions to these tests.

Headaches

Joseph Egger et al. in 1983 found that migraine headaches responded to an allergy-free diet in 93 percent of eighty-eight children.[2] Other associated symptoms that also improved included abdominal pain, leg aches, behavior disorders, seizures, hay fever, asthma, and eczema. They found sixty-four of the eighty-eight children had allergic relatives and that forty-eight of these children had classical allergic symptoms. (See Roger, Appendix E.)

A CHILD WITH EXCRUCIATING HEADACHES

Joseph

Joseph started to have headaches when he was nine years old, and he came to see us when he was ten. His face clearly reflected the intensity of his pain. His headaches were excruciating and tended to last all day. He would usually crawl into bed and ask to be left alone. They occurred about three times a week. His mother found that his headaches were particularly evident shortly after lunch.

In time we ascertained that he was drinking boxes of fruit juice at lunch and that his headaches were caused by the corn syrup that was in the juice. His mother also found that peanuts and peanut butter triggered similar headaches. He began P/N allergy treatment for foods, and his headaches subsided completely within two months.

Again, it is different foods for different children. Unfortunately the major culprits are often a child's favorite foods.

2. Joseph Egger, M.D., et al., "Is Migraine Food Allergy? A Double-Blind Controlled Trial of Oligoantigenic Diet Treatment," *Lancet* 11 (1983), pp. 865–869.

AN ADULT WITH CHRONIC DELAYED
HEADACHES DUE TO MILK

This adult, Sally, was never seen. She sent a letter to thank the *Don-ahue* show a year after our program about how foods can affect how children behave. The letter was typical in that her headaches started when she was very young. Once she thought about why they occurred, rather than what would relieve them, she no longer had her head-aches.

Sally

Sally had never been a cuddly youngster. Her mother said she did not sleep the first two years of her life. She was always irritable and depressed. As a child she absolutely loved milk and between the ages of twenty and thirty, she always ate lots of ice cream and cheese.

As an adult, Sally related, she could not recall *not* having head-aches. They routinely lasted three to five days and the usual home remedies did not help. In her late twenties, she noticed that her headaches seemed to become much more severe. Her pain tolerance seemed to be decreasing with each attack. There were times when she wanted to die because the pain was so excruciating. She had tried aspirin, ice, heating packs, sinus tablets, ointments on her forehead, and anything else she thought might help. The pain was so severe that Sally had to sit very still in a chair as soon as the headache began. She dared not move or exercise because the slightest movement caused her head to throb horribly.

When she saw a neurologist, he said that her headaches did not fit the migraine pattern, and he could not find anything wrong. Chi-ropractic adjustments were not helpful. Sally had her wisdom teeth pulled, as she thought they might be a factor. She saw a sinus spe-cialist, who also found nothing abnormal. But the pain persisted, always in the same spot, above her left eye.

Her headaches interfered more and more with ordinary living. If she made any plans, the possibility of a headache always had to be considered. Sally's life was filled with fear. She either dreaded that she would have another headache or she was suffering with one that she could not control.

In June 1988 Sally was ill at home with another headache. She happened to be watching television when we were on the *Donahue* show. On the program we discussed how almost any area of the body can be affected by food sensitivities and how these can cause both sudden and long-standing illness. As Sally reflected, she realized that the day before her present headache, she had eaten a full quart of ice cream. She realized from that television program that her persistent craving for ice cream could indicate an allergy to dairy products. She stopped all milk and dairy products for about three weeks, and then she drank one-quarter of a glass of milk. By the next morning she had her typical headache and realized she might have finally found the answer. She stopped milk for six weeks and then drank a little. The next morning, once again, she had her typical headache.

Similar to many other patients, Sally wondered why the diagnosis of food allergy had not been considered by any of the many physicians who had seen her in the past. Once again, I think the answer rests in our present medical education. Physicians are simply not taught the newer methods of detecting food allergy in general medicine or even in the specialties of otolaryngology (ear, nose, and throat), neurology, psychiatry, and—amazingly—allergy. This is unfortunate, but I am confident that the prevailing attitude will change. In time more and more physicians will appreciate that what their patients eat, breathe, touch, and drink can cause them to become ill.

One reason Sally's headaches were not recognized earlier was because several hours always elapsed between the time she ate ice cream or cheese and the onset of her headaches. A delayed food sensitivity can be elusive, and it may take years before a serendipity, such as a television talk show, provides the necessary insight. Fortunately most problem foods cause symptoms in less than an hour after they are eaten, so it is easier for parents to recognize cause-and-effect relationships. (See Eve, Chapter 13, and Roger and Linda, Appendix E.)

Tics or Habit Spasms

Tics are little involuntary jerks or twitches of various muscles of the body, often involving the face. In our office a solution to the problem of tics proved to be just one more pleasant surprise in a constant stream of many that began after we started to practice environmental medicine. There are, of course, many other causes for this type of medical problem, but during my first eighteen years in pediatric allergy it never entered my mind that tics could even remotely be related to an allergy. In some children such a relationship, however, apparently can exist. Dr. Albert Rowe wrote about this problem in the thirties in his book entitled *Food Allergy*.[3]

3. Albert Rowe, M.D., *Food Allergy: Its Manifestations, Diagnosis, and Treatment With a General Discussion of Bronchial Asthma* (Springfield, Ill.: Charles C. Thomas Publishing, 1972).

A Child With Tics and Hyperactivity

Julius

Julius was eight years old when he came to see us and subsequently to teach us. His parents were concerned mainly because he was hyperactive and had many school problems. Ritalin had been recommended, but his parents preferred to investigate alternative methods to control his hyperactivity. Julius had classical hay fever, as well as allergic puffy eyes, dark eye circles, and wiggly legs. Along with these symptoms, Julius had a facial tic, which we initially assumed was unrelated to his obvious allergies.

His facial and shoulder tics began at the age of eight years, in the rainy month of April. At the time of his first visit, his face and eyes twitched and jerked repeatedly and he constantly made little noises, called vocal tics. This happened so frequently that it would have been difficult to count each tic. The tics were understandably a source of embarrassment and concern for Julius. His parents noted that the tics seemed worse when it was damp outside, when he was outside during the pollen season, and when he was stressed or upset.

During P/N allergy skin testing for molds, dust, and tree and grass pollens, it was obvious that we provoked a marked increase in his tics. The tics decreased during testing but did not stop until a week after his correct neutralization allergy treatment was given. This was unusual because most children improve within a very few days if their medical complaint lessens during allergy testing.

It is of interest to note that in contrast to mold and pollen allergy treatment, his *food* allergy therapy never appeared to affect his tics in any way.

A brain-wave examination had revealed that he had had petit mal epilepsy at the age of four years. After appropriate drug treatment by a neurologist, his staring spells stopped, but that treatment did not prevent or relieve the tics, which began four years later.

Medical Complaints Began Early in Julius's Life

Once again we were impressed because his allergy problems dated back to infancy. He repeatedly vomited and spit up his infant milk formulas until he was given a soy formula.

Intestinal complaints, fluid behind his eardrums, overactivity, irritability, easy crying, and behavior and concentration problems were all evident by the age of three years. It took several more years, however, before his family realized that allergy might be related to his many diverse medical complaints.

He tended to wet his bed every year in the spring. In time we determined that unlike children who have lung spasm when the trees pollinate, Julius appeared to have bladder spasm at that time. After tree pollen treatment, he was dry at night for months.[4] (See Chapter 3 for more details about bed-wetting.)

Every few months, especially during damp weather or a pollen season, Julius's tics suddenly reappeared. His tics subside after he returns to our office for retesting and appropriate adjustment of his mold and pollen allergy extract treatment. It is essential to eliminate his tics as much and as soon as possible, so that his self-esteem can remain high.

The Multiple Food Elimination Diet revealed that many of his behavior problems became dramatically worse when he drank milk and to a lesser degree when he ate corn, wheat, and soy. In time his mother determined that his clucking throat sounds were due to milk. His headaches were associated with exposure to lawn spray.

How Is Julius Now?

Three years after ecologic and allergy care he remains about 90 percent improved. His school performance has improved along with most of his symptoms. When he suddenly develops tics, his parents usually know why. One typical example of this occurred about two years after we initially saw him. He visited a very moldy museum, and within forty-five minutes his severe tics suddenly recurred. They subsided within a half hour after he left the museum. The molds or dust in the museum were the likely causes, because so often in the past, skin testing for these items caused his tics to flare up and his neutralization allergy treatment relieved the problem. Molds in particular seem to be an allergenic substance that is often related to the occurrence of his tics.

Seizures

In 1904, there was one reference in the medical literature to foods causing reactions within the brain. In 1911, Dr. H. Batty Shaw reported that he had a patient whose convulsions were due to eggs and

4. G. Lagrue et al., "Food Sensitivity and Ideopathic Nephrotic Syndrome," *Lancet* 2 (1987), p. 277.

milk.[5] Numerous doctors have reported similar observations for the past sixty years. While foods appeared to cause many allergy-related seizures, others appeared to be caused by vaccines, pets, pollen, dust, and molds. Dr. M. Brent Campbell, M.D., reviewed the medical literature and reported that some investigators found that seizures due to allergies sometimes caused abnormal brain waves, whereas others remained normal.[6] To add to the confusion, the electroencephalogram can apparently on occasion be positive in some normal children who have no seizures and negative in others in whom seizures are a problem. Although helpful, the EEG unfortunately does not always provide definitive answers.

Dr. Hal Davidson reviewed the medical literature in 1952 and found that seizures were sometimes related to allergies to milk, egg, wheat, chocolate, beef, pork, veal, corn, citrus, cheese, nuts, potato, sugar, pineapple, pollen, and cats.[7] It was not uncommon to find that some epileptics also had allergies or allergic relatives. Some epileptics tended to have intestinal symptoms before their seizures, and some had other typical manifestations of allergy before or in association with their convulsions. Some had seizures only at the peak of the pollen season. Many of the patients he mentioned had their first seizure early in life, then after seeming to be well for years, they developed both allergies and epilepsy later on in life.

In 1985, Dr. Joseph Egger, head of a pediatric university hospital in Munich, collaborated with Dr. Jonathan Soothill from the department of neurology and immunology at the Hospital for Sick Children in London to study hyperactivity.[8] Their results were remarkably similar to the study I published in 1978.[9] They found that foods did affect the behavior and activity level of some children. During their hyperactivity study, however, they noted that a few epileptic overactive children stopped having seizures during the diet portion of their study. They therefore decided to study a group of epileptic children.

5. H. Batty Shaw, M.D., "Hypersensitiveness: The Parallelism in the Phenomena of Hypersensitiveness and Certain Clinical Manifestations of Obscure Nature," *Lancet* 1 (1912), pp. 713–719.

6. M. Brent Campbell, M.D., "Neurological Manifestations of Allergic Disease," *Annals of Allergy* 31 (1973), pp. 485–498.

7. Hal Davidson, M.D., "Allergy and the Nervous System," *Quarterly Review of Allergy and Applied Immunology* 6 (1952), p. 157.

8. Joseph Egger, M.D., et al., "Controlled Trial of Oligoantigenic Treatment in the Hyperkinetic Syndrome," *Lancet* (1985), pp. 540–545.

9. Doris J. Rapp, M.D., "Does Diet Affect Hyperactivity?" *Journal of Learning Disabilities* 11 (1978), pp. 56–62.

In that study they evaluated forty-five epileptic children who had associated headaches, hyperactivity, and abdominal complaints.[10] They found that twenty-five of the forty-five children in this group stopped having seizures, as well as their other medical complaints, after certain offending foods were removed from their diet. An additional eleven of the forty-five children had fewer seizures. Another group of eighteen children, however, who had epilepsy that was *not associated with other symptoms* showed no improvement with dietary manipulation.

Unfortunately, there was a delay of several years before these distinguished academic medical investigators were able to have the results of their double-blinded study accepted for publication. Finally, in the *Journal of Pediatrics* (January 1989), the pediatricians in this country could read about this well-conducted study that again indicated that foods can sometimes cause epilepsy.

AN INFANT WITH SEIZURES

Daniel

Most parents (or physicians) would not ever consider that epileptic seizures could be related to allergies. Daniel's parents, however, were exceptions. They brought Daniel to see us when he was sixteen months old because he began to have seizures when he was a year old.

Both parents were very allergic. When Daniel was in the uterus, he kicked more than normal. As an infant he had severe colic and excessive screaming from the age of two to six months. He was so overactive after birth that his mother said he was able to stand on his legs at two days and he walked at nine and a half months. He made clucking sounds until his mother stopped giving him milk. He developed a rash when he wore disposable diapers, but cloth diapers were well tolerated.

Daniel was given a milk formula during the first year of life. At one time he was tried on a soy formula, but he refused it. He had classical nose allergies by the age of four months and asthma by the age of sixteen months. He also developed hives from orange juice.

10. Joseph Egger, M.D., et al., "Oligoantigenic Diet Treatment of Children With Epilepsy and Migraine," *Journal of Pediatrics* 114 (1)(1989), pp. 51–58.

Daniel's First Seizure at One Year of Age

His first seizure occurred at the age of twelve months. He had one seizure a month for about eight months, then he had two to three a month. His seizures had a pattern. He would become irritable and cranky, then gag and vomit, and finally he would have his convulsion. These seizures tended to last only a few seconds, but on occasion they lasted as long as twenty minutes. His mother noted that the attacks repeatedly seemed to occur after he ate chicken, eggs, or dairy products. On occasion they were also associated with the odor of certain perfumes.

The family lived in a small town in New York near a cheese factory. His mother noted that her son did well provided she watched his diet very carefully and stringently avoided the suspected foods.

Then, for no apparent reason, he developed a series of seizures again. After some reflection she realized that his seizures began again the very first day after the local cheese plant began to dump its whey (milk residue) into the nearby creek at night. This caused the air in the area of their home to smell "foul and cheesy." Daniel would always complain of the odor before the rest of the family. (We wondered if this was another example of the enhanced sense of smell noted in so many allergic individuals to help protect them.) He was routinely the first one to alert the family when the plant resumed its dumping. The family would rush to shut the windows and use fans to cool their home. Daniel was not allowed to play outside very often that entire summer because his parents feared he would have another seizure. He continued to have seizures once or twice a week until the dumping stopped and the air quality improved.

In spite of his parents' many precautions to avoid the foods thought to cause seizures, unavoidable errors continued to confirm their suspicions. His latest attack occurred when he was two and a half years old. His mother cautioned the waitress that there must not be any cheese on a sub sandwich that she bought for Daniel. The girl, however, forgot and sprinkled it with cheese. Several hours later he had another seizure. That was the first attack in almost six months.

His IgE RAST blood test for egg or chicken allergy showed no reaction, and the milk IgE RAST showed only a questionably positive response. The less reliable test called IgG RAST surprisingly showed an extreme sensitivity to milk, and a moderate reaction to egg.

This again points out that the IgE RAST for allergy can be misleading and does not always give the final answers. These particular blood allergy tests certainly did not provide unequivocal evidence to help pinpoint Daniel's food sensitivities.

Repeated brain-wave tests and a CAT scan test were also negative. This again indicates that our tests to document certain medical problems are limited by the technology at this time. Future developments of more precise advanced methods to study brain function should enable us to confirm or negate that specific foods or odors cause his seizures in the next few years.

At the present time his seizures are infrequent unless he accidentally eats one of the foods that are thought to cause his epilepsy. His mother chose to treat her son by total avoidance of the foods she suspects cause his epilepsy rather than to use allergy extract therapy. She has been quite successful using this approach.

My Own Awakening About Seizures and Allergy

My own personal exposure to patients who had neurological problems due to allergy began in the late seventies. I was visiting Dr. William Rea's office in Dallas, Texas. His nurse was about to test a young woman who said that for five years she had had sudden "peculiar" spells during which she could not stand or walk normally. The nurse injected a drop of weed allergy extract into her arm, and in seconds this young woman began to walk in a most bizarre manner. She was quickly given a weaker dilution of the same allergy extract, and just as suddenly she was again walking normally. When she was fine, she went into the rest room. Unfortunately, someone had smoked a cigarette in that room a few minutes earlier. When she came out of the lavatory, she was again walking in the same strange manner. She was given her known correct neutralization dose of tobacco, and again she quickly returned to normal. She had repeatedly noted this type of response to tobacco odors in the past. Until she was treated, she was afraid to go outside her home because of this reaction. She told me about the many years of ridicule she had endured. Many medical specialists had been unable to relieve her progressively debilitating problem. She had been told repeatedly that her problems were purely psychological. Dr. William Rea resolved her unusual spells by diagnosing and treating her food and other allergies and by the recognition of her chemical sensitivities.

A few minutes later a refined, attractive patient was tested for dust. She lay on a blanket on the floor for the test because her medical history indicated that she had seizures. She was smiling when she was given her first injection of an allergy extract for dust. In seconds she stiffened and had a grand mal seizure. The nurse calmly and quickly gave her a weaker dilution of extract, and before my eyes, almost immediately, she was back to normal, smiling and talking again. Subsequent to her allergy treatment she had not had a seizure for two years.

I was bewildered and amazed by the many ways that the nervous system could be affected by a droplet of an allergy extract during that visit to Dr. Rea's clinic. Since then the specialty of environmental medicine has proven to be astonishing on many occasions. It seems truly amazing that one drop of a weak solution of a food or allergenic substance can suddenly cause a patient's medical complaint and a slightly weaker solution will just as speedily stop the response. Our bodies are truly created with an intricate magnificent sensitivity that deserves admiration and unending appreciation. There is certainly very much that we as physicians need to investigate and understand so that more people can be helped.

Could allergy or chemical sensitivities be part of the answer for some children or adults who have cerebral palsy, autism, multiple sclerosis, post-polio syndrome, tired-housewife syndrome, panic syndrome, or schizophrenia? Some specialists in environmental medicine, such as Dr. Marshall Mandell in Norwalk, Connecticut, and Dr. William Rea in Dallas, Texas, in particular, have studied patients who have these types of challenging problems. Some have appeared to be helped to varying degrees. Much more research is needed to help identify the subset of these affected individuals in whom allergy, chemical sensitivities, and nutrient deficiencies could be contributory and significant factors.

Post-Polio Syndrome

Recently a number of reports have indicated that some polio victims who had their illness forty-some years ago have redeveloped symptoms of their original polio, as well as nasal and sinus problems. Dr. Lawrence Dickey in 1971 reported one patient (his daughter) who improved after avoidance of environmental pollutants. Dr. William Rea and his associates in Dallas have reported long-term benefit in fourteen out of seventeen patients.[11] In one additional patient, however, the help was only temporary. He found fourteen out of seventeen had less leg weakness and eight out of seventeen had less pain when these patients followed a four-day rotation diet, ate organically grown foods, and made their homes more environmentally free of

11. William Rea, M.D., et al., "The Environmental Aspects of the Post-Polio Syndrome," World Conference on Post-Polio, 1986.

typical allergenic substances (dust and molds), pollutants, and chemicals. During P/N testing, they were sensitive to molds, foods, and chemicals, including the chlorine in swimming pools, and gas odors, tobacco, or formaldehyde in homes. Two of five patients improved with a P/N dose of polio vaccine. It was postulated that the overload of environmental pollutants had affected previously damaged areas of the nervous system. The heightened sensitivity to cold and odors also suggested that the environment was affecting these previously afflicted polio patients. Affected individuals should try to notice if chemical or pollution triggers sudden weakness or pain. Until more is known about how to help these individuals, allergy, sensitivities to chemicals, and the efficacy of their enzyme detoxification systems should certainly be evaluated in affected individuals.

CHAPTER 21

Delinquency—
Does It Start Early
in Allergic Children?

Key publications by Alexander Schauss and Stephen Schoenthaler and books by Barbara Reed and Schauss indicate that unacceptable, delinquent behavior can indeed be related to diet.[1] For example the final report of a one-year study of nineteen juvenile delinquents by one probation department in California (San Luis Obispo County) in 1979 indicated that diet did affect both the health and the behavior of these youngsters.[2] It concluded that the removal of sugar and dairy products from the youngsters' diets resulted in less stuffiness, fewer skin lesions, increased energy, and decreased hostility, aggressiveness, irritability, and depression.

In this study 80 percent of the juvenile delinquents appeared to be hypoglycemic, and about 90 percent had food and environmental allergies. Their early medical histories indicated that an inordinate number had a history of mouth breathing, crib rocking, colic, asthma, dark eye circles, bone aches, hyperactivity, prolonged bed-wetting, repeated ear and tonsil infections, fatigue, headaches, poor concentration, insomnia, irritability, excess thirst, and destructive behavior. Most of these complaints are typical of many allergic children, including the patients described throughout this book.

1. See Bibliography for details.
2. Kenneth Schmidt, et al., "Clinical Ecology Treatment Approach for Juvenile Offenders." For copy of article, write: Box 693, Atascadero, Calif. 93422.

We must ask if perhaps we should routinely evaluate more delinquent and adult offenders for possible allergy or unusual sensitivities to environmental factors.[3] Maybe this could explain some irrational, unacceptable behavior that results in unexplainable nonprovoked episodes of vandalism or crime. Published evidence certainly suggests that the recidivism (or return to jail) rate could be decreased if food sensitivities were detected and appropriately treated in some individuals who are unable to adhere to the mores and standards of our civilized world.[4] Incarceration has been shown to be ineffective in many ways, and it is certainly not the ideal, definitive answer to deter criminal behavior. Our aim should be the recognition and appropriate treatment of unsuspected allergies if this is a piece of the criminal pie. In this way this select group of individuals, who do not respect law and order, might be able to detect and eliminate the cause of their unacceptable behavior and activity so that eventually they could become more responsible, contributing members of our society.

Some verbally or physically aggressive children in our office seem to have a distinct pattern. Unlike many allergic toddlers who routinely hit, bite, or spit for a year or two, these few children continue to hurt others as they grow older. They punch and kick, in particular their younger siblings, their mothers, or their friends. The pictures they draw are black, dark, and often demonstrate some form of hostility (Figures 18.1, 18.2, 18.3, 18.4, 21.1, 21.2). After they receive allergy treatment, their drawings are typically in cheery colors and depict some happy scene. During reactions from provocation testing their drawings quickly change from bright to dark colors, and the content suddenly reveals aggression. After their neutralization allergy extract treatment, once again their pictures become pleasant and the colors selected are no longer black and ominous.

We have no idea how some of our patients might have been if their food and other sensitivities had been recognized during the infant or toddler period. The following youngsters, however, certainly appear to have been on a path leading to serious behavior problems or possible delinquency.

3. Stephen J. Schoenthaler, "The Effect of Sugar on the Treatment and Control of Antisocial Behavior: A Double-Blind Study of an Incarcerated Juvenile Population," *International Journal of Biosocial Publications* 3 (1982), pp. 1–19.

4. J. Satterfield, "Therapeutic Interventions to Prevent Delinquency in Hyperactive Boys," *Journal of American Academy of Child and Adult Psychology* 26 (1987), pp. 56–64.

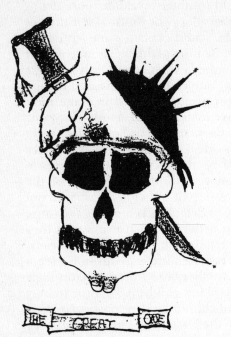

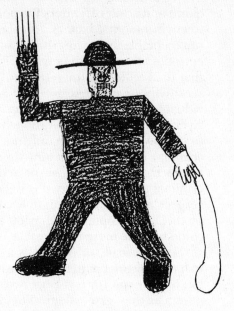

Figure 21.1. The hostility the young man has is evident in his drawings of skulls and knives.

Figure 21.2. This Freddy Kruger rendition was drawn by an aggressive youngster before allergy treatment.

AN EXTREMELY AGGRESSIVE AND DESTRUCTIVE YOUNGSTER

Jack

Jack was eight years old when we first saw him. His mother was distressed, disturbed, desperate, and badly bruised because of his recurrent episodes of violence. He frequently attacked her, as well as his younger brother and sister. He was known to stab his schoolmates with pencils and sharp rocks.

We documented one episode of extreme hostility and intolerable behavior shortly after Jack came to see us. During a provocative allergy skin test for strawberry, he proceeded to cover his mother's arms with bite marks. His face looked almost as if he were possessed. He glared at his mother, and in spite of our attempts to hold him and protect his mother, he jabbed and hit her in her eye. As she held her eye and quietly wept, he defiantly said, "Good." He cried at times, but his major activity during his reaction to strawberry was some form of aggression directed at his mother. After he received the correct dilution of a strawberry extract, he was again a normal, pleasant, cooperative youngster, in need of no outside restraint.

Unfortunately this was exactly the type of uncontrollable behavior he had often manifested in the past. Five days earlier he had eaten strawberry jam for breakfast prior to an unusually violent episode at school. That morning he refused to get dressed for school and kicked his brother. After he arrived at school, it was immediately apparent to his teacher that he was more uncooperative than usual. He was totally negative and refused to comply with any simple requests. In exasperation his teacher reprimanded him and sent him to the principal's office. He promptly grabbed as many papers as he could from the principal's desk and ripped them in half. Then he made one dramatic sweep with his arm across the desk, and everything else within reach was quickly propelled onto the floor. The security guards were called. They had difficulty restraining him. They urged that he be taken to the hospital because it appeared unsafe for his mother to drive alone with him in her car. His mother tried to give him his allergy extract under his tongue, but he spit it out. He did the same with his alkali. Finally she managed to give him his correct neutralization treatment dilution of histamine allergy extract. Within fifteen minutes he was quiet, calm, and pleasant. She had no difficulty taking him home. His behavior and activity were exemplary the rest of that day.

What were the clues that he might have allergies or that foods might be a factor related to his aggressive behavior? Let's start at the beginning.

Did he have allergic parents? His mother denied that she had an allergy but said that she frequently cleared her throat and "loved" cheese and ice cream. She knew that chemicals bothered her because automobiles, plastic, rubber, vinyl odors, or odors from grain factories all caused her to feel unwell. His father craved alcohol, and his allergy tests had revealed a very strong sensitivity to corn.

Jack as an Infant

As an infant Jack was calm and quiet. Aside from raw, bleeding buttocks on occasion, he seemed fine. He was breast-fed for the entire first year of life. However, ear problems began shortly after he started to drink milk. By the age of one and a half he needed to have tubes surgically placed through his eardrums because he had recurrent ear infections that caused fluid to form behind his eardrums.

Jack as a Toddler and Child

At fifteen months he ate candy for the first time. His mother said that Jack changed into a "Tasmianian devil." Later on he was so wound up at bedtime that he had problems falling asleep. As a young boy, his periods of hostility, hyperactivity, crying, and aggression were not rare. By the age of four he had added swearing and vulgarity to his repertoire. He would suddenly make karate-type chops at his siblings and mother. He would punctuate these with a few well-placed kicks, punches, and hits. The other children in school refused to play with him. He had no friends. He had many problems falling asleep at bedtime.

His mother had often noticed in the past that when Jack stopped eating because he had an infection, he became atypically pleasant, sweet, and loving. This made her wonder about a food allergy. When she asked her doctor if this could be an answer to his behavior problem, she was told that she should "learn to discipline him."

She was truly frightened by her son because he was so nasty and appeared to be so hateful when he became angry. He often stated he wanted to kill her. Although he was only eight years old, she was genuinely afraid when he attacked; he was extremely strong. His father's employment caused him to travel so frequently that he was usually not present to help control or discipline Jack.

A friend knew about her problems with Jack and sent his mother my previous book entitled *The Impossible Child*.[5] The friend had recognized a youngster who acted similarly to Jack on our 1988 *Donahue* show. In desperation his mother decided to try the two-week Multiple Food Elimination Diet. His Conner's Hyperactivity Score decreased from an abnormal high of 27 to a borderline normal of 15 within the first week. This improvement occurred even though his mother said he was very uncooperative during the first week of the diet. His mother concluded that his behavior improved about 20 percent, and his extreme halitosis subsided completely. During the second week of the diet, when milk was ingested, his karate chop activity recurred and he began to race around wildly and uncontrollably. At that time his halitosis also returned.

5. Doris J. Rapp, M.D., *The Impossible Child*. 1989. Practical Allergy Research Foundation (PARF), P.O. Box 60, Buffalo, N.Y. 14223-0060.

Handwriting ten minutes after drinking vanilla milkshake. At that time he became nasty and aggressive, and hit, screamed, and kicked.

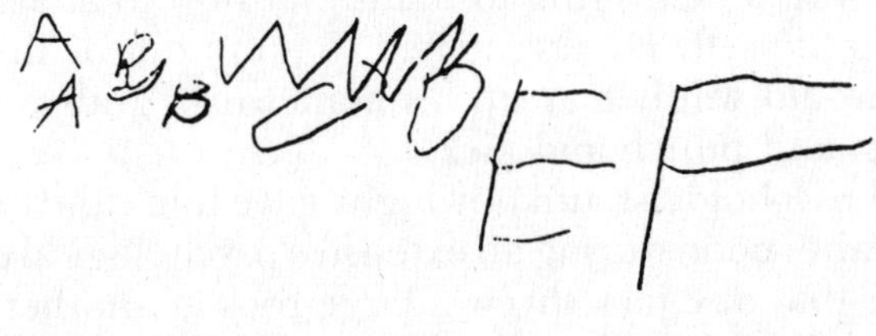

Handwriting twenty minutes after taking Alka-Seltzer antacid formula

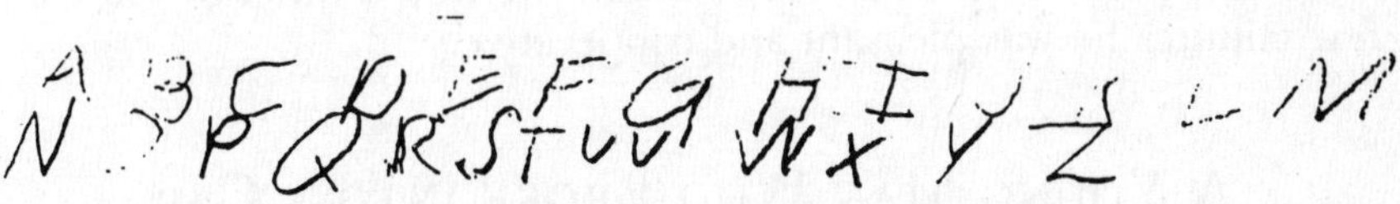

Handwriting twenty-five minutes after taking Alka-Seltzer antacid formula

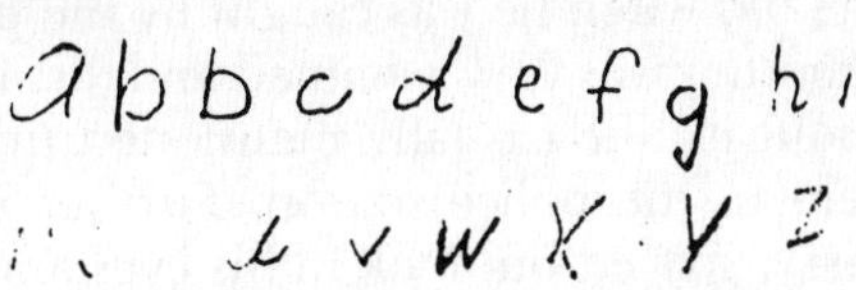

Figures 21.3–21.5. Jack would become noticeably hostile after drinking a vanilla milkshake. His handwriting and memory were also affected.

A vanilla milk shake a few weeks later caused another severe outburst of hostility. His mother found that an alkali often helped his unacceptable behavior to subside quickly. Figures 21.3–21.5 show samples of his writing before and after he received Alka-Seltzer Antacid Formula for his milk-shake reaction.

Jack's Response to P/N Treatment

After one month of treatment he was 40 percent improved, and after five months he was 75 percent better. Then he gradually stopped following his diet. He did not return for retesting and adjustment of his extract treatment doses because his family had problems with their insurance reimbursements and Jack did not want to return.

He began school in the fall without any treatment for ragweed. His school behavior was deplorable. At home he acted in an irrational manner. He would put his underwear over his head and then run around outside into the street. He frequently repeated that he was stupid and wished he was dead. On one occasion he ran wildly around the bedroom with a belt trying to figure out how to attach it so that he could hang himself. He threatened to jump out of the bedroom window. He would wildly tear up his homework, grab at other children's throats, and punch and kick.

His school psychologist, unknowingly, gave him candy corn in the morning and afternoon during an extensive psychological evaluation. By the end of that day Jack threw a large rock at another child. His mother had to chase him down the street, hold him down, and give him his allergy extract medicines before he would quiet down. In a few minutes he was pleasant and cooperative.

A YOUNG MAN WHO BROKE INTO A CAR

Martin

Martin was about fifteen years old when he was caught by the police after he broke into a car. His mother was very ashamed and disturbed when she called to tell us about it. She casually mentioned that he looked strange when she went to the police station. Further questioning revealed he had a glassy, spaced-out look in his eyes and red earlobes. He had apparently refused to eat breakfast that day and had skipped lunch. About an hour before the car break-in, at about 4:00 P.M., he ate for the first time that day. His meal consisted of several chocolate-covered peanut-butter cups.

We asked his mother to try to duplicate this diet the following weekend. He ate nothing that day until 4:00 P.M. and then he was given two chocolate peanut-butter cups again. He started to act up, so he was sent to his room. When his mother went to check to see how he was, she found her fifteen-year-old son eating toothpaste.

We decided to repeat the same diet once again the next weekend. He seemed fine before the candy. Afterward he again acted in an equally abnormal manner. He was kicking the walls of his home. He became very agitated. His mother could not believe how his personality changed and that his actions could become so unacceptable. We will never know for sure if this is why he broke into the car, but it appeared that chocolate peanut-butter cups certainly did alter his behavior in such a manner that he repeatedly acted inappropriately.

A DETERMINED YOUNG MAN WHO RESISTS BEING HELPED

John

John was only sixteen years old when he was asked not to return to school. He ran away from home, but fortunately his family found him. A few days after he returned home, his family was told that he had robbed a gun store a few months earlier. When the stash of hidden ammunition was found, he was placed in jail. This unfortunately was not the first time stealing had been a problem. His mother said that for years she had to lock up everything of value and hide her wallet. He had taken precious family items in the past and had sold them to play video games.

Let's try to answer some obvious questions. When did it all begin? Could anything have been done to prevent this problem? Can anything be done now to turn his young life around?

When Did It All Begin?

John's family had many allergic relatives. His mother drank an excess of milk each morning when she was pregnant, and John kicked very hard in the uterus, especially in the morning.

As an infant he broke his crib because he rocked so vigorously. He destroyed his high chair. He banged his head on things until he was black and blue. He screamed hour after hour, night and day, until he was three years old. His mother said she could not stand his crying and she would place him downstairs near the door of their farmhouse so that the screaming noises would go outside. She would then go upstairs to the most distant room so that she could hide her head under the blankets and cry. She said she was afraid she might lose control and hurt him. He only slept in short spurts and never ate well. He simply was not a cuddly, lovable baby.

By the time he was two years old, he had hay fever, asthma, and recurrent ear infections. He could not play more than ten minutes at a time. As a young child his parents described him as "intolerable" and "always difficult." Nightmares and temper tantrums were common problems for many years.

By the age of fourteen years his parents were concerned because he rarely smiled. He was hyperactive, restless, irritable, hostile, and argumentative. He complained of backaches, leg aches, and headaches. He was always worse near holidays, when he ate more sweets.

He was suicidal on occasion and had written a will by the time he was ten years old. His mother stated that at times he almost looked possessed. She was truly afraid of him when he developed a certain "terrible, hateful look in his eyes." He wore only black or gray clothing and he enjoyed drawing pictures of skulls, knives, lynchings, and blood. He did not respect other people's property and tended to take what he wanted. He never helped with any household or farming chores. He had many problems in school, and at the age of sixteen he was suspended three times in one month.

Could Anything Have Been Done to Prevent It?

When John was fourteen, he was initially seen in our office for evaluation of his allergies. He looked about eighteen and was totally disinterested in the visit, which his parents had insisted upon. He tended to breathe with his mouth open, had dark eye circles, and was so tired he slouched and could not sit upright in a chair. By the end of the first visit after P/N testing he was less wiggly and more pleasant. He was smiling and already breathing with his mouth closed. Within one month after comprehensive allergy treatment, which included diet and home changes, as well as allergy extract treatment, he was 70 percent improved. He continued to be happier and less negative. The Ritalin, which had not helped during the previous year, was discontinued. His school performance improved, although scholastically he continued to do poorly. He became more cooperative. He continued to be 70 percent better throughout the entire following year.

Then, at the age of fifteen, he decided that treatment was no longer required, refused to adhere to any diet, and rarely took his allergy extract correctly. Within the next few months his behavior gradually and progressively deteriorated. He was stealing and smoking. He became defiant and argumentative. By the age of sixteen he was detained in jail for several days after burglarizing a gun store.

Initially his attitude was unrepentant. He said that jail was a "riot" and that he enjoyed his stay. After several days, however, he reluctantly decided he would resume his allergy treatment if that might prevent a jail term.

Can Anything Be Done Now to Turn His Young Life Around?

The judge's decision concerning his future was influenced by the following:

His caring parents immediately brought him back to our office for reevaluation and retesting. He had a sour scowl on his face and he looked down or the other way when he answered questions. He drew a picture of a black skull with fanglike teeth (Figure 21.1). After the second allergy test for molds his face suddenly lit up and his parents noticed the first smile in about a year. He began to use colors in his drawings, and by the end of the day he was all smiles and even drew a smiling, animated object with several colors. His parents were delighted. That evening his behavior was remarkably improved. He could sit still and watch television without getting up every few minutes. He was pleasant and smiling. He went to sleep without difficulty. The next day he was still smiling and bought some white-and-red sneakers. They were not his usual black or gray!

After four weeks of comprehensive allergy treatment, his parents were elated. He was smiling more than ever, and his attitude was excellent. His room was cleaner than it had ever been. After his old carpet was removed and an air purifier was placed in his room, he breathed more easily and his nose was less congested. He also seemed less stuffy after he received his neutralization dose of allergy extract. He was more alert in the morning and looked forward to school. He wore brighter clothing, and his drawings showed much less aggression. His mood swings and depression were less evident. However, he continued to be disorganized.

Then he decided to stop the Practical Rotary Diet, and within a period of two weeks he began to smile less often and to become more argumentative, moody, and defiant. He returned for more allergy tests, and again he responded well and quickly. Once again, however, in a couple of months he was eating foods that adversely affected his behavior, stopped taking his allergy extract correctly, and refused to cooperate. He was caught stealing again and spent time in jail.

This young man's future is definitely in jeopardy if he chooses to ignore his allergies. He repeatedly backslides each time he manifests his independence.

If delinquency tendencies are to be prevented, parents, physicians, and educators should be aware of the *many early clues* that suggest that aggression and nonconformity may be related to allergies. Then measures could be taken much earlier to prevent possible delinquency. Many children, such as John, provide ample and repeated clues that allergy is one aspect of their problem and that the direction of their lives needs to be drastically altered. Even though we initially saw John at age fourteen, we could only help him on a temporary basis.

It is difficult to treat allergies in adolescence because the teenager's basic nature is often one of independence, denial, and self-assertion. We can show them the way, but we can't do it for them. Even if allergy is only a small piece of the total picture, appropriate treatment for that piece should help these children to some degree.

If you can recognize a basic allergic problem in your difficult child, preferably very early in life, you may be able to turn your youngster's entire future around. The typical clues are evident in one child after another, and are discussed throughout this book. Prevention is one key and that depends on earlier recognition and appropriate treatment.

CHAPTER 22

Could Allergy and Suicide
Be Related?

The Relation of Severe Depression to Allergy

Dr. Albert Rowe started writing about depression as a manifestation of allergy as early as the late twenties. Theron Randolph made similar observations in the forties.[1] Since we have been using the newer method of allergy testing called provocation/neutralization, we have definitely seen that we can "provoke" some children so that they suddenly act depressed from our allergy skin tests. We have repeatedly, dramatically, and quickly seen some children's despondency reversed. These children will appear normal during many allergy tests until they are tested with one specific offending item. Then they suddenly appear unhappy and begin to cry. Sometimes they curl into a fetal position, become withdrawn, scream, and pull away if anyone approaches them. After they are treated with the appropriate dilution of the same allergy extract solution, their joyful personality and affect quickly returns. We have videotaped these types of responses in older infants, toddlers, children, and adolescents. Their reactions are remarkably similar. (See Chapter 7.)

We routinely ask children to write and/or draw prior to the time we test them, during their reactions to our allergy tests, and again after the neutralization dilution of allergy extract has relieved their reaction. When their response is depression, they often refuse to write, write very tiny, push the pad away, heave the pencil and clipboard across the room, or break the pencil and crumple up the paper.

1. See Bibliography for details.

If they are depressed and angry, they often draw knives, blood, and skulls.

On occasion we see children in our office whose parents comment that they act just like a teenage brother, uncle, cousin, or father who committed suicide. Some parents also say that their three-, five-, or eight-year-old children repeatedly state that they wish they were dead or that they want to kill themselves. There are innumerable children who say, "Nobody likes me," "I hate myself," "I'm never good enough," and there are others who threaten to leave home. There are even some children who do more than talk; in some manner they actually attempt to kill themselves. A few children have tried to smother their faces in pillows, or they purposely sit in the middle of the road so that cars will hit them. Some have tried to jump out of windows or have taken knives into the bathroom with so much determination that their parents have had to feverishly break down the locked door to save them. Some have written wills.

Seasonally Suicidal Children

We are continually surprised to find children who have seasonal pollen or mold allergy that causes depression or withdrawn behavior rather than hay fever or asthma. Some parents have noted that their child repeatedly becomes suicidal at the same time every year. Some of these children act this way in the spring and summer when the trees or grass pollinate, others in the fall when the weeds are prevalent. Others act this way on damp, rainy days or whenever the outdoor or indoor mold spore count is high. This suggests that molds, fungi, or yeast may be factors in some children's depression. Their history of allergy-related illness rarely starts with a depression episode just prior to their first visit to see us. Similar to the other children in this book, the clues suggesting both the typical and the infrequently recognized forms of allergy, often with depression, date back to infancy or the toddler period. (See Bryan, Appendix E.)

A Son and Father, Depressed Every May

Bruce

The most suggestive evidence that a suicidal tendency might be related to seasonal allergy and be evident in families was noted in Bruce. He was initially seen in our office when he was twelve. His family lived in southern Pennsylvania.

Before he saw us, his mother had noted that each year in early May, Bruce seemed to become angry. At that time he walked in a slouched manner, stopped smiling, and developed headaches. In May 1988 this pattern was again apparent. He complained of headaches, acted depressed, and his behavior deteriorated, especially when he was outside. At times he acted gloomy, nasty, angry, and spaced out. His behavior and ability to pay attention were a definite problem in school.

In May 1989 he suddenly began to say, "It is the worst year in my whole life" and "I wish I was dead." He said, "I hope I will never wake up." Ironically I had called his mother the week before to find out how he was doing because I knew about his history of depression in May 1988. She assured me that he was acting fine and did not show a tinge of despair. One week later she called back to say he had suddenly become very depressed again. After P/N retesting for grass and tree pollen allergy, he resumed his usual happy nature.

Bruce's Father's History

His grandfather had two copies of a picture of Bruce's dad when he was about nine years old. They were identical except that one showed a halo pasted over the young boy's head, while over the other he had placed a pair of horns. As a very young child, Bruce's father would not stay dressed. He smashed all his toys, was unable to sit still, and could not concentrate. He had drastic mood changes and sometimes became violent. He tended to fight with everyone. Bruce's dad had a long history of disposition problems and was abusive to both his wife and his son, particularly every May. It happened year after year, and although his wife recognized the consistent pattern, she never understood why. His dad intensely disliked milk but craved cheese and ice cream, which strongly suggested a dairy sensitivity. He was also very fond of beer and junk food. Bruce's father had tried unsuccessfully to commit suicide at the age of eighteen. He succeeded, however, one May, when he was only forty-five years old. He had binged on dairy products and beer just before the tragedy.

Bruce's Early History

Bruce's history indicated that there were many allergic relatives on both sides of the family. His problems did not start at the age of twelve when he came to see us. When he was in the uterus, his mother thought he kicked and hiccupped more than normal. Later on, as an infant, he was never cuddly and his mother described him as "always on the go."

By the time he was three and a half years of age, he had a severe behavior problem. During his first session with the psychologist he kicked her in the leg and would not cooperate. His mother was urged to discipline him.

Bruce, Aged Six to Twelve Years

When he was six years old, his father committed suicide. Shortly after his father's death, Bruce was said to be borderline retarded and found to have an IQ of 80 during that evaluation. Four years later his IQ was gauged at 140. At age twelve it was gauged at 110 to 120.

When Bruce was seven, Ritalin was prescribed because he was extremely hyperactive. When he took it, however, he simply could not sleep. He paced all night, lost weight, and acted like a "zombie." This drug had to be discontinued. At that time his schoolwork was so poor that the teachers wanted to fail him. Although he seemed bright, there were times when he could not even complete a sentence.

By the age of nine he had frequent headaches and said, "I want to kill myself, like my dad."

Between the ages of seven and ten he was drinking an excessive amount of milk, and his hyperactivity and behavior were major problems. He also complained of the leg aches that are so commonly seen in younger children who have a milk allergy. His mother was told that she and her son were both "maladjusted and crazy." The doctors blamed Bruce's mother because he could not behave.

At the age of nine, because he was too active and always talking, behavior modification was tried again. It helped, but not nearly enough. By the age of ten he was failing in school and had been labeled by various experts as "retarded, handicapped, learning-disabled, and dangerous." He was also diagnosed as having ADD, attention deficit disorder. His mother was told that he was spoiled. She was urged to "be tougher" and to "beat some sense into the monster." He was seen by a psychologist, who said that Bruce was immature, lacked confidence, and had poor self-control. His mother was urged to retry Ritalin to control his overactivity.

By age eleven he was even worse. He was failing in school in every imaginable way. He had an impossible behavior problem, a reputation for fighting, and was unable to sit still. Although Bruce was in the fifth grade, he was reading at a second-grade level.

By the time he was twelve, Bruce was wiggly, irritable, clumsy, hostile, and unhappy. It was not unusual for him to pound the table, stamp his feet, and kick doors. He complained of frequent abdominal gas, belching, and diarrhea. After allergy diets and testing, it was determined that his intestinal problems subsided completely if he did not drink milk.

Bruce's Mother Has Two Choices

Early in 1988, his mother was advised to restart Ritalin after a two-week evaluation at a Pennsylvania state-subsidized institution. He lost total control and behaved most unacceptably shortly after he was given two glasses of an orange drink before one of his interview sessions. Only his mother recognized the cause-and-effect relationship. One doctor predicted that he had a 50 percent chance of becoming a drug addict, alcoholic, or criminal by the age of twenty. His mother was *assured* by the head physician that foods such as dyes and sugar could *not* cause behavior problems.

At that time, his mother happened to see our *Donahue* show, which discussed the relation of foods to childhood illnesses and behavior. She decided to remove milk and dairy products from Bruce's diet rather than to retry Ritalin. In one day he was better. In two days the change was so dramatic that the teacher called his mother. She said that his writing had suddenly became legible and that he was cooperative. He was so good, attentive, and quiet that his teacher thought Bruce was sick or taking some new kind of medicine to subdue him. His Conner's Hyperactivity Score decreased from an extreme abnormal high of 28 to a normal level of 3 within one week. He was able to sit still "for the first time in his life." His mother was astonished. In the next few weeks he stopped blurting out answers in class. His teacher said, "I can't say enough about the change I've seen in Bruce."

Bruce's Mother Finds Answers

When his mother evaluated other foods, she noted that, in particular, milk, apple, and egg caused him to develop dark eye circles and to go "berserk." He also began to talk excessively and became hyperactive and irritable. His voice even became higher in pitch if he drank milk. Within one hour after drinking milk, he had trouble spelling. He repeatedly whined "no," shook his hands, and pounded the table. He threw himself against a chair, tossed his pencil, and said he was stupid. His eyes became glassy. His head dropped, and when he was asked to sit down, he doubled up his fists and stood up, ready for action.

Six weeks later his mother said he was amazing everyone. Bruce stated that he was glad and relieved because for the first time he realized he wasn't crazy or dumb. His appearance was neater. His grades changed to all A's and B's. He continued to be cooperative.

Within a few months after allergy treatment Bruce won a coveted science award in school. His grades and behavior improved dramatically. His vocabulary and comprehension tests indicated an increase of two years during a one-year period. He finished schoolwork in about half the usual time and did it well. He had more friends. One year later his mother commented that whereas she could not stand to be around him before his allergy treatment, now it was pleasant to be with him, and they had quality time together.

Bruce was part of a pilot research study to monitor the changes in the brain and blood of children who react to foods. His neurometric brain waves showed only a minimal change in the posterior area of the brain during his reaction to red gelatin. His blood revealed that his serotonin levels rose progressively after he ingested food dyes. Tryptophan, our natural brain tranquilizer, makes serotonin in our bodies. Serotonin is released by blood platelets and tends to constrict blood vessels. This might have partially explained why his leg muscles cramped and hurt during and after the test. His blood was tested for thirty different amino acids. Thirteen of his were elevated before he was tested for food colors; during the reaction twenty-two increased; and after treatment only seven were raised. The changes in specific amino acids indicated increased tissue breakdown and stress, as well as changes in substances that can affect nerve transmission within the brain.[2]

A GIRL WHO BECAME DEPRESSED EVERY SPRING

Lalena

Lalena was only six years old when her mother came to see us from Michigan. Lalena's teachers noted that she seemed depressed each year at the time when the trees pollinate. She would act this way for

2. The above study was done in conjunction with David Cantor, Ph.D., a psychologist associated with the University of Maryland School of Medicine. J. Alexander Bralley, Ph.D., at MetaMetrix Laboratory in Norcross, Ga., kindly interpreted the amino acid data.

about two or three weeks and then seem fine again. Lalena had many other symptoms that were compatible with allergies, for example year-round nose symptoms, itchy and puffy red eyes, dark eye circles, severe coughing and wheezing during the fall and winter, excessive infections, eczema, bellyaches, irritability, easy crying, and behavior problems. Her well-read and -informed mother brought her in to see us mainly because she was particularly despondent and unhappy. At the age of eight, during retesting for tree pollen she wrote her name and drew the pictures in Figures 22.1, 22.2, and 22.3. On the first picture she wrote, "Jan is dumb." Jan was her allergy-testing nurse at that time. After her neutralization allergy treatment you can easily see that her picture reflected how much better she felt.

The next year at the same time she again acted morose, melancholic, and depressed. Her neutralization treatment dose for tree pollen had changed. After she was retested for tree pollen and the dose was corrected, she was fine. Since then we try to recheck her

Irritable, angry,
suicidal, uncooperative

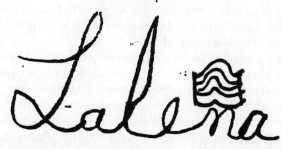

Ten minutes after pollen
treatment—pleasant

Figure 22.1. Changes in handwriting during a tree pollen allergy test in an eight-year-old girl

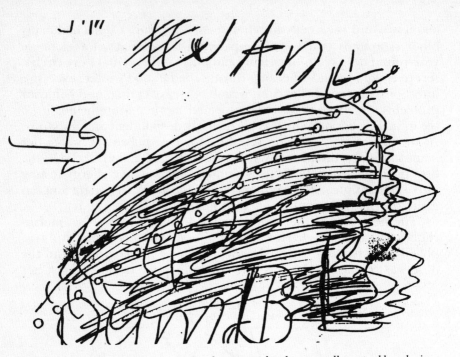

Figure 22.2. When Lalena was eight, she appeared to have an allergy problem during the tree-pollen season. In this drawing, her aggressive and unhappy nature is apparent.

tree-allergy extract dosage before each tree season, and she remains fine when the trees pollinate.

Allergy skin tests for airborne molds also repeatedly caused personality changes. Figure 22.4 clearly demonstrates how her writing changed during mold testing. She cried, became upset, and then refused to draw. Then she became very angry, said her hands hurt, and was very unhappy. Her disposition was explosive. When she was given a dose of mold extract that was close to her neutralization dose, she improved. Gradually she became less angry, stopped crying, and her hands became less painful.

Molds are accepted factors related to joint pain. It is well known that many arthritics are worse on rainy days and can predict damp weather. Maybe Lalena's inability to write because her hands hurt indicates a potential propensity to joint pain in the future. Can future arthritis be prevented with mold or other allergy treatment? We simply don't know. Some publications certainly indicate that diet does help some arthritics.[3]

3. See Bibliography for details.

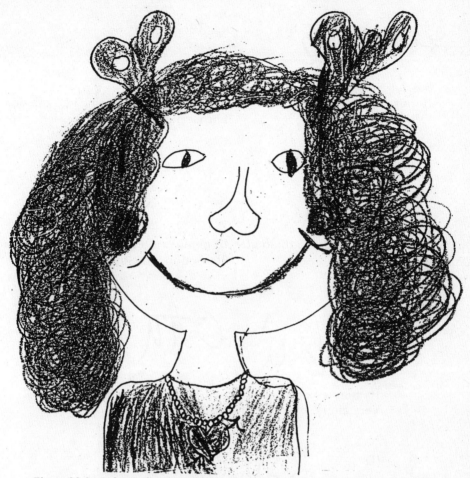

Figure 22.3. Lalena's drawing ten minutes after treatment with the correct dilution of tree pollen allergy extract

A GIRL DEPRESSED
EVERY FALL THROUGH THE WINTER

Erin

We saw Erin when she was six years old because she had hives and hay fever. Her mother was also allergic. She mentioned that Erin tended to become depressed shortly after school began each fall and that this change lasted until the following June. This had happened for the previous two years. Her mother was also concerned because Erin was a perfectionist. She had to do everything exactly right. She

(a)

Baseline
Happy

(b)

10 minutes after 0.05 ml 1:25 dilution
Throat hurt

(c)

(d)

10 minutes after 0.05 ml 1:125 dilution
Crying, upset

10 minutes after 0.05 ml 1:625 dilution
Refused to write or draw

(e)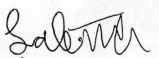

10 minutes after total 0.15 ml 1:125 dilution
Very angry, explosive, hands hurt, very unhappy

(f)

10 minutes after total 0.20 ml 1:125 dilution
Gradually stopped crying, less angry. Said throat
  and hands better.

(g)

17 minutes after total 0.20 ml 1:125 dilution
Much better. Smiling, back to normal.

Figure 22.4. Changes in writing during Lalena's allergy skin test for mold

seemed to be inordinately upset if her schoolwork was not absolutely correct. She also had some bizarre behavior patterns, which began with hives and progressed to hyperactivity and antsy behavior. Then she'd scream, thrash about, kick, and act "crazy." She developed a spacey look in her eyes, and at times she would even bite herself. Her mother described her as self-destructive during these episodes.

Initially she responded well to comprehensive allergy treatment. She remained improved through the rest of that next school year. The following fall, however, she began to have several episodes of hysterical behavior each week. One occurred after gym class, another after an exposure to a felt-tipped marking pen. She crawled on the floor and tried to get away from everyone. She acted in a bizarre manner, vacillating between uncontrollable crying and ridiculous silliness. She was totally unable to communicate verbally, and the school nurse described her actions as "incredible." During these episodes she also became very itchy. The latter clue suggested that her sudden changes in behavior could be related to allergy.

This recurrence of personality problems indicated that her allergy extract needed readjustment. During P/N retesting for dust, she became upset, cried, whined, and stomped her feet. We adjusted her allergy treatment, and her periods of inappropriate behavior disappeared.

The next fall, however, she returned once more because she had four more episodes of abnormal behavior at school within one month. She seemed worse at school and on damp days. She threatened to hurt herself. She climbed into a garbage can and on another occasion into a waste basket. She cried and said she hated herself. She fell apart because she could not play a new piece of music perfectly shortly after she initially saw it. These symptoms occurred when her school was being remodeled and shortly after the heat had been turned on. After retesting again, she began treatment with an updated allergy extract for molds, dust, and mites. We checked with her father during the winter of 1989 and he reported that she was doing very well. Once again she stopped exhibiting her previous aberrant, bizarre behavior and depression. This coming year we plan to retest her extract before the fall in an effort to prevent her winter flare-up of symptoms.

We are particularly concerned about each of the children just described and the many others who have similar problems. Their depression is frightening, and even the older youngsters may lack enough maturity to fully appreciate what could happen. If allergy is part of these children's despondency, they and their parents must realize that they may have to adhere to their diet, keep their home as environmentally clean as possible, avoid chemical exposures, maintain proper nutrition, and continue to properly use their allergy extract therapy. Sometimes this may be necessary for only a year or two, but some children may need comprehensive allergy care indefinitely.

A Near Miss in a Depressed Teenager Who Stopped His Allergy Care

Tom

One teenager recently was doing exceedingly well until he gradually stopped his rotation diet and didn't bother to take his allergy extract. He felt he was grown up and did not need treatment anymore. At the same time he stopped seeing his psychiatrist and discontinued the drug that had been prescribed. After three months he took an overdose of pills, but fortunately was unsuccessful in his attempt to commit suicide.

At present he is once again his delightfully positive and happy self. This change, however, did not occur until this teenager resumed his previous comprehensive allergy treatment program. He refused to resume the drug prescribed by his psychiatrist.

When he was retested for his allergies, it was obvious that his P/N allergy extract treatment needed many adjustments. Possibly this could have contributed to the onset of his noncompliance, which in turn snowballed into a potentially devastating situation.

When children need to have their allergy extracts corrected, they very often become negative. They begin to regress and behave in the manner they did before treatment was begun. Their food cravings return and they tend to binge on the very foods that they know cause undesirable changes in their personality. They adamantly deny that they feel or act different than usual and insist that they don't need more allergy tests or treatment. As a result their problems can spiral into a crisis situation, and even aware parents are often powerless to prevent it.

Although Tom's problems are not entirely due to allergies, he feels and acts fine when his allergies are well controlled. Prolonged psychological counseling and drug treatment did not resolve his depression when he was younger. His life did not turn around until his allergies were finally recognized and treated when he was twelve years old.

Older teenagers are special challenges. They want to make all their own decisions, but they are still incapable of taking full responsibility for their actions. At that age parents can't force them to eat the right foods, avoid known inciting odors or contacts, or order them to take their allergy extract correctly.

To my knowledge there are no well-designed scientific studies indicating that allergy can be a potential cause of adolescent or adult suicide. I feel certain, however, that some of the feeble suicide attempts ecologists see in young children could become tragic realities as certain depressed allergic children mature. Drs. Albert Rowe, Herbert Rinkel, and Theron Randolph all allude to this in their writings. Dr. Theron Randolph's book entitled *An Alternative Approach to Allergies* specifically describes in detail several suicidal adult patients, who were remarkably similar in many respects to the children we see.[4] Using the newer, more comprehensive approaches to controlling allergies and chemical sensitivities, there can be little doubt that some precious lives can be saved. It is imperative that severely depressed allergic children, who could potentially become suicidal adolescents or adults, receive psychological counseling. In addition it is hoped that they will somehow find their way to the offices of specialists in environmental medicine who can recognize their problems for what they truly are and offer more effective modes of treatment.[5]

One method for possibly confirming and relieving acute psychotic episodes related to allergy was described in medical journals by Dr. Randolph in the late 1940s. If intravenous sodium bicarbonate (baking soda) is appropriately administered by a knowledgeable physician, some patients improve remarkably. Within ten to thirty minutes after this is given, many patients will revert to completely normal, particularly if a food is the cause of their bizarre, irrational, or psychotic behavior. This might be particularly helpful for a physician to try, especially if a severely emotionally disturbed patient looked allergic, has had hay fever or asthma, or has close relatives who had typical allergies. If the bicarbonate helps, it suggests that the incident was possibly due to something the patient ingested a few minutes to an hour or so before the onset of the personality change. If an odor or chemical sensitivity triggers a psychoticlike episode, inhaled oxygen

4. Theron Randolph, M.D., *An Alternative Approach to Allergies* (New York: Harper & Row, 1989).

5. See Appendix D.

often helps to relieve some bizarre and inexplicable behavioral or physical complaints. One has to wonder why these simple and basically safe diagnostic and therapeutic methods are not tried routinely in emergency rooms and psychiatric hospitals if children look allergic, have had allergies in the past, and manifest a total personality change after a meal or exposure to some chemical.

A most gratifying opportunity awaits those clinicians or academic scientifically oriented psychiatrists, neurologists, allergists, or pediatric behavioral specialists. They need only to consider the possibility that dust, pollen, molds, foods, odors, and hormonal imbalances can cause or trigger depression and suicidal attempts to turn around the lives of some children and adults.

I firmly believe that many allergic children and young adults need psychological counseling, as well as recognition and treatment of their allergies. Most have had to withstand years of feeling unwell, rejection, and reprimands. These children, and especially the teenagers, often have decimated self-images and no realization of their true worth and unique personal gifts and capabilities.

One cannot help but ask why physicians are still not listening. Dr. Albert Rowe wrote about personality changes and depression due to foods and allergenic substances fifty years ago. Dr. Theron Randolph wrote extensively about this forty years ago and published excellent studies to verify his observations.[6]

On one occasion I showed a movie to a medical professor of an almost unbelievable personality change in an adolescent during a food test. After a tiny droplet of allergy extract was placed in this young woman's arm, her lips and eyes swelled, she swayed back and forth, and she then became withdrawn, untouchable, and screamed violently. During this reaction she tended to retract her body to an almost fetal position. Her speech reverted to that of a little girl and she asked for her "mommy." It was obvious that she could not think clearly or quickly. After the correct neutralization treatment she returned to normal and the swelling gradually subsided. This professor's only query after I showed this heartrending movie, which vividly demonstrated how we could turn on and off her exceptional behavioral changes with P/N testing, was to ask the make and model of the movie projector.

Similar testing for estrogen, as well as with many typical allergenic substances, caused similar marked personality changes. Previously we had demonstrated distinct neurometric brain-wave and endorphin

6. See Dr. Randolph's articles and books in the Bibliography.

changes during P/N tests for progesterone in this young woman at a brain research center.[7]

PMS Depression

In this regard it should be mentioned that many women suffer need-lessly during each menstrual period with premenstrual syndrome (PMS). Near the time of their menses they can be excessively de-pressed, fatigued, have crying spells, stare into space, and become irritable, withdrawn, and untouchable. Their behavior can range from hyperactivity to extreme depression and apathy, or at times border on hysteria. In Dr. Joseph Miller's book entitled *Relief at Last* he describes how a drop of a weak dilution of progesterone, for example, can sometimes provide immense benefit.[8] Women who are totally incapacitated, touchy, and unable to stand up because of in-tense cramps or bleeding often feel remarkably better after treatment with mini-neutralization doses of hormones.

The perplexing irony of this situation is that there is so little consideration or even curiosity about these methods by many in the medical profession. The prevailing attitude is one of total disinterest. It is the most exceptional physician who wants to personally observe the dramatic changes that I've described. Maybe if they don't see, they won't have to explain what is happening. The attitude is one of total denial, even when it is obvious that some perplexing and chal-lenging patients have dramatically improved.

Many specialists in environmental medicine have presented dra-matic movies or videos of patients before, during, and after allergy testing at medical conferences or psychiatric institutes. They have repeatedly demonstrated how a drop of allergy extract or eating a problem food can affect the drawing, writing, brain waves, and var-ious immune factors in the blood at the time of an obvious abrupt change in some children's or adults' behavior and activity. It is per-plexing that the attitude of total denial and disbelief prevails in spite of dramatic improvement in so many patients. Is there something to gain by keeping the census at psychiatric institutes at a high level? Is

7. Herbert Kaye, M.D., and Kenneth Bonnet, Ph.D., of the State University of New York. Study done at the Brain Research Center at New York University School of Medicine at Bellevue Hospital, 1980, New York, N.Y.

8. Joseph Miller, M.D., *Relief at Last* (Springfield, Ill.: Charles C. Thomas, 1981).

a simple, inexpensive two-week allergy diet too inconvenient to implement? If a patient's blood is monitored, why isn't intravenous sodium bicarbonate critically evaluated to see if it can relieve possible food-related psychotic behavior?

It is disappointing that the insurance companies are not actively encouraging this apparently beneficial way of treating chronically ill patients. These newer approaches could turn around the lives of many children and adults. In addition, enormous amounts of money presently spent for office or emergency hospital visits, endless consultations with various medical specialists, intensive clinic evaluations, and prolonged hospital stays might not be necessary.

One must also ask why our federal government is not leading the way in the evaluation of these newer methods to recognize and treat environmental illness. The ecologically minded national and provincial governments of Canada have spent an immense amount of time and money for preliminary evaluations and are now providing large amounts of funding for well-conducted scientific studies. Canada is also the only country in the world that has "clean" classrooms that are free of common allergenic substances and chemicals![9] Maybe the answer is related to their national health plan. Because of socialized medicine, their federal government has much to gain by recognizing the causes of illness so that Canadians can feel well and become productive citizens.

9. Contact: Brad Tucker, Waterloo County Board of Education, P.O. Box 68, Kitchener, Ontario, Canada N2G 3X5 (519–742–1751).

The Yeast, Candida, or Monilia Controversy[1]

What Is Yeast, Candida, or Monilia?

Yeast are microscopic egg-shaped organisms that make bread dough rise. Yeast are also found both inside and on the outside of our bodies. Body yeast are commonly called candida or monilia. Yeast are normally found on or in the skin, ears, or nails, and they can flourish in moist mucous membrane areas, such as the mouth, intestines, genitals, or rectum.

Yeast, molds, and fungi are all botanically related. We find that a number of children who act or feel worse when it is damp are also bothered when they eat bread or yeast-raised baked goods. They have yeast problems in addition to mold allergies. Yeast and mold sensitivities tend to occur together.

In our intestines we naturally have microorganisms or bacteria called lactobacilli, as well as yeast called monilia. They coexist in harmony unless we upset the natural balance by eating too much of certain food items or taking drugs such as antibiotics. Any type of significant imbalance of the normal flora or germs in any body area can lead to illness.

Yeast normally excrete a toxin that can travel via the blood to any site in the body. For example, an overgrowth of yeast in the vagina can cause a local irritation and discharge in the vaginal area. In

1. In this chapter I am not discussing the rare but serious yeast problems due to the invasion and growth of yeast in the body tissues called disseminated mucocutaneous candidiasis or systemic candidiasis.

TABLE 23.1
Medical Complaints Associated with
Yeast-Related Complex (YRC)

- Vaginal yeast discharges and infection
- White-coated tongue
- Redness around the anus
- Unpleasant odor to hair or feet
- Genital touching in infants and young children
- Skin rashes
- Behavior problems
- Chronic headaches
- Intestinal complaints (bloating, gas, nausea, constipation, diarrhea, heartburn, indigestion, abdominal cramps, excessive hunger, rectal itching, esophagitis, colitis, Crohn's disease)
- Fatigue, lethargy, weakness
- Depression
- Irritability and easy anger
- Anxiety
- Problems thinking clearly or remembering
- Menstrual irregularities
- Muscle aches; cramps in legs, arms, back
- Insomnia
- Hyperactivity
- Asthma
- Hives
- Bladder infection
- Ear infection
- Nail abnormalities
- Diaper rashes
- Thrush in infants (white patches inside mouth)

addition, yeast may cause depression and irritability, mainly in some adolescent girls and in women. The toxins from the yeast are thought to affect the brain area that controls disposition and mood.

The effects of a yeast overgrowth in a local area and a toxin at a distance appear to be able to produce a variety of symptoms, or an ill-defined medical illness, in some sensitive individuals. This illness has been called the yeast-related complex (YRC), candida-related complex, or the yeast-connection syndrome. This condition usually refers to a probable excess of yeast in the intestinal system or elsewhere (see Table 23.1).

The repeated or prolonged use of antibiotics in children and adults tends to kill the normal lactobacilli that are found in our intestines. Because the yeast are not killed by antibiotics, they begin to flourish. Antibiotics also reduce the normal bacteria in our stomach, which are needed to produce vitamin B_{12} and folic acid. Antibiotics create a problem that is in essence analogous to a lawn that has little grass and is overgrown with weeds: Normal balance needs to be restored; one needs to "kill off the weeds" and "reseed the lawn." The excess yeast or "weeds" can be killed or diminished by the judicious use of a wide variety of preparations, for example Mycostatin. The intestines, or "lawn," then need to be reseeded with some form of lactobacillus.

It is also thought that yeast overgrowth can weaken the immune system so that children become more prone to infection. A change in the balance of intestinal flora can weaken the mucous lining of the intestines. More yeast toxins can therefore enter the blood through the damaged intestinal lining, causing potential nervous system symptoms.

What Causes a Possible Yeast Overgrowth?

In addition to the use of antibiotics to treat repeated infections or persistent acne, other possible common causes of yeast overgrowth include the following:

- The excessive ingestion of sweets, candy, cookies, cakes, fruits, or fruit juices. The average person in the United States consumes one hundred pounds of table sugar each year! That is about two pounds per week. Much of the sugar we ingest is in hidden forms in such foods as ketchup, peanut butter, cereal, soup, luncheon meat, and so on. Sugary foods act like fertilizer for yeast. In addition, sugar also tends to paralyze the ability of our white blood cells to protect us. This observation has led to claims that too much sugar can increase our tendency to develop infections.

- The ingestion of low-calorie artificial sweeteners that contain aspartame (NutraSweet or Equal).[2]
- The excessive ingestion of yeasty and moldy foods such as mushrooms, cheese, bread, nuts, and fruits or vegetables. These foods contain molds not only on the outside but also throughout the inside, and this contributes to yeast problems.
- Poor nutrition due to a junk-food diet. This is a definite factor contributing to yeast overgrowth. For this reason nutritional supplements are thought to be helpful for people who seem to have yeast-related symptoms.
- The use of cortisone or steroid drugs.
- The use of birth control pills.[3]
- Repeated pregnancies.
- Diabetes.
- The use of chemotherapy or radiation for cancer.
- Anything that suppresses or damages the body's natural immunity, such as certain types of ubiquitous indoor or outdoor chemicals or pollution.
- Other predisposing factors, for example stress, inadequate stomach acid, and so on.

What Medical Problems Are Attributed to a Yeast Imbalance?

In some individuals chronic yeast imbalance or its toxins are suspected causes of the medical complaints listed in Table 23.1.

The more symptoms an individual has, the more likely that yeast may be a problem. Of course there are many other causes for each of these complaints, but a yeast imbalance or overgrowth should be considered if routine medical evaluations have not explained and relieved the symptoms. Physicians who diagnose these problems be-

2. Dennis W. Remington and Barbara W. Higa, *The Bitter Truth About Artificial Sweeteners.* 1986. Vitality House International, 3707 N. Canyon Road, 8C, Provo, Utah 84604.
3. Ellen Grant, *The Bitter Pill.* 1985. Practical Allergy Research Foundation (PARF), P.O. Box 60, Buffalo, N.Y. 14223-0060.

lieve that a yeast sensitivity represents only the tip of the iceberg. Much more needs to be understood about the relationship of yeast, allergy, immunity, infection, and the endocrine system. Many more details are provided in the books listed in the Bibliography.

Specific Clues Suggestive of Yeast Infections

In infants:

- Diaper rash that is worse in the skin folds. It has a deep red color, and little dots of red are often scattered just beyond the distinct outer margins of the scarlet areas.
- Thrush or white patches on the inner cheeks of the mouth.
- A white-coated tongue.
- Excessive genital touching.

In children:

- Thickly coated or patchy white tongue.
- Red ring around the anus or rectal area.
- Itchy genital area leading to frequent touching. Young children may not be able to verbalize that they have an itch.
- A chronic hair or foot odor.
- Bloated abdomen and bowel complaints.

In adolescents or adults:

- An excessive vaginal discharge or itching, particularly premenstrually or after eating sweets.
- Pelvic pain.
- Burning or white-coated tongue.
- Intestinal problems such as bloating, gas, and so forth.
- Itchy skin without a rash.
- Depression, fatigue, irritability.
- A distinct odor to the perspiration of the feet or hair.

Some women who are very yeast-sensitive may even quickly develop a visible faint white itchy skin rash and/or a vaginal discharge merely by touching the skin of an individual who has an overgrowth of yeast.

The Eight-Pronged Candida Attack

In general, an eight-pronged attack helps to relieve yeast-related problems. It should consist of the following:

1. Decrease yeast in the body. If excessive yeast are one aspect of an allergic problem, their numbers must be decreased to help restore a more normal balance of intestinal germs. Check with your physician about the following:

- For an intestinal imbalance: the drugs Mycostatin and Nystatin powder or tablets in essence make the yeast cells explode by damaging the outer membranes of the cells. These drugs are virtually nontoxic. Occasionally the side effects of large doses of these drugs include diarrhea, gastrointestinal distress, nausea, and vomiting.

  The dose for Mycostatin powder is gradually increased from a very small amount to ¼ teaspoon of powder four times a day. The powder must be swished in the mouth and then swallowed, to diminish yeast growth in the mouth as well as in the intestines. The powder has an unpleasant, but bearable taste. It occasionally causes diarrhea.

  One tablet of Nystatin equals about ⅛ teaspoon of the Mycostatin powder. If these colored tablets are preferred, allergic individuals should be careful. Rinse the color coating off the tablets with water to remove the food dyes before swallowing. Because these tablets are swallowed before the coating has dissolved, these pills do not control mouth yeast as well as Mycostatin powder. Individuals who are highly sensitive to corn or sugar could also be bothered by the cornstarch, which can be used as binders in tablet forms of medication, or the corn syrup, sugar, or dyes used in the liquid preparations.

- For the vagina: Suppositories can be placed directly into the vagina. One form is Monistat; another is called Terazol. Both are available as a suppository or cream. If a patient is sexually active, each partner must be treated.

- For the skin: Antifungal creams, ointments, and powders, such as Nystatin and Nizoral, are available. If the problem is severe, a dermatologist should be consulted.

- Ketoconazole, sold as Nizoral, is also helpful. Unlike Nystatin, it is absorbed into the bloodstream and on rare occasions it can cause liver damage. It is essential for a doctor to monitor each child's or adult's liver function with blood studies if this drug is used.

- Mycocidin, which contains castor bean oil, is a most effective antifungal agent. It seems to have fewer side effects than Nystatin or Mycostatin and appears to be well tolerated by many allergic children.

- A new form of high-potency and cost-effective short-chain fatty acid is called caprylic acid. It is sold in various forms as Mycopryl 680, Capricin, Caprylex, and Caprinex.

- Paracan is available in liquid or powdered forms. It is helpful for the treatment of parasites, as well as candida. Your doctor should prescribe and monitor this drug.

- Candida Cleanse is sold in health food stores. It appears to be well tolerated, relatively inexpensive, and helpful for some individuals.

- Preliminary reports of a new drug, fluconazole, called Diflucan by Pfizer Laboratories, sounds promising. It is now available in the United States. One dose is said to have the same therapeutic effect as five days on Nizoral and it is claimed to infrequently cause liver toxicity. The very early preliminary evaluation of the use of this drug to treat children indicates it appears to be safe.

- Garlic in the form of Kyolic (health food stores) is effective. This causes much less of a mouth odor than regular garlic. It appears to be outstandingly effective in some patients. In addition, it is inexpensive.[4]

- Broccoli, horseradish, kale, turnips, and cabbage naturally inhibit or kill yeast.

- Taheebo tea (Pau d'Arco), sold in health food stores, can be helpful. Check with a nutritionist and your physician if it is used on a daily basis. It is a diuretic and can cause a loss of certain essential trace metals and minerals in the urine. The used tea leaves can be placed in potting soil to decrease the growth of molds.

4. For garlic information, write to Wakunaga of America Co., Ltd., 23501 Madero, Mission Viejo, Calif. 92691 (800-421-2998).

Yeast therapy can be expensive, but at times it appears to relieve some patients' symptoms and restore a gratifying sense of well-being. Treatment failures are often attributed to resistant strains of candida, an inadequate duration of treatment, or the wrong diagnosis.

2. Increase a normal balance of intestinal flora. If an antibiotic or cortisone has decreased the normal level of lactobacilli in the intestines, the number of this bacteria should be replenished. Two brands, Vital-Dophilus and Vital-Plex (acidophilus), are sold by Klaire Laboratories.[5] Be careful to purchase *milk-free* lactobacillus if your child is sensitive to milk. A strain called *Lactobacillus bifidus* is recommended for children under five years of age. Some studies indicate that the *Lactobacillus bulgaricus* in yogurt is not as effective in replacing normal intestinal flora as the *Lactobacillus bifidus*. If you prefer yogurt as a source of lactobacillus, be sure to read the labels carefully. If it is pasteurized, it means the lactobacilli are killed, and our bodies need *live* lactobacillus organisms.

Lactobacillus food supplements appear to be well tolerated and safe to use. Many doctors suggest that a dose of 1 to 10 billion lactobacillus organisms be swallowed a day. If you use one of the two brands sold by Klaire Laboratories, the dose is ¼ teaspoon. This brand has almost no taste. If too much is taken, however, it can occasionally cause diarrhea. Other effective brands are also available.

3. Prevent future yeast imbalance. If your child has had a yeast problem in the past, ask your physician about the use of lactobacillus *every time* an antibiotic is used. Use the antibiotic exactly as recommended, but discuss your concerns about a secondary or subsequent yeast problem with your child's doctor. Some children might benefit from an antiyeast preparation and some lactobacillus for at least ten days during or after each course of antibiotics. If your child needs this form of therapy, you will notice that certain symptoms reappear each time your child takes an antibiotic. These will disappear after appropriate yeast treatment. In particular, watch for the clues listed in Table 23.1, which would suggest a possible yeast problem. These symptoms may persist for years if several courses of antibiotics happen to be given over a relatively short period of time.

Lactobacillus organisms may also help to decrease infection because they manufacture substances that help fight harmful bacteria and yeast. Dr. Khem Shahani, Professor of Food Science and Tech-

5. Contact: Klaire Laboratories, P.O. Box 618, Carlsbad, Calif. 92008 (619–744–9680).

nology at the University of Nebraska, observed that Vital-Dophilus appears to enhance immune responses in persons with yeast and other infections.

4. Limit drugs that increase yeast if possible. Antibiotics should be used in the correct amount and for the full period of time prescribed by your doctor unless there is a concern about some adverse reaction to the medicine. If the cause of repeated infections, however, can be determined, sometimes antibiotics won't be needed. This can sometimes be accomplished with appropriate allergy and/or nutritional therapy. If immunosuppressive drugs or cortisone must be continued, yeast growth can remain a potential concern and possible challenge. Consider an alternative other than antibiotics or birth control pills for acne.[6]

5. Limit yeasty foods. In general the recommended yeast-free diet is one that is low in carbohydrates. This diet suggests that the many foods that contribute to yeast problems should be avoided. These include cheese, sour cream, buttermilk, peanut butter, beer, wine, cider, mushrooms, soy sauce, tofu, vinegar, pickled foods, dried fruits, melons, frozen or canned fruit juices, commercial nuts, carbonated beverages, and any baked goods that use a raised dough. Some doctors also include grains in this list. The surface and inside of many vegetables, such as beets, are often moldy.

Foods that encourage yeast growth, such as sweets, must be discontinued. Some adolescent and adult women have such serious yeast problems that shortly after they eat candy, they notice an immediate vaginal itch or discharge. They just fed their yeast a meal. Others note a white-coated tongue or bad breath if they eat too many desserts in one day.

6. Try a modified yeast-free diet. Check with a nutritionist if a child's diet must be markedly curtailed to control a yeast overgrowth. It is essential that growing children receive an adequate diet. We want to starve the yeast, not the child. Low-carbohydrate diets tend not to be filling and can lead to constipation and possibly an elevated cholesterol. A combined yeast-free and four-day rotation diet are an almost impossible challenge. Strict adherence is not possible for some children if they are not growing properly. Mothers will need the help of an experienced nutritionist who is knowledgeable about both diets and allergy to help determine which diet to modify and how to do it.[7]

6. Ellen Grant, *The Bitter Pill* (see Bibliography).

7. Contact: PARF, P.O. Box 60, Buffalo, N.Y. 14223-0060 (716-875-0398).

7. Enhance your child's overall nutrition. If someone has yeast-related complex (YRC), an attempt must be made to make the body more healthy from the nutritional viewpoint. This in turn should strengthen the immune system and diminish the tendency to infection, allergy, and yeast overgrowth.

Many forms of B-complex vitamins are derived from yeast, and these can worsen some people's symptoms. Yeast-free varieties of B complex might be well tolerated. A yeast sensitivity is one major reason why some individuals are unable to take regular multivitamins. Patients can be sensitive to baker's yeast, brewer's yeast, and/or body yeast (candida or monilia). Even the odor of yeasty vitamins can bother some sensitive individuals.

8. Use allergy extract therapy. If your child has allergies, P/N testing and treatment for yeast should help to control or eliminate the yeast-related symptoms. If drugs that inhibit or kill yeast do not resolve the problem, then drugs *plus* a modified yeast-free diet and allergy treatment for candida might be needed. Candida therapy has also led to improvement in some patients' typical asthma, eczema, hives, and hay fever, as well as the other symptoms listed in Table 23.1.

Candida allergy extract treatment can at times be a challenge because certain patients must be treated with the exact species of candida that is causing symptoms. In addition allergy extract neutralization doses can change so frequently that repeated visits may be required for retesting.

Homeopaths and naturopaths claim that their remedies help some yeast-sensitive patients. I have had no personal experience with these particular forms of treatment.[8]

What Should You Watch for During Yeast Treatment?

The Die-Off Reaction

When yeast treatment begins, a large number of killed yeast suddenly burst and excrete their toxins. These cause most patients' symptoms to flare up and they become much more ill than normal. The "die-off" tends to occur within a day or two after treatment is started and can last for several days. If the antiyeast treatment is started more

---

8. For more information, contact: Robert Skiovsky, N.D., 6910 S.E. Lake Road, Malwakie, Ore. 97267, and the National Center for Homeopathy, 1500 Massachusetts Avenue, N.W., Suite 41, Washington, D.C. 20005 (202-223-6182).

slowly, with a smaller dose and given less often, this reaction will be less evident. Once the die-off flare-up is over, some patients appear to improve dramatically. Later on, the dose of antiyeast medication can be increased to tolerance, usually without difficulty.

If yeast therapy is not given for a long enough period, the original symptoms tend to reappear gradually within a week or two after therapy is discontinued. If this happens, it indicates that one or more months of yeast treatment may be required. Repeated prolonged courses of yeast therapy are sometimes required before certain patients no longer flare up shortly after their treatment is discontinued.

Why Is This Problem Difficult to Diagnose?

It is normal for candida to grow in many areas of the body. Finding them in the mouth, near the genitals, and in the rectal area, for example, is perfectly normal unless the laboratory indicates that there is an exceptional overgrowth. In contrast, if culture of these areas reveals no growth of yeast, then it is highly unlikely that yeast is causing illness in that body area. Yeast should never grow from samples of someone's urine, blood, or spinal fluid. This is abnormal and indicates a need for treatment by a physician.

Allergy skin tests for yeast are usually positive because we have all been exposed since early infancy. Ecologists, however, believe that yeast P/N allergy testing can be helpful. Sometimes this testing can reproduce the exact medical symptoms of which a patient complains. This not only suggests a probable cause-and-effect relationship but also indicates that yeast neutralization allergy extract should be a helpful adjunct for therapy. Usually yeast allergy extract treatment, however, must be combined with specific antiyeast drug therapy and/ or a modified yeast-free diet in any comprehensive medical approach to the YRC.

Since all humans are normally exposed to yeast, most people have antibodies to yeast. Many physicians, however, doubt that the level of candida antibodies are of value. A recent single-blind controlled study by Dr. John Crayton at the University of Chicago suggested that this test might be more helpful then initially anticipated.[9] A group of patients who had diverse types of medical and psychological symptoms associated with YRC were found to have significantly

9. John Crayton, M.D., "Anti-Candida Antibody Levels in Polysymptomatic Patients." Presented at the Candida Update Conference, Memphis, Tenn., September 16–18, 1988.

higher levels of various yeast antibodies than a group of healthy people.

At the present time, however, there appears to be no specific test or group of tests that will unquestionably pinpoint the YRC. Therefore, if a patient has several of the complaints listed on Table 23.1, and traditional medical therapy has not been effective in relieving the symptoms, a yeast problem should at least be considered. For example, some children have had extensive diagnostic bowel evaluations, but no answer for the intestinal problems has been found. Sometimes the problem is simply a yeast overgrowth. This is especially true if there are physical changes suggesting an excess of yeast (such as a white-coated tongue and red rectal area), as well as a past history of a prolonged need for many antibiotics.

Sometimes a clue for diagnosis is provided if a doctor simply makes a scraping or smear of the tongue, fingernail, saliva, vaginal mucus, or irritated skin areas. These samples can be examined under the microscope using potassium hydroxide. If a large number of yeast cells are seen, it suggests that a clinical trial of therapy might be indicated. If a person's medical complaints are significantly relieved within one to six weeks, this suggests that yeast is, in some manner, a factor related to that individual's particular medical problem. If the original symptoms recur a week or so after the treatment is discontinued, this again suggests the previous yeast treatment might have been helpful but that therapy was needed for a longer period of time.

All of this, however, is still only suggestive evidence. Maybe a rash was due to irritation from a strong laundry soap. If a milder soap happened to be used at the same time the yeast treatment was begun, one could falsely assume that the yeast therapy was the reason that patient improved. It is very easy to be fooled in medicine.

A TWO-YEAR-OLD WITH YEAST PROBLEMS

Mary

Mary's mother was concerned about her little girl's persistent yeast problem. On two occasions, before she saw us, yeast treatment with lactobacillus and Mycostatin had relieved her red anus; red, itchy genitals; and the odor of her feet within one day. She remained well while she took these drugs, but when they were stopped, her symptoms recurred within one day. In addition it was noted that her temper tantrums, biting, and screaming also diminished whenever she received her yeast treatment and that these returned shortly after that treatment was stopped.

Her mother's other concern was how to feed her child, because so many foods caused Mary to feel or act unwell. She already knew which foods were a problem.

Let us trace her food and yeast problems from their inception. Her history indicated that she had many allergic relatives. They were dairy farmers, so her mother drank and ate more dairy products than normal. This was especially true during her pregnancy. Before Mary's birth she kicked so hard, *particularly between 7:00 and 10:00 P.M.*, that her mother's ribs hurt. She was in tears because of the pain. The stage was already set for Mary to be a prime candidate for the development of obvious milk allergy after birth.

Mary as an Infant

The typical allergic infant pattern was evident shortly after she was born. She had extreme colic, as well as congestion and snorting, whenever she nursed. She spit up after each feeding. Each night, *again between 7:00 and 10:00 P.M.*, she would arch her back and wiggle so much that she could barely be held. This certainly suggests that this agitation was similar to that which occurred in the uterus when she was developing.

During the night, Mary would cry hysterically until she vomited several times. Fatigue, congestion, and allergies made her prone to develop one ear infection after another. The ear problems began at the tender age of five months, and she required repeated antibiotics. This in turn led to a probable imbalance of her normal intestinal flora and her eventual yeast problem.

At fifteen months breast-feeding was discontinued, and Mary's spitting and vomiting both stopped. Research has shown that the cow's milk that breast-feeding mothers often believe they must ingest can pass directly into the mother's milk. This could help explain why Mary's nose was congested. This swelling of the nose tissues, in turn, could indirectly have contributed to her repeated ear infections.

Mary was often overactive as an infant. She simply could not sit still. At five months she would crawl out of the shopping cart in stores and hang from the sides. She had to be held constantly. Her mother said that Mary clung excessively to her as an infant but that now, after allergy treatment, this tendency seems to be much less evident.

Throughout the infant period Mary was awake at least once an hour and at two years of age she continued to be up two or three times a night. She had diarrhea and abdominal gas every night until milk was totally removed from her diet. Her mother did not fully appreciate the significance of the milk problem until Mary entirely stopped all dairy products for a few days. This unmasked Mary's hidden milk allergy, and within twenty minutes after she was given a half cup of yogurt, her personality totally changed. She lay on the floor for about three hours, whining and acting abnormally quiet and subdued. No matter what her caring parents did, she could not be consoled.

Mary as a Toddler

Mary's personality tended to vacillate from whining and listlessness to anger, overactivity, and nonaggravated assault. Her mother finally saw clear-cut answers when Mary was placed on Part 2 of the Multiple Food Elimination Diet when she was two years old. Her mother said this diet helped her daughter about 65 percent. Corn and wheat appeared to cause her tantrums. Milk and egg caused her to become listless and tired. Pretzels, wheat crackers, and grape juice, in particular, seemed to cause her to bite.

At about that same time her mother also learned how to make Mary's room more allergy-free, and surprisingly she determined, on her own, that her daughter probably had a yeast infection.

Mary's Response to Treatment

Mary was approximately 90 percent improved after seven months of allergy extract therapy. She can now eat all the foods that previously caused symptoms without difficulty on a four-day rotation. She receives P/N treatment sublingually three times a day.

A 1987 study reported in *Clinical Pediatrics* showed a relationship between ear infections early in life, hyperactivity later on, and school failure.[10] That investigation found that 70 percent of hyperactive children, in contrast to 20 percent of normally active children, had over ten ear infections per year. The authors stated that 80 percent of these hyperactive children had more than ten ear infections before the age of one year. It would be of interest to know if these children had untreated milk or other allergies affecting their nose that pre-

10. R. J. Hagerman and A. R. Falkenstein, "An Association Between Recurrent Otitis Media in Infancy and Later Hyperactivity," *Clinical Pediatrics* 26 (1987), pp. 253–257.

disposed them to the ear problems. Did their excessive need for antibiotics lead to yeast problems? Did they eventually develop food or other unrecognized allergies prior to their hyperactivity and school failure? Mary certainly had this pattern. She had had ten ear infections before the age of one year, and at a very early age her hyperactivity was clearly evident. Her wise mother, however, probably prevented many problems by recognizing and treating her little girl's allergies and yeast problems long before she reached school age.

The original description of the candida problem appeared in a book by Dr. Orian Truss called *The Missing Diagnosis*.[11]

Dr. Billy Crook has become a vocal and visible expert to help educate the public in relation to the existence of the YRC. He has a hotline number—901-427-8100—available between 11:30 A.M. and 12:00 noon on weekdays, to answer questions related to yeast problems in children or adults.

How Is All This Related to Allergy?

As with many other children described in this book, both the yeast and the allergy problems can begin very early in life. Infants are exposed to yeast in the birth canal unless they are born by cesarean section. Yeast symptoms in a baby's mouth and diaper rash are common. If children have infections that require antibiotics later on, this sets the stage for yeast overgrowth.

How can allergic children who have repeatedly used antibiotics be helped? The answer is to ask your doctor to treat the yeast problem *as well as* the allergies if both are present. If allergy therapy is effective, the tissues should become more resistant to infection and remain intact. The end result should be a diminished need for antibiotics and therefore fewer yeast problems.

At times, for reasons not fully understood, some individuals surprisingly no longer have significant allergies after yeast treatment. This suggests an important gap in our knowledge and a need to explain the role of yeast in relation to immunity and allergy.

Specialists in environmental medicine are surprised at the skepticism of other doctors in relation to yeast problems, because this problem seems to be so prevalent and so gratifying responsive to treatment. In particular many environmentally ill women suffer from fatigue, depression, and irritability. These women may be unaware

11. C. Orian Truss, M.D., *The Missing Diagnosis*. 1985. The Missing Diagnosis, Inc., P.O. Box 26508, Birmingham, Ala., 35226.

that a yeast imbalance might be their basic underlying problem.

Those physicians who disagree say that YRC is presently both unscientific and unproven. They believe the patients who respond favorably have physical and emotional illness due mainly to psychological problems. They claim that doctors who help them have only treated their psyche and given their illness a respectable name. Rigid scientific studies to evaluate these issues are urgently needed. In the meantime patients should be sure that their treatment is strictly monitored by a physician or nutritionist, because yeast therapy and yeast-free diets can cause physical and nutritional problems in some individuals. For those who want to read more about yeast problems, there is a plethora of books discussing the many ramifications of possible yeast-related health problems.[12]

12. See Bibliography.

PART FIVE

TREATMENT REQUIRING THE EXPERTISE OF OTHERS

CHAPTER 24

The Practical Rotary Diet

Earlier in this book two simple, easy diets helped you detect unsuspected food allergies and the many common causes of allergies inside and outside your home. You are also now aware of the many ways that chemicals and pollution can affect the lives of your family.

In this part the Practical Rotary Diet will be discussed; it often helps children and families on a long-term basis. Some children improve so much that allergy treatment is unnecessary. Others need allergy extract therapy, not only to treat dust, pollen, and mold allergies but also to enable them to eat a greater variety of ordinary foods without developing symptoms. Prescription drugs to treat various medical complaints may not be required, or their need is often markedly diminished, if a diet changes in your home, and/or allergy extract therapy resolves your child's medical problem.

What Is the Practical Rotary Diet?

This diet simply means that each food is eaten at a four-day interval. It can be eaten more than once on that day *if* it is well tolerated.

The following table will give you a basic idea of what a Practical Rotary Diet is:

Day 1	Day 2	Day 3	Day 4
(Mon., Fri., etc.)	(Tues., Sat., etc.)	(Wed., Sun., etc.)	(Thurs., Mon., etc.)
Beef	Turkey	Pork	Chicken
Potato	Beets	Broccoli	Beans
Strawberry	Banana	Apple	Orange
Wheat	Corn	Rice	Oats

A "real life" sample of a four-day Practical Rotary Diet is given in Table 24.1. In that table, foods are purposely clustered or grouped in their botanical families so as to make eventual variations of this diet easier.

What Are the Advantages of This Diet?

The major advantage of this diet is that it does for *every* food what the Single Food Elimination Diet did for one. The result is that you can often quickly tell if a certain food your child eats is causing illness. Every time a problem food is eaten at a four-day interval, your child's medical, emotional, or learning problems repeatedly recur. The object is to see if a four-day pattern of symptoms is evident.

The second advantage of this diet is that it is thought to help prevent food allergies. If foods are eaten in moderation, but no more often than every four days, ecologists believe this diet lessens the tendency to develop new food allergies. We do not have scientific proof to document that statement. It is conjecture that is suggested by the observation of many patients.

The third advantage is that it quickly reveals a newly developed food allergy. If you crave a food and eat too much of it every four days, this diet will quickly reveal the effect of that excess. You will routinely become ill every four days when your craved food is eaten. In such a situation you may have to limit the ingestion of that food temporarily. For example, it may be necessary only to eat smaller amounts of the problem food less often, say every eight or twelve days rather than every four days. However, if the response to a food was very severe, it may be necessary to stop eating the offending food entirely for a few weeks or months before trying it again.

How Do Ecologists Treat Food Allergies?

Most ecologists treat children's food allergies with food allergy extracts, so children can eat most problem foods immediately or in a very short while. Most foods seem to be well tolerated at a four-day interval as soon as sublingual or injection neutralization food allergy extract is given.

Many new patients in our office become severe behavior problems after ingesting a little milk on cereal, a bite of a hamburger, or three bites of bread. By using the Practical Rotary Diet, as well as treatment with an allergy extract, these foods can typically be eaten without difficulty, in the usual amount, within a few weeks or months. With allergy extract treatment it definitely appears that the tolerance for many foods increases, at times, very rapidly.

A few excellent ecologists, however, strongly believe that most food allergies do not need to be treated with a food allergy extract. This attitude markedly diminishes the cost of food treatment. They urge patients simply to remove the foods that cause major problems totally from their diet for one or several months. They allow most other foods to be eaten at four- or five-day intervals. Sometimes this reestablishes the patient's tolerance to the food so that eventually some major formerly symptom-causing foods no longer cause symptoms. However, *some* foods may never be able to be eaten and well tolerated if there is an exceptional sensitivity to them.

What Can Be Done to Help Children Who Have Extreme Food Allergies?

Testing or treating individuals who have extremely severe sensitivities, for example to peanuts, egg, buckwheat, or fish, would rarely be attempted by most ecologists because it could be dangerous. This is particularly true if a youngster had a very high IgE RAST blood test to that specific food. An occasional child, however, has been successfully and safely tested and treated in a hospital setting when an accidental exposure to a certain food is not easily preventable. One outstanding retired pediatric professor, Dr. John Gerrard of Saskatoon, Saskatchewan, Canada, has documented successful treatment of life-threatening peanut allergy, for example, in this manner.[1]

In relation to exceptionally severe food sensitivities, it seems more logical and sensible to try P/N testing and treatment in a medical setting rather than to have parents try to resolve an unanticipated food-related health crisis all by themselves. At a minimum, parents of such children should at all times carry an antihistamine and know

1. John W. Gerrard, M.D., et al., "A Double-blind Study on the Value of Low-Dose Immunotherapy in the Treatment of Asthma and Allergic Rhinitis," *Clinical Ecology* 6 (1989), pp. 43–46.

exactly how to give an injection of adrenaline. It is almost impossible to protect some highly allergic children once they begin school because problem food substances are often hidden in mass-produced luncheon foods or mother-supplied party treats, such as cakes, cookies, and ice cream. School nurses need to have appropriate permission and instruction to care for food-related emergencies that could occur during school hours.

Some foods cannot be eaten at a four-day interval, even in the tiniest portion, without causing a reaction. Sometimes, however, if certain foods are completely omitted from a diet for several weeks or months, they can be gingerly added back into the diet without difficulty. The challenge is to start with such a small amount that it does not create a medical emergency. A speck might be too large an amount for the initial feeding of certain food items to some children. Even the odor of some foods can cause a life-threatening crisis in some children (see Chapter 8). For this reason, check with your doctor.

If at any time during the buildup period a certain amount causes symptoms, that food must be stopped. When the child is back to "normal," the previous amount that was well tolerated can be given for several weeks, and then a more gradual buildup is attempted again. In other words, if eight teaspoons caused symptoms, but four caused no problem, the child should eat no more than three or four teaspoons every four days for one or two months. Then try five teaspoons every four days. After a few weeks try six, etc. In this way, with your physician's guidance, some moderately problematic foods eventually may be able to be ingested in normal amounts without difficulty.

Special Problems Related to Diet

Attempts to control the cause of allergies often present challenging problems for working parents. If baby-sitters care for children in their own homes, how can they be asked to comply with a strict rotation diet and to keep their home allergy-free? Will the child's school be able to cooperate with the child's special diet and realistically be able to decrease exposure to common highly allergenic substances? Can a school that does not have a full-time nurse handle an allergic emergency? There are no easy answers to these questions. Do the best you can. If you adopt a positive attitude, you may be pleasantly surprised. Perhaps your baby-sitter or the school principal also has allergies, so they will not only cooperate, they will understand.

The Details of the Practical Rotary Diet

Examine the four-day Practical Rotary Diet in Table 24.1 for a few minutes before you read further. This diet corresponds to our office companion diet booklet entitled *Rotary and Other Allergy Diets Made Easy for Children*, which contains basic recipes for everyday use, such as muffins, waffles, cookies, and loaf cakes made with different grains and sweeteners.[2]

Some of the recipes in this booklet were specifically created for our patients by Ann Miller using ingredients specified in the Practical Rotary Diet detailed in this book. These recipes rotate sweeteners such as cane sugar, corn syrup, pure maple syrup, and honey. Each sweetening agent is eaten, but only on a four-day interval, and only combined with the other food items allowed on each specific day.

Ann Miller's recipes usually rely solely on natural fruits and vegetables as sweeteners.[3] Ideally this is certainly best and preferred, but sometimes a diet that is too stringent in relation to sweeteners is difficult for mothers because the children simply won't eat the baked goods. While natural sweeteners from fruits and vegetables are certainly preferable for many reasons, more typical sweetening agents need to be used initially, at least during the transition period. Therefore, the recipes in our office companion booklet for the Practical Rotary Diet are basically transitional and include as sweetening agents: cane sugar on Day 1, corn syrup on Day 2, pure maple syrup on Day 3, and honey on Day 4.

General Tips Concerning the Practical Rotary Diet

1. All the foods you may eat are listed in four separate columns in Table 24.1, one for each of the four days of the diet. Each column contains different fruits, vegetables, meats, grains, condiments, sweeteners, oils, nuts, and beverages that are *not* included in the other three lists.

The menu for each day is selected from the food items listed as allowed on that day. On Monday, for example, one would eat any

2. Doris J. Rapp, M.D., *Rotary and Other Allergy Diets Made Easy for Children.* Practical Allergy Research Foundation (PARF), P.O. Box 60, Buffalo, N.Y. 14223-0060.
3. Ann Miller, *Who Needs Wheat?!: A Guide for Successful Wheat-Free Baking.* 1990; and *Organic Annie's Booklet Series.* Organic Annie's Wholefoods, P.O. Box 751, Baldwinsville, N.Y. 13027.

TABLE 24.1
Practical Rotary Diet

Day 1	Day 2	Day 3	Day 4
		Grains*		

Wheat:
  Flour
  Bread
  Rolls
  Graham
    flour
  Bran
  Wheat germ
  Farina
  Seminola
  Gluten flour

Potato:
  Flour,
  Starch,
  Bread

Barley:
  Pearl barley
  Barley flour
  Barley
    flakes

Corn:
  Starch
  Cornmeal
  Grits

Rye:
  Flour
  Bread
  Crackers
  Noodles

Millet:
  Flour,
  Cereal

Amaranth:
  Cereal
  Flour
  Puffed
    amaranth

Artichoke:
  Flour

Rice:
  Flour
  Cakes
  Noodles
  Snaps
  Puffed rice,
  Cream of
    Rice
    cereal

Buckwheat:
  Noodles
  Kasha
    (toasted
    buckwheat)

Quinoa:
  Cereal
  Flour

Oat:
  Oatmeal
  Oat bread
  Oat flour
  Oat cakes
  Puffed oats

Soy:
  Flour
  Pea flour
  Mung bean
  Noodles

Flaxseed

*Grains are all in one family, but if tolerated, try a different one each day.

Meats

Day 1	Day 2	Day 3	Day 4
Beef	Turkey	Pork	Chicken
Beef liver	Turkey liver	Bacon	Chicken liver
Lamb	Turkey eggs	Ham sausage	Chicken eggs
Veal	Duck		Peafowl
Rabbit	Duck eggs		Pheasant
Venison	Goose		Quail
Moose	Goose eggs		

Unusual ingredients not readily available can be obtained from Frontier Cooperative Herbs, Box 299, Norway, Ia. 52318. Wholesale to companies only (319-227-7791); retail division (sells to individuals), Herbs and Spices (800-365-4372).

Day 1	Day 2	Day 3	Day 4

Fish

Day 1	Day 2	Day 3	Day 4
Abalone	Crab	Cod	Whitefish
Squid	Crayfish	Haddock	Yellow perch
Clams	Lobster	Ocean perch	Catfish
Mussels	Prawn	Flounder	Lake trout
Oysters	Shrimp	Halibut	Lake perch
Scallops	Salmon	Plaice	Bass
Red Snapper	Herring	Sole	Smelt
	Sardines	Turbot	Pike
	Anchovies	Monkfish	
		Roughy	
		Tuna	
		Mackerel	

Fruits

Day 1	Day 2	Day 3	Day 4
Strawberry	Muskmelons:	Grape	Citron
Raspberry	Cantaloupe	Raisin	Orange
Blackberry	Honeydew	————	Lemon
Boysenberry	Watermelon	Apple	Lime
————	Casaba	Apple butter	Grapefruit
Breadfruit	————	Pear	Kumquat
Figs	Blueberry	————	Tangerine
————	Huckleberry	Rhubarb	————
Mango	Cranberry	————	Persimmon
————	————	Guava	————
Papaya	Prickly pear	————	Pomegranate
————	————	Kiwi	————
Pineapple	Banana		Currant
	Plantain		Gooseberry
	————		————
	Apricot		Avocado
	Cherry		
	Nectarine		
	Peach		
	Plum		
	Prune		

Unusual ingredients not readily available can be obtained from Frontier Cooperative Herbs, Box 299, Norway, Ia. 52318. Wholesale to companies only (319-227-7791); retail division (sells to individuals), Herbs and Spices (800-365-4372).

Day 1	Day 2	Day 3	Day 4

Vegetables

Day 1	Day 2	Day 3	Day 4
Potato	Carrot	Turnip	Peas
Tomato	Celery	Cabbage	Beans*
Eggplant	Parsley	Radish	Lentils*
Peppers,	Parsnip	Kraut	Soybeans*†
Green	———	Watercress	Bean sprouts
Red	Beet	Cauliflower	Alfalfa
Chili	Swiss chard	Broccoli	Fenugreek
———	Spinach	Brussels	Carob
Asparagus	Lamb's-	sprouts	———
Garlic	quarters	Kohlrabi	Cucumber
Leeks	———	Rutabaga	Squash
Chives	Corn	Kale	Zucchini
Onion	———	———	Pumpkin
———	Okra	Sweet potato	Acorn and
Lettuce		———	seeds
Endive		Olives	———
Escarole		———	Water
Romaine		Bamboo	chestnuts
Artichokes		shoots	
Salsify (scorzonera)			
Dandelion			
Burdock			
Cardoon			
———			
Yam			
———			
Mushroom			
Yeast			

*Beans are all in one family, but if tolerated, try a different one each day.
†If soy/peanut day is okay, try to split soy and peanut so that one is on Day 2 and the other on Day 4.

Beverages

Day 1	Day 2	Day 3	Day 4
Cow's milk	Cranberry	Grape juice	Orange juice
Papaya juice	juice	Apple juice	Grapefruit juice
Pineapple	Aloe vera	Pear juice	Lemonade
juice	juice	Sesame seed	Soy milk:
Sunflower	Prune juice	milk	Nursoy
seed milk	Apricot nectar	Alfalfa tea	Liquid

Unusual ingredients not readily available can be obtained from Frontier Cooperative Herbs, Box 299, Norway, Ia. 52318. Wholesale to companies only (319-227-7791); retail division (sells to individuals), Herbs and Spices (800-365-4372).

Day 1	Day 2	Day 3	Day 4
Chamomile tea	Banana milk	Kukicha twig tea	I-Soyalac
Hops tea	Sarsaparilla tea		Comfrey tea
Wintergreen tea			Fennel tea
Chickory tea			Red clover tea
Rose hip tea			Licorice tea
			Coconut milk

Sweeteners

Day 1	Day 2	Day 3	Day 4
Cane sugar	Corn syrup	Pure maple syrup	Honey
Molasses	Beet sugar	Maple crystals	Date sugar
Sucanat	Sorghum	Rice syrup	
Turbinado		Buckwheat honey	
Barley syrup			
Malt powder			

Nuts and Seeds

Day 1	Day 2	Day 3	Day 4
Cashews	Almonds	Walnuts	Peanuts†
Filberts (hazelnuts)	Brazil nuts	Pecans	Caraway seeds
Pine nuts	Chia seed	Butternut	Chestnuts
Sunflower seeds		Hickory nuts	Anise seeds
Poppy seeds		Sesame seeds	Pumpkin seeds
Pistachio nuts		Tahini	Macadamia nuts
		Psyllium seeds	Cumin seeds
			Fennel seeds

†If soy/peanut day is okay, try to split soy and peanut so that one is on Day 2 and the other on Day 4.

Snacks

Day 1	Day 2	Day 3	Day 4
Ice cream	Popcorn	Rice Dream	Peanut butter
Cheese	Corn chips	Rice crackers	Carob
Yogurt	Corn muffins	Rice cakes	Tofu
Cashew butter	Corn bread	Pecan butter	
Pistachio butter	Tortillas	Walnut butter	
	Almond butter	Tahini	
	Rye crackers		

Unusual ingredients not readily available can be obtained from Frontier Cooperative Herbs, Box 299, Norway, Ia. 52318. Wholesale to companies only (319-227-7791); retail division (sells to individuals), Herbs and Spices (800-365-4372).

Day 1	Day 2	Day 3	Day 4
		Oils	
Butter	Corn oil	Canola oil	Soybean oil
Safflower oil	Cottonseed oil	Sesame oil	Peanut oil
Sunflower oil	Almond oil	Walnut oil	Flaxseed or
	Pumpkin seed	Olive oil	linseed oil
	oil		Coconut oil
		Thickeners	
Wheat flour	Cornstarch	Cream of	Oat flour
Potato flour	Agar-agar	tartar	Tapioca
Beef gelatin	Irish moss	Guar gum	Kudzu
		Psyllium husk	Gum acacia
		powder	Taro
		Arrowroot	
		Spices	
Chili pepper	Black pepper	Horseradish	Cinnamon
Cayenne	White pepper	Mustard	Bay leaf
Pimiento	Basil	Ginger	Nutmeg
Tabasco	Oregano	Turmeric	Mace
Garlic	Marjoram	Cardamom	Sassafras
Chives	Rosemary	Cloves	Cumin
Wintergreen	Sage	Allspice	Anise
Tarragon	Spearmint	Paprika	Fennel
	Peppermint		Asafoetida
	Chives		(Indian
	Parsley		spice—garlic
	Fennel		flavor)
	Dill		Caraway
		For Infants	
Cow's milk	Alimentum	Goat milk	Nursoy Liquid
		Good Start	I-Soyalac

Unusual ingredients not readily available can be obtained from Frontier Cooperative Herbs, Box 299, Norway, Ia. 52318. Wholesale to companies only (319-227-7791); retail division (sells to individuals), Herbs and Spices (800-365-4372).

of the Day 1 foods; foods from the same list would be eaten again on Friday. In other words:

- Day 1 foods are eaten on Monday and Friday of one week and on Tuesday and Saturday of the next, and so on.
- Day 2 foods are eaten on Tuesday and Saturday, and then on Wednesday and Sunday, and so on.
- Day 3 foods are eaten on Wednesday and Sunday, and the next week only on Thursday and Monday, and so on.
- Day 4 foods are eaten on Thursday and Monday, and then again on Friday and Tuesday, and so on.

2. *Start slowly*. At first rotate only the fruits at a four-day interval. Then after about eight or sixteen days, if those four different fruits cause no problem, continue to try to rotate the fruits while you begin to rotate four vegetables. After another eight or sixteen days, add four different meats. In other words, ease into the diet. *If you try to rotate everything at once, watch out for Days 5 through 8!* It means that all the foods in your diet will be added back at the critical four-day interval, so exaggerated allergic responses to problem foods would be the expected response. This means that if any member of your family has many food allergies, any of these foods potentially could cause some form of illness. Remember, adding foods back at four-day intervals unmasks food allergies. This diet helps reveal unsuspected foods that can cause your family to become ill. On this diet you will readily see that problem foods cause the same medical complaint every four days.

3. You may not see any pattern in your child's response to the Practical Rotary Diet until it has been used for about a month. In other words, you won't notice that your child regularly tends to wet the bed on the "milk day" or that his or her joints ache on the "wheat day" until you have followed the four-day rotation for a few weeks.

4. After your child or cooperative family members are eating four fruits, vegetables, meats, and grains without difficulty, continue to expand your diet with more fruits and vegetables, but try to adhere stringently to the four-day addition pattern. For example, on Day 3, if apple was no problem, then also add pear to the foods eaten in the "apple day." They are clustered on Table 24.1 because they are botanically similar. Therefore, if one is well tolerated, the rest in that grouping usually (but not always) should also be all right.

5. Give the foods and beverages for each day a specific colored

label. For example, label all Day 1 items red. Put stickers on these items or place them on a red-labeled shelf in the cupboard and re-frigerator. Day 2 can be labeled blue, Day 3 orange, and Day 4 green. Then children can be told that today is the "red day" and that they can eat whatever has a red label or is on the "red shelf." This makes it easier for everyone to comply with the diet.

6. If a food causes difficulty, try an alkali such as Alka-Aid (available in health food stores). In some patients, but not all, it helps to relieve symptoms quickly (see Chapter 8).

If you have a neutralizing dose of allergy extract for histamine or for the specific problem food that caused the symptoms, either or both might be helpful in aborting or stopping the food reactions. You merely give the allergy extract sublingually or by injection.

7. The same food can be eaten more than once a day, but *only* if that food is well tolerated. In other words, if milk is not a problem once a day, try it twice, and if it is still all right, try it three times. Children can generally, initially, or later on, eat normal-sized portions of most foods on each specific day of the cycle. If a child binges, however, too much and too often, expect the symptoms to recur. Even if milk is well tolerated, common sense is necessary. Most allergic children, even if they are treated for their sensitivity, can't eat a half gallon of ice cream, drink six glasses of milk, and eat cheese all on the same day.

8. Use four fruit juices from the four different allowed fruits on each of the four cereal days. On Day 1 put strawberry juice in wheat cereal. On Day 2 put banana "milk" or apricot nectar on corn cereal. On Day 3 put apple or grape juice on rice cereal. On Day 4 put orange juice on oat cereal.

On Day 1, you can use cow's milk. On Day 2, use banana milk (made in the blender from a mix of banana and water). On Day 3, you can even try goat's milk if it causes no difficulty. Some children can drink goat's milk without difficulty even though they can't tolerate cow's milk. On Day 4, you can use soy milk. Check with your doctor if you are concerned if any of these milks are not well tolerated.

The attitude of parents will determine many children's response to novel approaches to eating. If you act elated about purple (or colorless) grape juice on cereal, your child may also be delighted with this new idea. Remember Dr. Seuss and his green eggs and ham? Young children would be delighted to try eating these after reading these stories. If either parent is negative, however, expect the child to adopt a similar attitude.

9. If the Practical Rotary Diet is tried by the entire family, other family members are often helped even though they never realized they had allergies. It is not uncommon for a number of relatives to have the same sensitivities. Once a family understands the scope of the problem, they can often even help distant relatives who have "learn to live with it" types of chronic illness. Sometimes chronic heart, bowel, joint, or emotional illnesses can be due to unsuspected allergies. If milk bothers several family members, tell your sick relatives. Maybe a fringe benefit of your Practical Rotary Diet will be that you'll help them. In general, if several close family members have a milk sensitivity, it is certainly possible that other more distant relatives also have this problem.

Sometimes fathers or older children refuse to adhere to the diet. Do your best. Breakfast and dinner can sometimes be controlled, and if done skillfully, they may not even notice that every food is rotated. If they insist, they will eat what they want for lunch or anytime. If they make the wrong decisions, their food allergies may remain hidden, but we live in a world of choices. In the future, when they see how well other family members feel and behave after they adhere to the diet, they may also decide to try it.

10. Food families are very important in rotation diets. They are clustered together on Table 24.1 and listed on Table 24.2. For example, oranges, grapefruits, lemons, and limes are in the same botanical family. If you find that oranges are not a problem, you can rotate other citrus at a two-day, rather than a four-day interval. If grapefruit is also not a problem, then you can try oranges and limes on one day, and two days later try grapefruit and lemons. This is one way to expand your diet and have more variety. In other words, if a botanical family causes no symptoms, half can be eaten every two days. This means that no item in a botanical family is eaten more often than every four days, but it also adds more variety to the diet.

If, however, orange is a slight problem, then you must wait a full four days to eat grapefruit or any other citrus.

11. Try to keep beef and milk on the same day; similarly chicken and egg should be eaten on the same day. Although many allergists disagree and there are no definitive scientific studies, we often find that when patients are sensitive to one, they frequently cannot tolerate the other. Some even claim capon is less of a problem than a hen.

12. You can change your four lists of foods to suit your family's preferences. The suggested Practical Rotary Diet is not written in stone. Each day's list should contain foods your family really likes. If you have one day that is wonderful and one day your family hates,

Table 24.2
Botanical Families for Major Food Groups

Fruits, Vegetables, Nuts, Herbs, Seeds, and Spices

DAY 1

Berries: Blackberry, boysenberry, dewberry, loganberry, raspberry, strawberry

Birch: Filbert (hazelnut), oil of birch (wintergreen)

Cashew: Cashew nuts, pistachio, mango

Composite: Artichoke, burdock root, cardoon, chamomile, chicory, endive, lettuce, salsify, sunflower seeds and oil, tansy, tarragon

Conifer: Juniper (gin), pine nut (pinon, pinyon)

Fungi: Mushroom, truffle

Lily: Aloe vera, asparagus, chive, garlic, leek, onion, sarsaparilla

Mulberry: Breadfruit, fig, hop, mulberry

Papaya: Papaya

Pineapple: Pineapple

Potato (Nightshade): Chili, cayenne pepper, eggplant, green and red pepper, potato, tomato, paprika, pimiento, tobacco

Yam: Chinese potato (yam)

DAY 2

Banana: Banana, plantain

Cactus: Prickly pear

Carrot: Anise, carrot, caraway, celery, coriander, cumin, dill, fennel, parsnip, parsley

Goosefoot: Beet, lamb's-quarters, spinach, sugar beet, Swiss chard

Grass: Bamboo shoots, citronella, corn, corn products, lemon grass

Heath: Blueberry, cranberry, huckleberry

Mint: Applemint, basil, bergamot, catnip, chia seed, clary, dittany, horehound, lemon balm, marjoram, oregano, pennyroyal, peppermint, rosemary, sage, spearmint, savory, thyme

Mallow: Althea root, cottonseed oil, hibiscus, okra

Sapucaya: Brazil nut, sapucaya nut (paradise nut)

Stone fruits: Almond, apricot, cherry, nectarine, peach, plum, prune

DAY 3

Buckwheat: Buckwheat, garden sorrel, rhubarb, sea grape

Dillenia: Chinese gooseberry (kiwi)

Ginger: cardamom, arrowroot, ginger, turmeric

Grape: Cream of tartar, grape, raisin, Welch's unsweetened grape juice

Morning Glory: Sweet potato

Mustard: Broccoli, brussels sprouts, cabbage, cauliflower, horseradish, kale, kohlrabi, mustard greens, radish, turnip, watercress

Myrtle: Allspice, clove, eucalyptus, guava

Olive: Green or ripe, olive oil

Pedalium: Sesame seed and oil, tahini

Pomes: Apple, apple cider, apple pectin, apple vinegar, pear, quince, rose hips

Walnut: Black walnut, butternut, English walnut, heartnut, hickory nut, pecan

DAY 4

Beech: Chestnut, chinquapin

Citrus: Citron, grapefruit, kumquat, lemon, lime, orange, tangerine

Ebony: American persimmon, kaki (Japanese persimmon)

Gourd: Acorn squash and seeds, cucumber, cantaloupe, melon, pumpkin, squash, zucchini

Laurel: Avocado, bay leaf, cassia bark, cinnamon, sassafras

Legume: Alfalfa (sprouts), carob, carob syrup, chick-pea (garbanzo), fenugreek, gum acacia, kidney bean, kudzu, lentil, licorice, lima bean, mung beans (sprouts), pea, peanut, soybean, soy flour, soy milk

Nutmeg: Nutmeg, mace

Palm: Date, cabbage, coconut, palm, sago starch

Pomegranate: Grenadine, pomegranate

Saxifrage: Currant, gooseberry

Sedge: Water chestnut, chuta (groundnut)

Meat, Fowl, Fish, and Seafood

DAY 1

Bovine: Beef, butter, cheese, goat, goat's milk, goat cheese, ice cream, lamb, milk, veal gelatin, yogurt

Mollusk: Abalone, clam, mussel, oyster, scallop, snail, squid

Red Snapper: Red snapper

Other: Moose, rabbit, venison

DAY 2

Crustacean: Crab, crayfish, lobster, shrimp

Duck: Duck, duck eggs, goose, goose eggs

Herring: Herring, sardine

Salmon: Salmon, trout

Turkey: Turkey, turkey eggs

DAY 3

Codfish: Cod, cusk, haddock, hake, pollack

Flounder: Dab, flounder, halibut, plaice, sole, turbot

Mackerel: Albacore, bonito, mackerel, skipjack, tuna

Swine: Bacon, ham, lard, pork, pork gelatin, sausage, scrapple

DAY 4

Pheasant: Chicken, chicken eggs, peafowl, pheasant, quail

Grass, (Grains and Cereals)

DAY 1

Barley: Barley flour, malt, maltose (malt is also derived from both wheat and corn)

Sugar Cane: Cane sugar (white sugar, brown sugar, raw sugar), jaguary sugar made from sugar cane, molasses, turbinado sugar (this is not really a grain, but it is in the grass family)

Triticale: A cross between wheat and rye, it was developed for hardiness and high protein content.

Wheat: Bread, bran, buns, Cream of Wheat, gluten flour, graham flour, macaroni, noodles, pasta, Red River cereal, rolls, spaghetti, wheat germ, wheat germ oil, white flour, whole wheat flour, vitamin E from wheat germ oil

DAY 2

Corn: Corn meal, corn oil, cornstarch, dextrose, fructose (derived from corn and causes reactions in many corn-sensitive people), glucose, grits, most vegetable oils, corn oil margarine, syrup, popcorn

Millet: Very similar to wheat

Rye: 100 percent rye bread, rye flour, Ry-Krisp

Sorghum: Grain syrup (used as an alternative to sugar)

DAY 3

Rice: Rice flour

DAY 4

Oats: Oatmeal

Some very grain-sensitive people must avoid *all* members of the grass family, especially when grass is pollinating. If an individual is less allergic, cereal grains can be rotated so that a different one is used each day. That is, wheat on Monday, corn on Tuesday, rice on Wednesday, and oats on Thursday. Sometimes individuals are so exquisitely sensitive that a different single grain is eaten only once every four days. For example, on Day 1, wheat can be eaten, on Day 5, corn, on Day 9, rice, and on Day 12, oats. No grains are allowed on the other days because of the extreme grain sensitivity. If each grain is eaten more frequently, symptoms develop.

---

they will never follow the diet. Move the goodies around so that every day has foods everyone enjoys eating. If this is done, however, then the recipe booklet that makes the diet practical may also have to be altered.[4]

13. Yes, you can break the diet on special occasions. If you adhere to the diet most of the time, you can bend once in a while and still remain well. If you break the diet all the time, however, certain family members may remain ill and no cause-and-effect relationships will be obvious.

14. Every individual is different, and although in general many patients appear to feel better on the four-day Practical Rotary Diet, it is not the answer for everyone and for every food. Some allergic children need to rotate certain foods at an eight-day interval, whereas other foods that seem to cause less difficulty can be eaten more often than every four days. Individuals who have difficulty with the rotation diet definitely need the help of a doctor or an experienced dietitian or nutritionist who is knowledgeable about rotary diets. The diet is truly easy once it is understood and used for several weeks, but many parents need some personal help when they first try the diet.

4. Doris J. Rapp, M.D., *Rotary and Other Allergy Diets Made Easy for Children.*

15. Check with your physician about a calcium substitute. Children over eighteen months of age do not need extra calcium *if they are eating a well-balanced diet.*[5] If in doubt, about 250 milligrams of calcium is roughly equivalent to one glass of milk. Appendix A lists possible sources of milk. Pregnant, lactating, or postmenopausal women need extra calcium. (For sources of calcium, see Chapter 27.)

16. If your child likes soda pop, use carbonated soda water and pure fruit juice. You can also make popsicles from fruit juice.

17. If your child craves a particular food, find a doctor who can treat food sensitivities (see Appendix D). If your child is already treated but she or he is sneaking the problem food again, the treatment dose for that food needs to be rechecked. Food cravings tend to diminish after appropriate food treatment.

18. School lunches simply *can't* be eaten by children on the Practical Rotary Diet. The lunch for each day must be packed with much thought and sensitivity. Your children *must* have foods they love to eat every single day. Check with a nutrition consultant who is familiar with the Practical Rotary Diet if this is a problem.[6]

19. The teacher or school nurse must have a special party-time snack for school children on this diet. The snack should be kept at school and might include a pure fruit juice and pure potato chips fried in a single oil.

20. Remember that grass is in the grain family. Grain-sensitive individuals tend to have more symptoms when grass pollen is in the air. In other words, some children can't eat as much bread or as many pastries if the grass pollen count is high. Treatment for grass pollen *and* grains helps to eliminate some summer symptoms.

21. Once a month check your child's vitamins and toothpaste at a four-day interval. If a sensitivity develops to these items, you will have to change to another brand or try to rotate these items.

22. Remember, when you go on the Practical Rotary Diet, you will find the spikes, the nails, and the thumbtacks in relation to your food allergies. The major foods that cause the worst problems are the spikes, and you'll easily recognize these. Later on you will find the nails. When you also detect the thumbtacks, some discouraged

---

5. Frank A. Oski, *Don't Drink Your Milk*. Mollica Press, Ltd., 1914 Teall Avenue, Syracuse, N.Y. 13206.
6. Contact: Practical Allergy Research Foundation (PARF), P.O. Box 60, Buffalo, N.Y. 14223-0060.

parents finally see the true blessing their child really is. Some parents comment that it is almost like "having a new child in the old body."

23. Some excellent, experienced environmental medical specialists, such as retired John Maclennan, M.D., of Hamilton, Ontario, believe that a five-day rotation diet is superior to a four-day rotation diet. One outstanding book, for which he acted as a consultant and advisor, is entitled *Why 5? A Complete Food Allergy Guidebook*, by Donna Powell.[7] They believe that this rotation diet is one of the best preventative measures to use on a long-term basis for patients who have multiple food sensitivities.

What Is the Major Problem With the Practical Rotary Diet? Unequivocal Answer: Grains!

Grains include mainly wheat, millet, rye, rice, corn, oats, and barley. Wheat, millet, and rye are so similar that some allergists consider them to be essentially the same grain.

The major problem in relation to the Practical Rotary Diet is that grains are classified in the same botanical family. This means theoretically that only one grain should be eaten every four days. On Monday you can feed your child wheat, but then no grains are allowed on Tuesday, Wednesday, or Thursday. On Friday you can give corn. Then no grain is given for the next three days. You can easily see that this would be impossible for most children. They not only want grains, but many simply need grains to feel full and to grow normally. Fortunately most allergic children do not need to be that strict.

A few adults certainly must eat this way, however, if they have a total grain sensitivity and want to feel well. For example, some adults delete all grains for a week, and suddenly their knee and back pains are gone, their vaginal itch subsides, or they suddenly have energy and don't feel hungry all the time. Unlike children, extremely food-sensitive adults can quite readily manage a four-day grain rotation providing they have some help from a dietitian and nutrition specialist.

Because a true four-day grain rotation can be a challenge, many ecologists suggest that although it is not ideal, it is practical to com-

7. Donna Powell, *Why 5? A Complete Food Allergy Guidebook*. 1989. Donna Powell, Box 25, Waterdown, Ontario, Canada LOR 2HO.

promise a bit so that children can eat a different grain each day. So, on Day 1, for example, wheat would be allowed; on Day 2, corn; on Day 3, rice; and on Day 4, oats.

What Can Your Child Use for Lunch at School?
—If Sandwiches Are a Must

You might be concerned about the desire of your child to eat sandwiches for lunch. The answer is not as difficult as you think.

The answers are not as difficult as you think. Breads which are totally wheat or pure rye are readily available, so two of the four-day diet lunches are no problem. Another common variation for the third day which is readily available and acceptable to most children is rice wafers, crackers, or cakes. For the fourth day, or if your child refuses to eat rice cakes, contact Ener-G Foods, Inc. They can make your life much more pleasant because they sell rice, tapioca, poi, and potato-rice bread plus a variety of cookies, pizza shells, cereals, donuts, buns, and flours made from different grains.[8] It is truly easy to create sandwiches made from different grains for each of the four days on the rotation diet.

But Are Sandwiches Really Necessary?

No. Many children accept and enjoy some fruit, celery, cucumber, carrots, peanuts or other nuts, raisins, potato or corn chips, pretzels, and the "meat of the day" wrapped in a cellophane bag. They can have the homemade "soup of the day" in a thermos. With some creativity many children adjust and seem quite content.

Another variation is to consider using a single-grain loaf bread such as banana nut bread. When sliced, it looks similar to a half slice of bread. Place sliced home-cooked chicken, for example, between two slices and your child will have a sandwich that is similar to the other children's. You might also consider using flat breads, pitas, or square waffles made from different grains to replace regular bread.[9]

8. Ener-G Foods, Inc., P.O. Box 84487, Seattle, Wash. 98124-5787 (800-331-5222 or 206–767–6660).
9. Doris J. Rapp, M.D., *Rotary and Other Allergy Diets Made Easy for Children* (see Bibliography).

How Can You Encourage Your Child to Eat Unusual Baked Goods?

It is immensely helpful if parents of children on the Practical Rotary Diet learn to bake. If you can also teach your children to help with the culinary creations—the cookies, loaf cakes, muffins, waffles, and breads suggested in the booklet—it will make everyone's life sweeter. Younger children are more apt to eat such foods if they help cut out or decorate the cookies, for example.

If you don't want to purchase single-grain baked goods and can't bake, for many reasons, consider the following: Some busy parents might consider asking a grandparent to help prepare the four-day snacks and breads. Others hire a neighbor or friend to do the baking and then label and store the goodies in the freezer so that they can be used as needed. Some even put an ad in a local paper and find some grateful woman who would enjoy being paid to bake in her own home.

How Long Should You Stay on a Practical Rotary Diet?

Theoretically, it would certainly be best if children who feel unwell or can't act appropriately because of major food allergies maintain their Practical Rotary Diet indefinitely. But in real life this is seldom done unless it is found to be absolutely necessary. Some find that every time they stop the diet, their child's symptoms recur. These families have little choice. They have to maintain the diet in order to stay well. Most parents purposely stop the diet as soon as children feel and act well to see if it is really necessary. Others choose to maintain the Practical Rotary Diet so that their children do not continue to need repeated allergy testing or treatment.

In general, I would say that most children who are seriously ill with allergies should usually maintain the Practical Rotary Diet for at least six months or a year while they are being treated for their food allergies. After that period of time parents may sometimes choose to stop their allergy extract treatment for foods. Others prefer to become more lax in relation to their food rotation. For example, they may continue to rotate milk and wheat if those were two major causes of illness, but not attempt to rotate any other foods. Foods that cause only minor problems probably will not have to be rotated forever, particularly if a child receives food allergy treatment.

It is unique to find a patient whose problems are entirely due to one food. Most children and adults appear to have multiple food sensitivities, as well as allergies to dust, molds, and pollens. Most also appear to have chemical sensitivities.

Can a Food-Allergic Child Be Helped When the Allergy Extract Therapy Is Based Solely Upon Blood Test Results?

The answer is yes, but this, too, has definite limitations. If only a few of many allergenic foods are treated with an allergy extract, that child may not improve as much as possible. IgE RAST blood tests do not appear to be nearly as reliable as P/N testing and treatment.

A Child Helped by Eliminating Problem Foods

Sally

Sally's mother had seen an allergist about one and a half years before she came to see us. He had performed some RAST blood tests and found that four-year-old Sally was sensitive to dairy, yeast, orange, and corn. When Sally stopped eating these foods, the change was remarkable. Four weeks after the RAST-positive foods were totally removed from her diet, Sally's hyperactivity score decreased from an extremely high level of 28 to a remarkably low normal level of 6½. Her mother was amazed because Sally could sit down and color with crayons. In the past she could only scribble. Her behavior was unbelievably better. She was happier, less whiny, and less clingy.

Sally Before Her Allergy Treatment

Prior to this diet Sally was "uncontrollable, off the wall, and wild." She cried easily and often, could not concentrate, and ran from one thing to another. She was extremely active from morning to night and was in constant motion. She had dark eye circles. She needed antibiotics frequently for "constant" ear infections, which had been a problem since she was nine months old. On two occasions she had needed surgery to place tubes through her eardrums.

Diet Helped, But Not Enough

The results of the allergy tests on her blood revealed some important problem foods. Sally certainly improved after these were eliminated, but she was still not as well as her mother wanted her to be.

In time, her mother recognized that there were other things that bothered Sally. She hoped that newer allergy testing and treatment methods, namely provocation/neutralization, might detect other problem foods. In particular, her mother desired a treatment that would enable her child to eat a more normal diet. She wanted Sally to be able to eat some of her RAST-positive food items. These aims were not unrealistic.

Results of Comprehensive Allergy Treatment

Within two months after she was placed on the Practical Rotary Diet and allergy-treated for many other items that were positive during P/N testing, her attention span was better. She had less diarrhea, was even happier, less active, and for the first time could play by herself for extended periods. After four months of treatment she was 75 percent better, and although she still had a few stubborn episodes, she no longer had recurrent ear infections. Seven months later she was 85 percent better, delightful, and cooperative. An elderly baby-sitter was also truly amazed by Sally's improved disposition. Her mother stated that she was "in a state of shock" because Sally was so good. In essence, P/N treatment enabled her to have her cake and eat it too.

Remember that routine RAST tests detect only the IgE piece of the allergic pie. Many children have a negative RAST to foods or other allergenic substances that can be the cause of some form of illness. Using P/N testing and treatment, another piece of the allergy puzzle can be detected. Some children improve dramatically by using a combination of the Practical Rotary Diet and P/N allergy treatment. These enable many children to tolerate a significant number of foods that previously repeatedly caused significant symptoms. We are truly fortunate to have such methods available. As with many diagnostic procedures, however, P/N allergy testing, too, can indicate sensitivities when none exist or miss some that are a problem. In general, however, this method appears to provide some critical but missed answers needed to help many children improve. Foods continue to be a major unrecognized cause of many illnesses, with chemical sensitivities being an alarming and ever-increasing second unsuspected factor. P/N testing also helps to detect and verify some of these chemical problems.

Again let me stress, these methods are not applicable for foods that cause severe incapacitating illness, such as extreme asthma or loss of consciousness, but they certainly relieve many of the more common types of less serious food-related medical complaints.

Allergy Extract Testing
and Therapy

How Is the Diagnosis of Allergy Made?

In Chapter 1, certain aspects of the diagnosis and treatment of allergies were discussed. The current chapter will discuss allergy testing and treatment in more depth. One major and most reliable method for diagnosing an allergy is for the physician to take a detailed history and to do a thorough physical examination. The physician must decide if the medical complaints are compatible with an allergy problem.

Of course allergy treatment is not the answer for every child. Only some children have physical illness or emotional, behavioral, and learning problems partly or mainly related to allergies or environmental exposures. Other children's various complaints are totally due to unrelated medical problems. Because of the complexity of the many variables that must be considered, a thorough environmental allergy history and physical examination can take as long as two hours directly with a physician to evaluate the many facets of an ecologic illness.

If a patient's family has many allergic relatives, this certainly is one more factor to consider when information is being gathered to make a diagnosis of allergy. Certain blood or allergy skin tests also help to confirm a suspicion of allergy and sometimes newer testing methods (P/N testing) can actually pinpoint a specific cause of one particular symptom. The allergy test results, however, represent only one possible piece of the total allergy puzzle. Multiple factors must be considered, and the skill of a physician rests in her or his ability to interpret the many variables and come to the right conclusion. The skin and blood test results, by themselves, provide essential, helpful confirmation, but even these can be misleading at times. They surely are not the sole factors involved in either making or negating a diagnosis of allergy in a child.

For example, it is possible for both the blood and skin allergy tests to be positive and yet the patient may have no symptoms. The tests may represent a past or future allergy. It is equally possible for a patient to have classical allergy symptoms with totally negative blood or skin tests. Allergists feel most secure in their diagnosis if:

- The history of illness suggests allergy.
- There is evidence of allergy on the physical examination.
- The patient has allergic relatives.
- Special blood tests indicate an allergy.
- The nose, eye, or chest mucus show evidence of allergy.
- Dietary challenges at four-day intervals confirm that certain foods repeatedly cause specific symptoms.
- The skin tests for allergy indicate specific allergies.

Even with all this you can be fooled. Let me give you one example discussed by Dr. Jonathan Brostoff, from London, at a recent medical meeting.[1] He discussed a marathon runner who found that if he ate no shrimp or oysters, he could run well and not develop hives. If he ate shrimp or oysters, he did not develop hives. If, however, he ate shrimp or oysters *and then ran,* his hives were so severe, he had difficulty completing his run. Similarly, a child might eat chocolate and have no symptoms. A hot bath might cause no problems. But if that same child ate chocolate and then took a hot bath, hives would be evident.

Tests to Confirm an Allergy

There are several kinds of tests used to confirm the presence of allergy. The Prist blood test measures the total amount of immu-

1. Jonathan Brostoff, M.D., *Food Allergy and Intolerance.* 1989. Bloomsbury Publishing Limited, 2 Soho Square, London, England W1V 50E.

noglobulin E. If this is elevated, it is thought to indicate a *general* allergy.

The RAST blood test (radio-allergo-sorbent test) helps to pinpoint *specific* allergies, for example to dust, mold, ragweed, milk, dog, and so on.

In general, if the Prist test is positive, so are certain RAST tests. It is possible, however, for the Prist test to be negative while several RAST tests are positive or vice versa. It is even possible, however, for both the Prist and RAST tests to be negative even though a patient, for example, might have typical pollen-related seasonal allergic symptoms that respond favorably to pollen allergy extract therapy. This means, again, that although the results of these tests usually correlate with the child's history, they can, at times, be misleading.

A third kind of blood test involves an examination of a patient's blood for eosinophils. This is a type of white blood cell that characteristically increases in the blood or nose mucus of patients who have allergy. It is often found in excess in the nose mucus of patients who have seasonal hay fever. In other typically allergic patients, however, the eosinophil level may not be elevated, even though obvious allergy is present.

A blood examination is also possible for substances called chemical mediators, such as histamine. One common, but certainly not the only, cause for an elevated histamine level in the blood is an allergic reaction.

The so-called gold standard for the diagnosis of food allergy is to observe what happens to children when they ingest capsules that contain different food items. One set of capsules would contain a dehydrated suspect food; the other set a placebo or something that does not cause an allergy. Both capsules must look and taste alike. This type of evaluation is more scientific than simply eating a food and noting what happens, because it helps to remove bias due to a child's, parent's, or doctor's preconceived ideas. The gold standard evaluation of problem foods in capsules, however, can be misleading for the following reasons:

- This accepted method allows the food to be encased in a capsule until it reaches the stomach. This excludes ordinary absorption of the food from the mouth, which surely can cause some allergic reactions.
- There is a limit to how many capsules of food a child can or will swallow.

- The quantity of a suspected food that can be placed inside a tiny capsule is obviously limited. The amount of food that a child can ingest in capsule form may be far less than the amount a child normally eats on a daily basis. As with pollen allergies, each patient has a threshold. If the pollen count is low or if the patient eats only a very little of an allergenic food, it is possible that no symptoms develop. If the pollen count or the amount of a food that is eaten reaches a certain critical level, however, symptoms are evident.

- In an attempt to give a child a larger quantity of food, the suspected allergenic foods, which are placed in capsules, are usually dehydrated. This means that the tested food is not in its natural form. Dehydration, or drying a food, can alter some allergenic factors in foods to such a degree that a true food allergy could be missed.

Ideally, foods to be tested should be cooked and eaten in the normal amount, in their *usual* form. If one food is the major cause of an allergic reaction, then the best way to test that food is at a four-day interval as outlined in the Single Food Elimination Diet. On the fourth day, swallow only the food-filled capsules on the empty stomach.

Suppose a child is allergic to ten foods, however, which cause symptoms most of the time. Feeding one of these foods in capsular form, while the other nine are also eaten, might demonstrate very little change in how the child feels or acts. The symptoms from eating nine problem foods might be very similar to eating ten such foods. This is why the Multiple Food Elimination Diet is so important.

From the foregoing it is clearly evident that although food capsules are one method for confirming some food allergies, they certainly do not provide foolproof evidence. If the test is positive, a food sensitivity probably exists, but if the child shows no response to the capsules, it is still possible for a normal amount of a favorite food in its usual form to cause symptoms.

Options for Allergy Testing and Treatment

There are several types of allergy extract testing and therapy presently used in the United States. Traditional allergy testing was initially performed in this country in about 1914. The two major types are called scratch and intradermal tests. In addition one newer method, called provocation/neutralization (P/N), is also being used by a growing number of physicians in this country and abroad. Two major differences between the traditional and P/N allergy testing are that the latter is more precise and much more time-consuming. Many details about P/N testing are included in Chapter 1. One newer helpful method to detect and treat allergies, not discussed in this book, is called Intradermal Serial Dilution Titration or End-Point Titration.

What Is Traditional Allergy Extract Testing and Treatment?

Traditional Testing by Scratch or Prick Tests

The scratch test is performed by simply placing a drop of allergy extract on top of a slight indentation that was previously made on the surface of the skin. The indentation is made with an instrument that leaves an impression on the skin that is similar to the mark that an ordinary fingernail would make if it was pushed firmly into the skin. A toothpick is then used to scratch this area. This is called a scratch test. If the skin test site beneath a drop of allergy extract is pricked with a needle, this is called a prick test.

Over forty of these tests can be done at the same time on the back or arms. If the skin test site becomes red and looks like a mosquito bite within fifteen to twenty minutes, it is called positive. This suggests the presence of an allergy to the item tested. If the skin test site remains unchanged, it is interpreted as a negative skin test, and this suggests there is no allergy to that item. This method of testing is most effective in detecting extremely strong sensitivities to pollen, dust, molds, pets, or foods.

There is little disagreement among allergists, however, that this testing method is not always reliable. Sometimes there is a large skin reaction but the patient appears not to have symptoms from that item. This is particularly true in relation to food-allergy reactions. At other times the scratch test site remains unchanged although a definite allergy exists. At times there is no immediate skin reaction, but several hours later a red spot appears that indicates that a different, delayed type of allergic response has occurred.

When I learned scratch testing thirty-five years ago, I was frequently perplexed. Some children would have many large positive reactions to foods, but when parents excluded these foods from the child's diet for several weeks and then added them back into their child's diet, those suspect foods infrequently caused symptoms. It took eighteen years in practice before I found out why food skin test results and the child's history appeared to give a mixed message: *If too many days elapse between challenges with a suspect food, it is easy to be misled into thinking that there is no allergy to that food.* At that time I simply did not understand that if a food sensitivity is to be detected, that suspect food must be eaten a minimum of every four days (for example on Monday and then not eaten again until Friday) or at a maximum of about fourteen days.[2]

Intradermal Allergy Tests

Many allergists prefer to do intradermal testing by injecting ten to twenty possible allergenic items, all at one time, into one or both arms. Using this method, a tiny amount of each allergy extract is injected into the outer layers (intra) of the skin (dermal). In ten minutes the tests are interpreted in the same manner as scratch or prick tests. A large mosquito-bite-like reaction indicates a strong allergy, and a small red spot with a tiny raised white center indicates a lesser allergy. Allergists routinely start testing with weak dilutions of allergy extract. If those skin reactions are negative, they repeat each test with progressively *stronger* tenfold dilutions of allergy extract, for example from 1:10,000 to 1:1,000 to 1:100, and so on.

At the present time this form of allergy testing is somewhat less popular than it was previously. The major emphasis of some physicians' allergy-training programs today for doctors training to become allergists is the proper use of a wide range of newly formulated improved antiallergic drugs. This is combined with a thorough understanding of the basic physiologic, pathologic, and immunologic changes that occur during allergy reactions. The detection of allergy by skin tests, diet, or the evaluation of home factors is often not the major focus of some allergy residency programs.

Traditional allergy testing can sometimes be deceptively inaccurate for the detection of multiple food allergies unless a patient has an exquisite sensitivity to only a few major foods. Most patients who have severe, incapacitating or life-threatening food allergies already know they will become desperately ill or need to be hospitalized if they eat or smell foods such as peanut, egg, fish, or buckwheat. Skin testing those patients is not only not required, it can be dangerous. Typical IgE RAST blood tests, in general, easily and accurately con-

2. Herbert Rinkle, Theron Randolph, and M. Zeller, *Food Allergy* (Springfield, Ill.: Charles C. Thomas Publishing, 1951).

firm such extreme sensitivities. Traditional allergy testing is usually reliable for the detection of dust, mites, mold, pollen, and pet sensitivities.

Traditional Allergy Treatment

A typical allergy extract is usually a combination of tree, grass, and weed pollen; molds; dust; and mites that caused positive reactions by scratch or intradermal testing. Each allergist must decide exactly how much and how strong each item should be when each patient's treatment solution is prepared. This decision depends upon the concentration of the extract used to test a patient, the intensity of each skin reaction, and each patient's particular history. For example, if a person had many symptoms during the pollen season but only a little stuffiness in the winter, that extract might contain relatively more pollen than dust. If a patient had slight hay fever in the summer but seemed worse in the winter while living in a damp, moldy house, that extract would be weighted more heavily with dust and molds, rather than pollen.

Most patients receive their extract subcutaneously, or under the skin, three times a week for several weeks or months. This is called a build-up period because the patient receives either a larger amount of extract or a stronger concentration of extract with each injection. After an arbitrary top dosage (often 1 cc of a 1:10 dilution) is reached, the patient receives that top-tolerated dose as a booster injection at weekly-to-monthly intervals until the symptoms of allergy have not been evident for two or more years. It is not unusual for some patients to require these treatments for many years.

The Advantages and Disadvantages of Traditional Allergy Testing and Treatment

The major advantage of traditional allergy testing and treatment is that it helps many individuals. Parent reimbursement from insurance companies is rarely a problem.

Scratch or intradermal testing is fast. It takes less than a half hour to place the extract on or in the skin and to interpret the results. After several months of allergy treatment this form of therapy appears to help many patients who have dust, pollen, or mold allergies. They often have fewer symptoms and require less medication.

The disadvantages related to traditional allergy treatment include the following:

- Traditional treatment can routinely require several months before any benefit is apparent. During that time patients continue to need drugs to control their symptoms.

- It is not unusual for some patients to develop a hot, swollen, sore arm after each injection treatment of traditional allergy extract therapy. Sometimes, but not always, this problem can be diminished by giving a smaller or weaker dose of extract.

- Although this method certainly helps many patients, it is not unusual for some patients to continue to need daily drugs to control their remaining symptoms. In other words, they are improved but not entirely well.

- It is difficult to detect accurately certain mild-to-moderate food allergies using the traditional allergy-testing methods.

- Allergy extract treatment is not recommended for either food or pet allergies. Patients are usually told to avoid foods that are a problem and not to have pets.

- Traditional allergy testing does not routinely include a provocation challenge to detect most chemical sensitivities.

- Traditional subcutaneous allergy treatment, on very rare occasions, can cause an alarming, severe allergic reaction requiring immediate medical attention. For this reason it is prudent to receive this type of extract therapy only in a physician's office.

- Some patients appear to be sensitive to phenol, which is routinely used as a preservative in many allergy extracts. This can cause a wide range of ill-defined symptoms, ranging from a sore arm to dizziness, headache, fatigue, weakness, personality changes, or irritability *every time* an allergy extract is received. (See Joan, Chapter 6, and Rick, Chapter 15.)

What Is Provocation/Neutralization (P/N) Allergy Testing and Treatment?

Carleton Lee, M.D., originated the idea of provocation/neutralization testing and treatment. He applied some basic concepts of allergy testing suggested by Herbert Rinkel, M.D., and found he could produce and eliminate symptoms of allergy. Then Joseph Miller, M.D., in Mobile, Alabama, began to write books and teach physicians how to do P/N allergy testing. As it is presently done, P/N testing is simply a much more precise and time-consuming method of doing traditional allergy testing. It is more precise because 1:5, rather than 1:10, dilutions are used for testing, and because each allergenic substance is tested separately. The same stock allergy extract is used by both traditional allergists and those physicians who do P/N testing.

This method is called P/N testing because it can at times provoke or cause miniature symptoms of the type that bother an individual. The test can precipitate sudden stuffiness, asthma, or personality changes if that is a child's problem. Many times, however, the only change that occurs during testing is that the area of skin where the extract was injected becomes red, swollen, and itchy, exactly as it does during traditional allergy tests.

During P/N testing each patient is tested every seven to ten minutes with progressively *weaker* dilutions of the same test item, for example 1:100, then 1:500, then 1:2,500, and so on. The object is to find the correct treatment dosage, one that no longer causes a significant skin or body reaction or the one that will neutralize or relieve a child's symptoms.

Specific medical complaints or inappropriate behavior patterns can often be both reproduced and eliminated at will by single-blind P/N allergy testing with common allergenic substances, such as dust, pollen, molds, or foods. It is not unusual for provoked symptoms to be totally eliminated with weaker dilutions of the same allergy extract.

It is possible, for example, to provoke sudden intense itching episodes during P/N allergy testing in patients who have eczema or hives. The itch can often be relieved with a weaker dilution of the same allergy extract that caused it. In very young infants or children who respond favorably, the extensive eczema can sometimes improve so much that the intensely distressing itching subsides and the skin heals dramatically within a few days. Although patients with eczema seem to need frequent retesting and adjustment of their extract treatment, it is gratifying to see how favorably some respond to neutralization allergy therapy. (See Katie, Chapter 4.)

How Effective Is Sublingual or Subcutaneous Extract Treatment?

A detailed example of how P/N testing is done is included in Chapter 1. Scientific studies to verify the efficacy of sublingual and subcutaneous treatment have been repeatedly published since 1978.[3]

In spite of this, there is a marked difference of opinion about the benefit of sublingual allergy extract treatment. No one doubts that under-the-tongue nitroglycerin tablets relieved heart pain or angina for many years. Most allergists agree that pollen allergy treatment is effective in treating hay fever if pollen extract is placed inside the nose. For some strange reason, however, many allergists, quite often those who have never personally used or seen this technique, doubt that sublingual allergy extract can be effective.

With neutralization treatment, in time, the drops under the

3. William King, M.D., et al., "Provocation/Neutralization: A Two-Part Study. Part 1. The Intracutaneous Provocative Food Test: A Multi-Center Comparison Study," *Otolaryngology Head Neck Surgery* 99 (1988), pp. 263–277; Jonathan Brostoff, M.D., et al., "Low Dose Sublingual Therapy in Patients With Allergic Rhinitis Due to House Dust Mite," *Clinical Ecology* 16 (1986), pp. 483–491; Marshall Mandell, M.D., et al., "The Role of Allergy in Arthritis, Rheumatism, and Polysymptomatic Cerebral, Visceral, and Somatic Disorders: Double-Blind Study," *Journal of International Academy of Preventative Medicine*, 1982; J. O'Shea et al., "Double-Blind Study of Children With Hyperkinetic Syndrome Treated with Multi-Allergen Extract Sublingually," *Journal of Learning Disabilities* 14 (1981), p. 189; D. King, "Can Allergic Exposure Provoke Psychological Symptoms? A Double-Blind Test," *Biological Psychiatry* 16 (1981), pp. 3–19; Doris J. Rapp, M.D., "Food Allergy Treatment for Hyperkinesis," *Journal of Learning Disabilities* 12 (1979), pp. 42–50; Doris J. Rapp, M.D., "Weeping Eyes in Wheat Allergy," *Trans-American Society of Ophthalmology and Otolaryngology* 18 (1978), p. 149; Doris J. Rapp, M.D., "Double-Blind Confirmation and Treatment of Milk Sensitivity," *Medical Journal of Australia* 1 (1978), pp. 571–572; Gerald Ross, M.D., et al., "Confirmation of Chemical Sensitivity by Double-Blind Inhalant Challenge," Presented at the International Conference on Food and Environmental Factors in Human Disease, Buxton, Derbyshire, England, July 3–6, 1990; Gerald Ross et al., "Environmentally Triggered Hypertension Part II: Environmental Health Care—Dallas Treatment Experience," Presented at the 8th Annual International Symposium on Man and His Environment in Health and Disease, Dallas, Tex., February 22–25, 1990. (not in print); William King, M.D., et al., "Provocation/Neutralization: A Two-Part Study. Part 2. Subcutaneous Neutralization Therapy: A Multi-Center Comparison Study," *Otolaryngology Head Neck Surgery* 99 (1988), pp. 272–277; Marvin Boris, M.D., et al., "Antigen-Induced Asthma Attenuated by Neutralization Therapy," *Clinical Ecology* 3 (1985), pp. 59–62; William Rea, M.D., et al., "Elimination of Oral Food Challenge Reaction by Injection of Food Extracts: A Double-Blind Evaluation," *Archives of Otolaryngology* 110 (1984), pp. 248–252; Doris J. Rapp, M.D., "Food Allergy Treatment for Hyperkinesis," *Journal of Learning Disabilities* 12 (1979), pp. 42–50; Joseph Miller, M.D., "A Double-Blind Study of Food Extract Injection Therapy," *Annals of Allergy* 38 (1979), pp. 185–191; J. Gerrard et al., "A Double-Blind Study on the Value of Low-Dose Immunotherapy of Asthma and Allergic Rhinitis," *Clinical Ecology* 6 (1989), pp. 43–46; William Rea, M.D., et al., "Elimination of Oral Food Challenge Reaction by Injection of Food Extracts: A Double-Blind Evaluation," *Archives of Otolaryngology* 110 (1984), pp. 248–252; D. King, "The Reliability and Validity of Provocative Food Testing: A Critical Review," *Medical Hypotheses* 25 (1988), pp. 7–16; Doris J. Rapp, M.D., "Environmental Medicine: An Expanded Approach to Allergy," *Buffalo Physician* (2/1986), pp. 15–24.

tongue or the injections should be needed less and less often. For example one to two eggs can probably be eaten every four days without causing a headache shortly after either sublingual or injection therapy is begun. Initially, sublingual therapy is needed three times a day. Later on it might be needed only on a weekly or monthly basis, *providing eggs are eaten no more often than every four days*.

Similarly, subcutaneous neutralization treatment with allergy extract appears to be very helpful. At first it is needed daily for maybe a week, and then twice weekly. In time, the injections may be needed only once every two to four weeks. Again, repeated scientific studies since 1979 indicate this form of therapy is beneficial.

What Are the Advantages of Provocation/Neutralization Allergy Testing and Treatment?

P/N helps parents pinpoint specific cause-and-effect relationships. It often enables parents dramatically to see exactly which allergenic substances are causing each of their child's individual medical complaints. One item might cause obvious hay fever during testing, another asthma, a third depression, and a fourth a rash.

Some patients improve *immediately* during their first office visit, others within a few days or months. If this method is helpful, it is not unusual for many children to improve 50 to 85 percent within a few weeks or months. Of course not every patient is helped, but the improvement quite often appears to be surprisingly rapid and beneficial.

If patients do not improve significantly within three to six months, the reason must be sought. Typical questions to ask would include the following:

- Are the neutralization treatment doses in the extract correct? If the doses for certain substances are incorrect, the child could become worse, not better, with each treatment.
- Were all the suspected items tested and treated? If you have ten nails in your shoe and remove five, you will still limp. Maybe some major allergenic items were missed.
- Did the parents change their home, do the Practical Rotary Diet, and use nutrients to enhance their child's immune function as advised? Halfhearted compliance can be rewarded with halfhearted improvement.

- Is the child avoiding offending chemical odors or pollution?

- Is the problem only partially due to an allergy? Many children have a complex medical problem that requires the expertise of several medical specialists. This is especially true for some children who have hypoglycemia or a wide variety of learning disabilities or emotional problems.

- Is the problem totally unrelated to allergy? Some children need a totally different type of medical specialist and evaluation to resolve their health problems.

One must not assume that a child does not have environmental illness until all the foregoing factors have been considered in depth. If a doctor suggests that the allergy extract be given three times a day, but the patient takes the extract only once every two days, the patient may not improve, even though the treatment is correct.

This treatment is so safe that it can be administered sublingually or injected in the arm by a parent. This means that most patients do not have to return repeatedly to their physician for each treatment. Ideally this factor should enhance its popularity among patients and their physicians.

P/N testing often reveals the cause of complaints that were never thought to be due to an allergy. The child who writes upside down and backward during a grass allergy skin test could do well all year in school but routinely write this way during final examinations that happen to occur at the peak of the grass pollen season. With proper treatment this problem might be resolved. The child who is depressed and suicidal on damp days can curl into a tight ball in some dark corner or under the furniture, become untouchable, and cry during the mold allergy test. Some parents are all too familiar with this type of response in their child but never dreamed it could be due to an allergy. Such bizarre behavior usually ends in a referral to a psychologist, not an allergist or specialist in environmental medicine.

Using the P/N method, it is possible to treat many food allergies and some allergies to pets.

P/N testing helps some parents determine why their child wheezes. Some asthmatics, but certainly not all, are improved after only one or more days of testing. Lung function is at times measurably better within minutes after the correct neutralization dosage of dust, molds, milk, or other common allergens has been found. Surprisingly a correct neutralization dose can sometimes relieve wheezing more quickly than an injection of adrenaline, which is a standard recommended treatment for severe asthma attacks.

What Are the Disadvantages of Provocation/ Neutralization Allergy Testing and Treatment?

The major disadvantage of this method of testing is that it is *very time-consuming*. It can require as much as three to six *full* days of constant testing and supervision to complete the necessary initial allergy evaluation. Many children need fifteen or more foods tested plus dust, mites, molds, yeasts, and pollens. In some offices a maximum of about eight new items can be tested in one day.

It is difficult for parents to watch their child, especially their infant, be repeatedly skin-tested every few minutes for several hours. Apprehensive, frightened children should be tested for short, rather than long, periods of time. Caring nurses can often test so well that children truly enjoy coming to the office, and many children cry only when they are reacting severely to some specific allergen. One comforting observation is that many children who feared needles initially are no longer afraid of them by the end of the first day's testing.

Another disadvantage is the need to retest or fine-tune the neutralization doses. Retesting, however, is much less time-consuming than the initial P/N testing. Sometimes up to twenty-five items can be retested in a single all-day office visit.

A parent can tell when retesting is needed because the extract no longer helps as much as it did before. A child may do well and eat a food without difficulty for weeks or months, and then in spite of continued treatment, that food may again appear to cause slight or moderate symptoms. This often indicates that the neutralization dose needs to be rechecked because it has changed. Most patients need retesting possibly four times during the first year and, depending upon how well they respond to therapy, less often from then on. Yearly retesting is often needed before or during each pollen season in very pollen-allergic patients. On *rare occasions* a few children unfortunately need weekly or monthly retesting, especially if they have an exquisite mold sensitivity and are continuously exposed to a moldy environment.

This need for retesting can present a major problem if parents have to travel long distances to see their doctor. For this reason it is best to select the nearest physician who is well trained in environmental medicine whenever possible (see Appendix D). The relative paucity of physicians, however, who are expert in methods similar to P/N testing can make this difficult in many areas of the country.

Other challenges are related to differences in youngsters. Some children are difficult to test because they appear to be exceptionally sensitive to almost every item tested. Some children may test well and easily for many items on one day, but for unknown reasons are very difficult to test on another day. Some children test well in the morning and early afternoon but it is difficult to find a neutralizing dose later in the day. Individualized testing schedules are the key for youngsters of this type.

Every once in a while it is difficult to stop a reaction once it has started. It can occasionally be difficult to find a particular neutralization dosage. Sometimes it can require two or three hours to find one answer in an exquisitely sensitive child.

For example, on rare occasions a child becomes very hyperactive from a skin test and the correct neutralization dosage can't be found. This type of problem is most apt to occur late in the day, when the child, and possibly her or his immune system, is tired. Usually an alkali (see Chapter 8) or the child's histamine neutralizing dose helps. Fortunately, frightening allergic reactions are exceedingly rare when doing P/N testing.

If parents have major-medical insurance and do not have a restricted group health insurance plan, 80 percent of the costs of P/N testing are presently covered. If parents have limited insurance, the parents may have to pay for the entire cost of the testing and treatment.

Amazingly, a few insurance companies have recently ruled that they will not reimburse patients for food allergy testing. In addition, they will not pay for either sublingual allergy extract treatment or injection therapy *if* it is administered by the parent or patient. Why would they want to pay to have it administered in a physician's office? It will needlessly raise the cost of medical care. This form of P/N treatment is not harmful.

Initially P/N therapy can be more expensive than traditional allergy therapy. In time, however, the reward is often a well child who learns better in school, has friends, and needs fewer or no drugs. These children's need for routine medical attention, hospital visits, prescription medications, and possibly even surgery can decrease. If parents follow the diet and home suggestions urged by environmentally oriented physicians, the need for retesting and allergy extract therapy and drugs is often markedly diminished as time passes.

Another disadvantage of some health care plans is that the family's physicians must be selected from a specified list. If parents select a doctor who is not on the list, their insurance will not cover the cost of the evaluation. Ironically, they will sometimes pay if parents have their child evaluated by an allergist who is not specifically trained in environmental medicine or food allergy detection and treatment. If a physician who knows environmental medicine but is not on the list is seen for an allergy evaluation, the visit may have to be entirely paid by the parents. This is true even if the physician is a board-certified, well-trained pediatric allergist and if the child responds favorably and quickly. Some children need to be evaluated by a doctor who is knowledgeable, experienced, or successful using P/N or the newer concepts of allergy therapy. A growing number of ear, nose, and throat specialists, as well as pediatricians and family practice physicians now know or are learning these techniques. It puts an unnecessary burden on the family if the insurance company refuses payment for methods that are helpful but ironically will pay for treatments that have repeatedly not been beneficial in the past.

One last disadvantage is that there is a relative paucity of physicians who are qualified, trained, and knowledgeable in doing this newer P/N testing. At least two thousand physicians, mainly ear, nose, and throat specialists, use a method called End-Point Titration. This provides a similar but faster method to find the correct treatment doses with allergy extract for pollens, molds, and dust than P/N, but it is less helpful in the detection of food sensitivities. In addition this treatment requires a series of build-up injections as well as treatment every few days to maintain a high level of tolerance to allergenic exposures. Many specialists in environmental medicine successfully combine the use of Intradermal Serial Dilution, or End-Point Titration, for inhaled allergenic items with P/N testing for foods.

When Is Provocation/Neutralization Treatment Indicated?

Although both traditional and P/N allergy extract treatment are helpful ways of treating some allergic children, they are not always needed. Remember, you only need to lower a child's *total* allergy load. Many parents determine by observation or diets that a particular food is a problem. They merely omit that food from their child's diet and sometimes the physical illnesses, behavior problems, or learning difficulties subside. Other parents only make their child's bedroom allergy-free and more ecologically sound, and the medical problem is resolved. At times it is remarkably easy. Replacing an old mattress with a new one or replacing a feather or urethane pillow with cotton towels in a cotton pillowcase can entirely relieve some children's congestion, asthma, or repeated infections. Sometimes parents find that their old dusty, moldy home or their new chemically enriched home is the cause of their child's chronic medical and emotional problems. A temporary or permanent move to a different home may be the answer. This is especially true if a child became ill shortly after a move or is routinely worse within a few hours after returning home from a vacation.

But...if changing your home or diet, avoiding pollution and chemical exposures, or traditional allergy extract therapy has not helped a child, it is possible that provocation/neutralization therapy might help.

Who Might Be Helped by P/N Testing and Treatment?

The following are some typical examples of the types of children who sometimes benefit from this newer, more precise form of allergy testing and treatment:

- Some children appear to be allergic to many foods and can eat only a few foods without becoming ill. Concerns about their nutrition, growth, and the emotional impact of not being able to eat normally is paramount in their parents' minds. P/N testing at times enables children on very limited diets to eat many more foods without difficulty. I vividly recall one two-year-old who existed solely on a Nutramigen infant formula. He was so hungry, he tried to eat the putty off the windows. Within three to six months after P/N testing and treatment he was eating six, then ten, and then twelve foods. In less than six months many of his symptoms were 80 percent better. His allergy extract was given by injection every twenty-eight hours. If his treatment was as much as four hours late, his symptoms recurred.

- Some strong-willed teenagers cannot withstand peer pressure. They eat whatever they want, even though they know that certain foods bother them. They go into areas they know will make them ill because they want to do whatever their friends do. They need help and relief of their symptoms, regardless of their attitude, denial, or negativity about changing their diet, bedroom, or life-style.

- Clever children sneak and hide foods and swap lunches. Those tendencies, combined with a persistent determination, mean that a diet cannot be effectively carried out. No matter how hard parents try, P/N treatment for food allergies may be the only practical and helpful answer. If children cheat on their diets, but are treated for their food sensitivities, they often have less difficulty when they eat some problem foods.

- Children who must continue to live in dusty, moldy homes often require P/N allergy extract treatment because cleaning cannot compensate for an extremely allergenic environment. Many parents want to move but simply can't afford to do so. In our experience molds seem to cause many more problems than house dust.

- Many allergic children are sick and misbehave all year long but are considerably worse in the warm months, when pollens or molds are in the air. These children often have multiple factors causing their allergies, and although their parents can make changes in their diet and home that diminish their illness, the children will probably also need some form of allergy extract therapy. Seasonal allergy pollen problems can be lessened with room or home air purifiers, but if the child's symptoms interfere with normal living, some form of allergy extract therapy would be indicated. With seasonal allergies, many parents prefer drug therapy for a few weeks. However, they should be aware of the side effects of every drug they give their children, especially if they opt to use cortisone (see Chapter 26). You don't use nuclear arms to kill a fly when a swatter is handy. Ask your doctor, druggist, or librarian to let you read about all your child's drugs in the *Physicians' Desk Reference* (PDR).

- Children who have had asthma or hay fever treatment for years are sometimes helped to a greater degree when they receive P/N testing and treatment. Many children improve significantly with traditional allergy treatment, but some children continue to need daily medicine to control their symptoms or require repeated nose, sinus, or ear surgeries. Sometimes P/N can help detect missed food or chemical sensitivities, for example, which might have been unknowingly contributing to a child's problem. With appropriate food P/N treatment or chemical avoidance to supplement some children's dust, mold, and pollen allergy treatment, it is sometimes possible to decrease or eliminate the need for drugs.

- Some children have been told they must not return to school because they are too hyperactive and disruptive in the classroom. Some of these children can be helped by specific P/N allergy extract therapy. Some parents have been told that their children "must" be placed on the Class–2 controlled addictive substance Ritalin. Parents should be aware that there are alternatives to addictive drugs and that a few safer and possibly more helpful types of other mood-altering preparations do exist (see Chapter 18).

- Some children simply cannot live a normal life because they are too fatigued, too depressed, or have unusually severe medical problems such as uncontrollable asthma, hives, recurrent intestinal complaints, or seizures. Sometimes, but certainly not always, P/N treatment helps to resolve these problems when other measures have repeatedly failed.

- Children who have difficulties because of odors within certain moldy, dusty old houses or classrooms can sometimes be helped by allergy extracts. These can be prepared from the air in a particular offending school or home. P/N testing with such extracts will often reproduce a child's exact illness or disruptive symptoms and can sometimes provide an effective form of treatment. The response to a home or school air extract, however, is not always satisfactory, so at times, the only and better choice may be a switch to another school or a move to another home or area.

- Children of parents who find the Practical Rotary Diet too challenging or complicated may need P/N allergy treatment. The same is true of children in families where one parent realizes that diet changes help, but an opposing, skeptical parent adamantly refuses to comply. Not uncommonly relatives or baby-sitters feel sorry for the "deprived" child, so they purposely give him or her the exact goodies known to cause illness or personality changes. More than one father or grandparent has purchased a gallon of ice cream to give some milk-allergic children a special treat, only to find that they have caused a drastic deterioration in the child's behavior or well-being. After P/N treatment, however, most skeptical fathers, relatives, teachers, and doctors can see the difference. Even more encouraging, after they respond favorably to treatment, some of these children may be able to eat these same goodies without having symptoms.

- Some single parents can control their child's diet nicely when the child is at their home, only to watch the child repeatedly return home from visits with the "other parent" ill with physical or other allergy-related complaints. The solution to angry, estranged spouses who routinely welcome well children on Friday afternoon only to repeatedly return sick children by Sunday night might not be impossible. One answer is to try injections of a P/N allergy treatment just before the child walks out the door on Friday. Injection treatments often relieve symptoms for two to three days, in comparison to sublingual treatment, which can be required one to three times a day. Be certain to have your child's physician document all details if this scenario occurs in your family. The doctor may have some other practical ideas about how to help prevent such problems. The physician's records might provide some legal benefit in making the reluctant spouse enforce the necessary suggestions regarding diet and avoidance of common allergenic environmental factors.

- Some children have working parents who simply do not have the time to do a diet. Many really don't have the energy, desire, or finances to change their diet or home. Many mothers in today's world can barely handle their routine daily stresses, one day at a time. Some parents want and need pills for immediate relief of their children's symptoms. Often they are not concerned or knowledgeable about the possible complications or side effects of drugs commonly used to treat allergies. They may not be aware of the long-term results of possible smoldering chronic illness that appears to respond favorably to intermittent or daily drug therapy. Some drugs merely mask illness so the disease process progresses with only a temporary paucity of physical complaints. Extensive P/N allergy testing and extract therapy may possibly provide more permanent relief for some of these children.

- Single working parents often need a series of baby-sitters or relatives to help care for their allergic children. They may find it is impossible to keep the children well without extract treatment. Some allergic children cannot tolerate several hours in a home that is dusty or moldy. Many become ill because of unavoidable tobacco or chemical exposures. Realistically it may not be possible to teach any or all caretakers about the many aspects of allergy that contribute to some children's illness.

- Children who have atypical unrecognized allergies can grow up to be maladjusted and nonproductive adults, even though they have great potential. The earlier children receive comprehensive ecologic care, the sooner their lives can sometimes be turned around.

- Children in families who live in highly polluted cities or in areas that are naturally very damp and moldy may need P/N extract therapy. P/N treatment for molds, in particular, can be most helpful. Such testing can sometimes be most challenging and difficult, however, because mold treatment doses tend to need to be rechecked repeatedly in a minority of patients.

Questions That Need Answers

Why do many scratch and intradermal allergy tests done at one time rarely precipitate a child's symptoms whereas a single provocation skin test can cause symptoms?

It is difficult to say. Traditional testing can certainly precipitate asthma and hay fever on occasion in some patients, but the obvious personality and emotional changes so commonly noted with P/N testing are rarely seen. In part this may be due to the fact that parents, patients, and medical personnel are usually not instructed to watch as carefully and constantly as they are during P/N testing. However, this is certainly not the total answer.

I personally think that when many items are tested at one time, it sort of jams the biological nervous system circuitry, with the result that various types of reactions are neutralized. For example if one food that makes a child tired and another that makes the child hyperactive are tested simultaneously, no change may be evident. Maybe the sudden influx of numerous offending items through the skin causes some as yet undefined defense system to come into play and protect the body. Maybe as some chemical substances are depleted during a reaction, other balancing compensatory ones are produced to protect it. Maybe one favorable bioneurological system overrides another that is less advantageous for the body. At this time we are guessing. It is doubtful that anyone really understands what happens.

How can a child's body apparently respond to one single P/N antigen test after another over a period of several hours so consistently and accurately?

We really don't know. One would theorize there would be an additive effect when different dilutions of the same allergenic substance are injected repeatedly. There is some evidence to suggest this can happen and this merely underscores how much we simply can't explain.

Why are the treatment doses of allergy extract for some children unstable?

There must be something different about their immune systems. This problem seems to be inordinately evident in relation to molds in extremely ecologically ill children.

Why do some children respond poorly to sublingual treatment while the very same dose and strength of allergy extract by injection is extremely helpful?

Sometimes children tend to have an excessive amount of saliva so the treatment under the tongue is diluted, but this is not always a factor.

Why Are the Majority of Allergists So Negative About These Newer Testing Methods?

The answer to this is most difficult. The majority of allergists doubt that testing single allergenic items can cause certain types of specific symptoms such as hyperactivity. The medical literature early in this century, however, clearly indicates that foods can cause symptoms in many areas of the body other than the nose, eyes, lungs, and skin. Skeptical doctors also doubt that a reaction can be eliminated by giving a patient a weaker dilution of the same extract.

Because of the number of scientific articles that document what is included in this book about P/N allergy testing and treatment, it is difficult to understand many doctors' reluctance to at least consider this form of therapy.[4] Anyone who spends an afternoon in the offices of most physicians who do P/N testing will clearly see that the observations are not exaggerated. They are merely not explained. There are many movies and videos available of infants, children, and adults demonstrating the startling changes that can occur in minutes as a response to a tiny droplet of allergy extract in the arm or under the tongue. One preliminary pilot study suggests that in some patients certain discrete areas of the brain are altered at the same time that immunological and metabolic changes occur in the blood. These appear to correlate with the physical changes that occur when some, but certainly not all, patients react to testing.[5]

There is little disagreement that we need more large-scale, well-designed scientific studies conducted by unbiased academic medical scientists. We need these studies not only to help understand why so many patients improve, but also to encourage more dedicated physicians to become interested in providing this type of medical care.

It is unfortunate that many physicians remain unfamiliar with the over twenty double-blinded studies that either strongly suggest or clearly demonstrate the efficiency of P/N allergy testing.[6] An August 1990 article by Dr. Don Jewett et al. in the prestigious *New England*

4. Ibid.
5. The above study was done in conjunction with David Cantor, Ph.D., a psychologist associated with the University of Maryland School of Medicine. J. Alexander Bralley, Ph.D., at MetaMetrix Laboratory, in Norcross, Ga., kindly interpreted the amino acid data.
6. See material listed in Note 3, except King et al., "Provocation/Neutralization."

Journal of Medicine claimed that provocation testing for foods was of no value.[7] The selection of patients and methodology surprisingly revealed flagrant errors in design, execution, and interpretation. Important details regarding testing were omitted, so valid interpretation of certain salient factors is unfortunately impossible.

Superficial reading of this article by those who have no in-depth knowledge about the technique might lead to the erroneous conclusion that provocation allergy testing is of no value. Many aspects of that study, however, do not withstand careful scrutiny:

- In this study, patients were injected with twice the amount of allergy extract that is routinely used for testing, or the authors were so unaware of the usual amount that is routinely used that they wrote the wrong amount in their article.

- As this book has indicated repeatedly, after a patient is given a neutralizing treatment dose (N/D) of a food, that child can frequently eat that food without difficulty. In this study, if some patients thought they reacted to an injection of either a placebo or a food, they were given the N/D. This means it would be most unlikely that they would subsequently react when they received a skin test for the real allergenic item in an unlabeled syringe. They had already been treated!

- Many patients do not feel any different during P/N testing. The skin test site was consistently concealed during this study. In some patients the reaction in the skin test site may be the *only* change that reveals the presence of an allergy. This study did not allow this essential visual marker to be observed.

- The article did not state how long the patients had been on treatment. Once again, well-treated patients would not be expected to react to either an overdose or underdose of a food allergy extract.

- In addition, some children or adults cannot breathe well, their pulse increases, they can't write clearly, and they become irritable and aggressive during testing. Some of these clues of a possible allergic reaction may not be noticed or acknowledged by the patient but would be evident or detected by any experienced nurse in the office of any well-trained doctor who uses provocation. For example, it is not uncommon for children or adults not to realize that they are wheezing but routine mon-

7. Don Jewett, M.D., et al., "A Double-Blind Study of Symptom Provocation to Determine Food Sensitivity," *JAMA* 323 (7) (1990), pp. 429–433.

itoring of lung function during testing would clearly document such a change. In other words, the interpretation of properly conducted P/N testing depends on much more than what the patient feels or notices. This study was erroneously based solely on the latter.

- According to one of the investigators, this study was further biased because seven of the subjects were mistakenly told they were to receive three injections of a substance to which they were sensitive and nine injections of a placebo. This information would enhance the anxiety levels of the patients and certainly jeopardize the study's reliability.

- The reference section quoted less than 5 percent of the scientific studies that indicate that P/N testing is effective, but mentioned most of the negative studies. This suggests immense bias, certainly not a balanced, fair presentation of facts.

Such poorly designed studies as this one would assure false negative responses to a food allergy extract. With all the errors in the execution of this study, negative results should be expected.

It is indeed regrettable that articles such as this are accepted for publication by highly respectable journals, for they provide insurance companies and the federal government with the "evidence" that is needed to disallow or deny payments to parents whose children are desperately in need of environmental medical care.

Any experienced and knowledgeable physician and nurse can produce and eliminate P/N reactions quite easily. The challenge is not to do it, but to explain why a strong dilution of an item causes a child or adult to feel unwell or to act inappropriately while a weaker dilution of that same allergy extract eliminates this response. Theories abound, but as yet we really don't have the answer. We only know the bottom line: These methods appear to safely and quickly help many patients who have not been helped by other measures.

Lastly, some wonder if part of the reluctance to accept this form of medical care is in some way related to the powerful pharmaceutical, food, and/or chemical industries. The bottom line, unfortunately, appears possibly to be vested interests. The drug industry often subsidizes research for the powerful decision-making academic allergists who in turn dictate policy and medical practice. They select speakers for medical conference presentations, make recommendations to insurance companies, and select the articles for medical journal publications. The pharmaceutical industry pays for the medical journal

publications with their ads for their drugs. Because of this, many
physicians in practice have never heard or been exposed to "the other
side" of these important newer approaches to help resolve allergies
on a long-term basis.

Proof for Parents

The effectiveness of P/N testing is easy for parents to prove shortly
after this form of P/N treatment is begun. At that time parents are
urged to purposely feed their child a food that routinely causes mild
to moderate symptoms when it is eaten at a four-day interval. If the
P/N test was positive, that food should cause symptoms within an
hour. When symptoms recur, the P/N treatment should provide relief
within a few minutes. As a double check give that same treatment
dose of extract *before* the test food is eaten and see if it prevents the
symptoms. A correct neutralization dose should prevent or relieve
symptoms depending upon whether it is given before or after an
offending food is eaten.

But . . . There Can Be Exceptions

If you see no difference when you feed your child a food that appeared to be positive by P/N testing, it suggests that that food is not
a problem. One can easily be fooled, however. Remember the barrel
effect? If "the barrel" is full, that is to say, if your child has been
exposed to an overload of allergenic items, a little of anything to
which the child is sensitive can produce symptoms (see Chapter 2).
If, however, your child sleeps in a pristine, clean bedroom, avoids
chemicals, adheres to an allergy diet and a nutritional program, and
has received allergy extract therapy for a while, the barrel may be
half empty. A little of some allergenic item, under those circumstances, might still produce a positive P/N test but not produce symptoms.

It might be easier to relate this to grass pollen. P/N testing for
grass pollen may cause a decrease in your child's ability to breathe,
which is relieved by the neutralizing dose of a grass-allergy extract.
If the pollen count reaches 20, your child can appear well, but when
the level of pollen in the air reaches 60, your child may wheeze. Your
child was allergic when the pollen count was less than 60, but the
barrel wasn't full. After treatment the pollen count may have to reach
300 before symptoms are evident again. P/N treatment essentially
appears to give a patient a larger barrel. If a patient has responded

well to treatment, the same exposures that previously caused symptoms may no longer cause any difficulty. This is the ultimate aim of such therapy.

Parents can also evaluate the effectiveness of dust or mold P/N treatment. Expose your child to a dusty or moldy area that routinely causes a headache or some other obvious but not incapacitating physical complaint. See if the P/N dose of dust and mold allergy extract will prevent or eliminate the symptoms.

The bottom line for parents must rest with their own observations. After P/N testing and treatment, ask yourself the following:

- Is my child now able to eat a food that routinely caused symptoms in the past?
- Can my child be exposed to pollen and dust without developing hay fever, asthma, or other symptoms?
- Does my child need less medicine? Have my drug bills decreased?
- Does my child feel so much better that we don't need to visit the doctor as often as before?
- Have others commented about how much better my child is in relation to behavior, activity, or ability to learn?

Some children may have a type of medical problem that no one knows how to relieve. There are many illnesses that physicians can help only on a temporary basis with drugs. Unfortunately there are times when we simply do not know why someone develops a certain sickness. What is truly astounding about environmental medicine, however, is the scope of medical illnesses that appear to be helped by the newer comprehensive diagnostic and therapeutic approaches to allergy care.

ALLERGIES IN A MOTHER AND HER SEVERELY ASTHMATIC CHILD: BOTH RECEIVED TRADITIONAL AND THEN P/N ALLERGY TREATMENT

The Bardon Family

Megan came to see us when she was four and a half years old. Her medical history surprisingly dated back to her mother, and possibly to her grandmother.

Megan's Grandmother's History

Megan's grandmother was an avid milk drinker, and when she was pregnant with Megan's mother, Mrs. Bardon, she vomited much more than normal. At that time Megan's mother hiccupped excessively in the uterus, especially during the evening and nighttime.

Mrs. Bardon's History

In spite of traditional allergy care as a child, Megan's mother was perpetually ill. Mrs. Bardon was my patient twenty years ago when I practiced traditional allergy.

Megan's grandmother was given information about how to make their home more allergy-free. In those days this involved giving allergy extract therapy for dust, molds, and pollen plus detailed information about how to clean the bedroom thoroughly. I suggested no pets and that a plastic mattress cover be placed over a synthetic mattress. It took several more years before I realized that the odor of a plastic mattress cover or that a synthetic polyurethane pillow or mattress could make some children wheeze. Ironically, although I tried diets that helped, because of the delayed manner that I was taught to reintroduce foods into a diet, I rarely detected food culprits. My allergy training had thoroughly indoctrinated me with the misconception that food allergy was uncommon and the only way to treat a food allergy was avoidance.

With my traditional allergy care, Mrs. Bardon did not improve significantly during her childhood. Although the severity of her headaches and nose symptoms lessened, she continued to have hay fever. She would still awaken with her eyes glued together in the morning. She was so congested that she had to sit upright during the night. She always had a pile of tissues next to her bed in the morning, but after traditional allergy treatment she gagged less on the mucus during the night. She routinely vomited her nightly accumulation of mucus each morning before she left for school. During the night she sporadically wheezed and coughed. She had fatigue, depression, and trouble concentrating in school. She cried easily and often. She was totally incapacitated during the grass pollen season because of the severity of her hay fever, asthma, and headaches.

Until the age of twenty-five, when she initially brought Megan to see us, she continued to feel poorly. After putting Megan, along with the rest of her family, on a rotation diet, and making their home more ecologically sound, she noticed a dramatic improvement in her own health and capacity to cope. It is ironic that twenty years later we were finally able to help Mrs. Bardon while helping Megan, by using the newer approaches to diet and environmental allergy care.

Megan's History

When Megan's mother became pregnant, she feared she would have an allergic child. She took every possible precaution. She even sought the advice of an allergist before Megan was born. He recommended that Megan be totally breast-fed for at least six months.

Megan's mother had always craved milk and was in fact a perpetual milk drinker. She drank three to four gallons of milk each week and ate cheese and ice cream every day. During her pregnancy she vomited eight to nine times every day and night for the first five months of her pregnancy and then sporadically throughout the remaining four months. She was so ill that at one point she was placed on total bed rest for four weeks. This history strongly suggests a milk sensitivity in Mrs. Bardon, which we eventually confirmed. During her pregnancy, Megan tended to hiccup frequently, but she was not an overactive baby in the uterus.

Mrs. Bardon breast-fed her new infant in an effort to prevent allergies. In less than twenty-four hours, however, Megan began to wheeze. By six months of age she had persistent, unyielding asthma. As soon as one bout of asthmatic bronchitis was under control, another infection began. The mother saw her pediatric allergist repeatedly and he treated Megan with daily asthma drugs, as well as frequent courses of cortisone and antibiotics. She seemed to become more seriously ill, however, as each month passed.

As a toddler Megan had a bloated abdomen; dark, sunken eyes; clammy skin; and she always seemed tired. She fought a never-ending battle. She never felt well and she was never able to breathe easily. Newer and better asthma drugs and cortisone were repeatedly tried, as well as various medicated aerosol mists. However, Megan continued to have unyielding asthma and constant nausea. Her behavior and moods vacillated up and down. She would switch suddenly from happy to sad, from wildly hyperactive to uncontrollably aggressive, and from bright and attentive to withdrawn, apathetic, and dull.

Two pediatricians and three private board-certified allergists could not find the answers. Megan's mother finally decided to have the hospital doctors treat Megan. At least once a month for seven months Megan was in the hospital emergency room for uncontrollable asthma. As her asthma became more resistant to treatment, she had to be hospitalized every two weeks over a period of two to three months. On those occasions she was given more intravenous asthma medicines, cortisone, and antibiotics. In spite of vigorous and appropriate accepted treatment with the latest and best drugs, Megan perplexed the staff because her attacks continued to be debilitating and increasingly difficult to control. Her mother truly feared that Megan would die. Her child became more frail and worn out as each week passed. It had become a vicious circle. It was a struggle for her to keep any food or medication down, and without either one, she had no strength left to fight for breath. When Megan's lung collapsed while she was in the hospital receiving the best traditional comprehensive allergy treatment that was available, her mother realized that something else simply had to be done to help her daughter.

In her search of answers to help her daughter, Mrs. Bardon questioned each of the private and hospital physicians continually about the possibility of Megan coming to our office. Megan's grandmother always believed that Megan might be helped by our care, but the continued opposition of the doctors "scared" Mrs. Bardon. She was told that I was using "different" and "clinically unproven methods" to treat allergies. Finally, in anger and desperation, her mother felt she had no choice and made an appointment. During her first visit to our office her mother was pleased and relieved to find that our approach emphasized attempts to determine *why* Megan wheezed rather than which new drug might better control her wheezing.

During Part 1 of the Multiple Food Elimination Diet, her breathing did not improve greatly, but she did not have any of her typical major wheezing crises during that week. After only seven days on the diet her nausea, bed-wetting, wild nightmares, depression, aggression, and hyperactivity all dramatically improved. Her mother was truly afraid to add foods back during the second week of the diet because Megan was so much better. After only two days of Part 2 of the diet, Megan's mother discontinued the diet. Severe symptoms were produced each time a new food was reintroduced. Her asthma, nightmares, bed-wetting, severe nose symptoms, and wild, tearful, "weird" behavior returned with the reintroduction of milk. Severe stomach pain, nausea, asthma, bed-wetting, nose symptoms, and uncontrollable aggressive behavior were produced with the reintroduction of wheat. There was no reason to purposely precipitate more illness by adding more test foods back into her diet. Her mother justifiably feared the reactions that might occur. Her mother realized now that foods were one major missing link that accounted for her daughter's persistent ill health. If Megan was simply treated for her food allergies, would this diminish the severity and frequency of her asthma?

Megan responded well to our newer, more expanded approach to allergy care. Within weeks after her initial P/N testing she was much improved. Over the course of several years, with neutralization injection treatment for molds, dust, pollen, and foods, her asthma, nose symptoms, intestinal symptoms, bed-wetting, sleep problems, depression, personality changes, and constant chest and sinus infections have either been absent or well controlled. Her face, skin, eyes, and abdomen now appear normal. Her family moved out of their polluted neighborhood, gave away their pets, gradually made their home as ecologically sound as possible, and adhered to a strict rotation diet.

During the one-month period before we saw her, she had had three emergency-room visits, two requiring hospitalization. When we first began to treat Megan, she still intermittently needed to visit the emergency room. During the first three months of our allergy treatment she required emergency-room treatment maybe two times in a three-month period. At the present time she has not been to the emergency room for over two and a half years. She has not needed hospitalization since she began our treatment. Asthma medicine is needed only once a day during the wet fall and colder winter months. During the summer her asthma is controlled solely with her neutralization allergy extract treatments twice a week. No cortisone has been required for five years.

If she has a drop in her ability to blow into a peak-flow meter (PFM), indicating an incipient asthma attack, Megan's knowledgeable mother knows exactly what to do. She checks to determine what Megan ate, touched, or smelled that could have caused the drop. She can usually find the answer without much difficulty. Selective provocation retesting usually resolves the problem. Especially in the humid or cold months Megan may still need frequent retesting, for molds in particular.

For example, in damp mid-February 1990, after the snow had melted and the molds on last year's grass were prevalent, her PFM fell. She developed severe headaches, became "wild," bit her brother, and her grades fell from 85 to 35 percent. We retested her for molds, and within a few hours her behavior and activity level were back to normal. Her schoolwork improved, and within a week she was doing well again academically.

If Megan is given too much of any food, she becomes ill. As her mother so aptly put it, "Megan found out it was better to eat a food every four days and breathe than to eat a problem food every day and gasp for air." Megan was sick of not feeling well and was most anxious to cooperate with a comprehensive allergy program. Without her neutralization extract therapy, however, the majority of Megan's symptoms such as asthma, hyperactivity, and aggressive behavior will quickly reappear.

With increased knowledge and the newer approaches to allergy care, Megan and her entire family now have much less illness. Megan's parents are less apprehensive and fearful about her future than they were before. At this time, Megan and her mother both continue to be significantly improved. It is truly a pity that her mother's food sensitivities were not recognized by myself many years earlier. How different her childhood and early adulthood would have been if I had learned how to more accurately detect and treat food and chemical sensitivities when I was initially trained as an allergist.

CHAPTER 26

Drug Therapy

When Are Drugs Needed?

It is the hope of all ecologically oriented physicians that drugs would not be needed by their patients. Of course this is not always possible but it is a worthwhile goal. Most new patients require prescriptions, because children are usually ill when we initially see them. It takes a while for parents to carry out our suggestions. It takes time to complete the allergy testing and prepare allergy extract treatment. In the meantime drugs must be available to control each child's symptoms.

Later on, drugs must be available for emergencies or if a child's allergy extract therapy does not remain helpful. If an extract helps but only on a temporary basis, this often indicates a need for allergy retesting and additional reevaluation of the home and diet factors related to a child's illness.

Some patients' responses are not significantly better, for a wide range of reasons, and those children need medication of various types to control their symptoms. Sometimes a family cannot move from a moldy home or a chemically contaminated area of a city. Sometimes both parents work, so they cannot do the rotation diet or keep their home ecologically clean. And lastly, ecologically oriented physicians sometimes cannot find and eliminate the cause of a child's illness. Environmental medicine is not a panacea. It is merely a giant step in the right direction to help relieve some allergic children's medical, emotional, and behavioral problems.

If possible try your child on new medicines when they are not needed to determine if there is any problem with the medication. For example, try a new asthma drug when your child is not wheezing to see if it causes nervousness. Try an antihistamine on a weekend to be sure it doesn't cause drowsiness, which could interfere with school work.

Special Problems With Drugs Used by Allergic Children

Some children appear to be sensitive to sugar, corn, dyes, artificial flavors, and artificial sweeteners such as aspartame found in many children's chewable or liquid medicines. Other colorless liquid drugs are sweetened with corn syrup, which can cause symptoms in corn-sensitive children. However, for some children, these are preferable to those that contain dyes or aspartame. Whenever possible, ecologists urge that allergic children be given colorless liquids, white granules, or crushed white tablets. Be wary, because specific flavors of a single product can, at times, cause symptoms.

For example, one six-year-old boy took fluoride tablets without difficulty when they were unflavored. When only the artificially pineapple-flavored but dye-free tablets were available, he routinely wet the bed every time he took one. The artificial pineapple flavor was not tolerated by this child. This means that different variations of the same product can cause symptoms.

The white contents of colored capsules can be put into mashed potatoes, jelly, or peanut butter, providing these foods do not cause illness. The colored empty capsules can be thrown away. Young children will often take medicines readily if they are given in this manner.

One must wonder why pharmaceutical companies do not use natural food colors (beet, carrot, grape, cherry, chlorophyll) and natural flavors and sweeteners in children's medicines and vitamins. Many FD & C colors were banned in the sixties and seventies because they caused cancer. Why is FD & C Red 4, for example, still in maraschino cherries when there is evidence that it causes brain damage?[1]

If your child requires an antibiotic because of fever, green or yellow mucus, or obvious infection, see Table 26.1 for choices that your doctor can consider when he or she prescribes medicines.

---

1. Joseph Beasley and Jerry Swift, *The Kellogg Report* (see Bibliography for details).

Aerosol Drugs

Aerosol drugs are often used to treat asthma, nose, and skin allergies. In addition, aerosol cans are used for dispensing insect repellents, furniture polish, deodorizers, lubricants, adhesives, de-icers, etc. All of these contain some form of chemical propellant which is ejected under pressure from the spray can, along with the medicine or chemical for which the aerosol is being used. The propellant chemical is a halocarbon, which contains chlorine or fluorine. These halocarbon vapors accumulate in homes. Some aerosols also contain ether, acetone, or clorinated hydrocarbons which, along with the halocarbons, can be dissolved and stored in our fat. These chemicals can act as local eye, skin, or respiratory irritants, and in addition, they can enter the blood stream and dull the nervous system.

There is no biological cycle to degrade or get rid of halocarbons. When they accumulate in the atmosphere they contribute to the breakdown of ozone. The ozone in the upper atmosphere protects the earth from the nuclear radiation of the sun's cosmic rays. These rays in turn can lead to skin cancer, to name only one sequelae for disregarding the health of our planet.

How to Swallow a Pill

Method 1: Druggists sell cups that are constructed with a special inside pill pocket. You merely put the pill in the pocket and when the child swallows the water from the cup, the pill goes down along with the water.

Method 2: Carefully place the pill in the center and back of the tongue and then ask your child to drink a liquid. The pill should easily pass over the back of the tongue and into the stomach.

Method 3: Wait until your child is about to swallow a big mouthful of any chewed food. Ask your child to open his mouth and put the pill into the center of the chewed food.

Some Dye-Free Drugs Are Available

If your child appears to be sensitive to dyes or artificial flavors, when you visit your doctor ask for white or colorless liquids. If sugar or corn is a problem, ask for medicines that do not include dextrose or glucose. You can also request white tablet medications and crush them yourself.

TABLE 26.1
Dye-Free Drugs

Liquids

Antiasthmatic	Antihistamine	Antibiotics	Eye Medicine	Cough Medicine
Slo-Phyllin GG	Ryna		Opticrom	Codiclear
Marax DF	Tacaryl		Chloroptic	DH syrup
Quibron	Tavist		ophthalmic	
	Rhinosyn		solution	
	Neo-Synephrine		Estivin with	
	nose drops		ephedrine	
	Otrivin pediatric		Collyrium-Fresh	
	nose drops		Cortisporin	
			ophthalmic	
			solution	
			Neosporin	

Tablets

Antiasthmatic	Antihistamine	Antibiotics		
Alupent	Tavist	Spectrobid		
Marax	Tavist-1	Bactrim DS		
Bricanyl	Tavist-D	(Trimethoprim-		
Proventil	Seldane	Sulfameth-		
Theo-Dur	Hismanal	oxazole)		

Brethine	Rynatan (long-	Pentids	Tessalon
Respbid	acting)	E-Mycin 333	Cough-Gard
Uniphyl	Sudafed (white)	Penicillin	Expecto-Gard
Slo-Phyllin	Actifed	Amoxicillin	
Theochron		Ceftin 125 mg	
Theolair-SR			
Sustaire			
Tedral			
Ventolin			

Capsules

Theo-Dur	Isoclor	Keflex
Sprinkles	Benadryl	Amoxil
Slo-bid	Novafed A	Tetracycline
Slo-Phyllin	Bromfed	
Theo-24	Hista-Gard	
	Nasalcrom	

Asthma Medicines

The secret of treating asthma is to prevent the attack whenever possible, or to treat it early and vigorously, before the airway spasm becomes severe. Increased fluid intake is essential to help thin the lung mucus so that it is easier to cough up. A wide array of asthma medicines is available, which includes sprays, tablets, capsules, and injectables. An injection of short-acting adrenaline lasts only twenty minutes, while a preparation such as Sus-Phrine provides both immediate and delayed asthma relief. It can help in minutes, and the effect can last for as long as twelve hours. This would be preferable for controlling nighttime wheezing or for treating hives in select patients.

In general, asthma medicines are divided into two major groups. One group is called beta-adrenergic drugs (these are similar to adrenaline) and the other is theophylline. Both these drugs help relax the muscle spasm in the lungs and diminish the swelling and mucus production inside of the air tubes.

Indications for the Use of Adrenaline/Epinephrine for Asthma and Other Medical Emergencies

- Sudden, severe asthma attacks when a doctor or emergency room is not readily available or, for example, when traveling or if you live far away from a hospital or doctor. An injection of adrenaline could be most beneficial for a sudden asthma attack (see Table 26.2 for dosage).

- Sudden reactions to foods or odors that cause a tight throat, tongue swelling, a change in voice such as hoarseness, or a blue color to the lips or fingernails. An adrenaline spray might be best, or an injection of adrenaline could be lifesaving.

- Reactions to stinging insects that are not confined to the area of the sting, such as a sting on the foot that causes a tight throat, nose allergies, wheezing, or hives on some other area of the body. These are all indications that your physician or an emergency room doctor needs to see you. Adrenaline is usually the drug of choice for such emergencies, and anyone who is old enough and has such a reaction should know how to give adrenaline.

TABLE 26.2
Dosages of Adrenaline*

The dose, based on the patient's age and weight, is 0.005cc/lb, or 0.01cc/kg (1kg = 2.2 lbs).
For example, 0.2cc/40 lbs (0.005 × 40 = 0.2cc).
Do not use over 0.35cc in an adult unless prescribed by a doctor.
The dose for Sus-Phrine is 1/2 the dose for adrenaline.
(.01 mg = .01ml.)

Age	Adrenaline Dose is 0.0005cc/lb	Sus-Phrine Dose is 1/2 dose of adrenaline	Weight (in pounds)
1–2 years	.10cc	.05cc (not 0.5)	19–28 lbs
2–4 years	.15cc	.07cc	29–38 lbs
5–6 years	.20cc	.10cc	39–49 lbs
7–8½ years	.25cc	.13cc	50–60 lbs
9–10 years	.30cc	.15cc	61–72 lbs
11 years	.35cc	.18cc	73–82 lbs
Adolescents or adults	.35 to 0.5cc	.15 to 0.25cc	83 lbs and up

*Always check dose with doctor before use.

Inhaled Adrenalinelike Drugs

As shown in Table 26.3, a number of liquid drugs, such as Ventolin, Alupent, Brethine, and Bronkosol, can be placed in devices that produce an aerosol or spray of the medication. This helps young asthmatic children breathe the medicine directly into their lungs and tends to decrease shakiness, a rapid heart rate, and nausea.

Spacing Devices

Young children often cannot learn to use an inhaler correctly. It is difficult for them to push the lever on the plastic medicine container so that the asthma medicine is sprayed into the mouth at the correct time. The spray must be coordinated so that the child breathes it in deeply and at the same time holds his head back. To help young children, there are a variety of cylinders in which the medicated mist can be placed so that it is breathed from an enclosed small space in the chamber rather than directly from the mouth. The chemical odor of certain chambers, unfortunately, can cause symptoms in some children.

Aerosol-Mist Therapy for Infants and Children

These are machines that deliver a spray mist of asthma medicine. The spray is produced in a machine and sent through some tubing

TABLE 26.3
Asthma Medicines*

Trade Names	Generic Names	Tablets	Syrup	Inhaled
Ventolin Proventil	Albuterol sulfate	2–4 mg every 6–8 hrs.	1–2 tsp. every 6–8 hrs.	1–2 puffs, maximum 2 per 4–6 hrs.
Alupent Metaprel	Metaproterenol sulfate	10–20 mg every 6–8 hrs.	1–2 tsp. every 6–8 hrs.	1–2 puffs, maximum 2 per 4–6 hrs. Nebulizer 0.3cc in 2cc saline
Brethine Bricanyl	Terbutaline sulfate	2.5–5 mg every 6–8 hrs		
Brethaire (inhaler)				1–2 puffs, maximum 2 per 4–6 hrs.
Bronkometer (inhaler)	Isoetharine HCL			1–2 puffs, maximum 2 per 4–6 hrs.

Bronkosol		Nebulizer 0.25–0.5cc in 2.5cc saline
Isuprel Medihaler	Isoproterenol HCL	1–2 puffs, maximum 2 per 4–6 hrs. Nebulizer 0.25–0.5cc in 2.5cc saline
Tornalate	Bitolterol Mesylate	2 puffs spaced 1–3 min. apart every 4–8 hrs.

*Check all dosages with your physician before use.

to either a nose or a mouth piece. A plastic mouth piece delivers the spray directly into the mouths of older children. A plastic mask that covers both the nose and the mouth is used for infants. Ceramic masks are available for children who are bothered by the odor of plastic.

Adrenalinelike or Beta-Adrenergic Drugs

Three major types of these adrenalinelike drugs are available. All have advantages and disadvantages. Most are available in tablet, liquid, and spray forms (see Table 26.3). In general, the newer preparations have fewer side effects, such as jitteriness, tremor, flushing, headaches, or a rapid or irregular heart rate. Some act longer, so they can be taken every twelve rather than every four hours. Sometimes the side effects of these medicines decrease after the drugs have been used for a few days. The object is to find the dose of a drug that does not make a child shaky but still helps a child to breathe more easily.

In general, spray drugs tend to be overused. If they do not help, children must be warned not to continue taking them. Overuse sometimes causes the air tubes to go into spasm, making the asthma worse, not better.

The major categories of beta-adrenergic drugs include the following:

- Metaproterenol (Alupent and Metaprel). The liquid and tablet forms of these drugs are usually not suggested for children under six years of age. The advantage is that this drug can help for six hours. The most undesirable common side effects of these drugs are shakiness, twitchiness, tremulous muscles, and an increased heart rate. This sometimes diminishes or stops after a week or two of use.

- Albuterol or salbutamol (Proventil or Ventolin). This group of drugs is similar to the metaproterenol drugs. They are thought to be more effective in dilating the air tubes and less apt to cause cardiac stimulation. The spray lasts for four hours and seems to cause fewer side effects than the tablet medication. At times, side effects such as tremor, nervous tension, headaches, dry mouth, and flushing are noted.

- Terbutaline sulfate (Brethine, Bricanyl, and Brethaire). This drug is available in liquid, tablet, or inhaler form. It is similar to Metaprel or Proventil. Terbutaline is not recommended for children under twelve years of age. This drug also tends to cause cardiac stimulation, shakiness, headaches, and muscle cramps but is thought to have less effect on the heart rate than metaproterenol.

Theophylline Preparations

Theophylline drugs are in vogue at the present time. They are often used with beta-adrenergic drugs because each has a different mechanism of action. Although they certainly are helpful, they can cause intestinal complaints in some children. Check with your physician if nausea and vomiting, in particular, occur when this drug is used.

Theophylline relaxes the air tubes and prevents the release of histamine, which causes asthma. The right dosage is often difficult to determine because many individuals appear to utilize the drug in such a way that they require either less or more than the "usual" amount. Unlike most drugs you cannot always calculate the right dose for a child according to her or his weight or age. As a result this drug should be monitored when it is used so that the proper blood level is maintained. The object is to use the smallest dose that is effective.

Side effects include nausea, an increased need to urinate, shakiness, diarrhea, headache, insomnia, depression, an increased or irregular heart rate, and leg cramps. It is available in slow- and long-acting forms, in liquids, capsules, and tablets.

Intal or Cromolyn Sodium

If you are vacationing and your child is five years or older, Intal spray may prove very helpful and safe. The liquid form is better than the powder because the latter contains lactose, or milk sugar, which could bother milk-sensitive children. Intal should be used to *prevent* asthma attacks. Use it *before* a visit to the relative's dusty, moldy home. Use it for two days *before* and during your entire vacation so that the hotels, different foods, excitement, exhaustion, and new exposures do not precipitate an upsetting attack of asthma that ruins a holiday. Use it *before* the party or celebration, because the junk foods, perfume, and cigarette smoke can cause symptoms. Use it *before* exercise or exertion. Intal often helps to prevent asthma providing it is used *before* an offending exposure occurs.

It can also help if it is used after someone is already wheezing, but this may require several days to weeks.

It has one other advantage, in that it makes the air tubes less reactive, so they are less apt to go into spasm causing asthma. It must be used on a daily basis to have this effect.

If the contents of several capsules of Intal are dissolved in water and then taken twenty minutes before meals, this drug can effectively prevent many mild food-related reactions.

In general, Intal is remarkably free of significant side effects. A few patients complain of throat irritation, headaches, hives, abdominal pain, diarrhea, vomiting, insomnia, depression, coughing, and a runny nose.

Antihistamines for Nose, Eye, and Skin Allergies

Antihistamines help a stuffy or watery nose; itchy, red, watery eyes; and itchy skin or hives. Many antihistamines, however, tend to make children or adults very sleepy. If this is a problem, that drug should be avoided, particularly before tests in school. This side effect can be helpful, however, for hay fever or itchy skin, which is associated with insomnia.

If drowsiness or sleepiness is noted, but the drug relieves the nose, eye, or skin allergic symptoms, use the medicine at bedtime. During the daytime try half the recommended dosage and it may be effective without causing drowsiness. If this does not help, check with your physician, and another chemical type of antihistamine can be prescribed. Sometimes when an antihistamine is first taken, it causes sleepiness, but after a few days this no longer occurs. Some newer varieties of antihistamines, such as Tavist, Hismanol, or Seldane, appear to cause less drowsiness.

Other common side effects from antihistamines are that they can alter one's coordination, so they should not be taken before a child engages in competitive sports. Exercise will frequently clear a nose temporarily, so this medication might not be needed. Antihistamines can also sometimes cause nervousness, tremors, stomach upsets, a dry mouth, and blurred vision.

Nose Drops and Sprays

Nose drops such as Neo-Synephrine, for which no prescription is needed, can be used for a stuffy or runny nose or for ear problems due to nose congestion. There is one strength for infants, another for children, and a third for adults. Many physicians do not recommend them because children and adults tend to overuse them. Normally they should be used for no more than two to three times a day or for no longer than two to three days. If they are used too often or too long, they can irritate the membranes or tissues inside the nose. This can cause swelling in the nose, which can interfere with breathing. The tendency to overuse nose drops occurs at this point, and thus a vicious circle begins: The inside of the nose swells from allergy; then the same area swells because of irritation from using the nose drops too long. This is called rhinitis medicamentosa. For this reason, they should be used only in selected instances, when the nasal problem is severe. An example would be if a child cannot sleep because of extreme nasal obstruction or stuffiness. The ultimate answer is to find out why the nose swells and eliminate the cause whenever possible.

Nose drops are considerably more effective if used in the following manner: Have your child lie on his back sideways on a bed. The head should hang over the edge so that the nostrils face the ceiling. Put one or two drops in one nostril. (If you are using a spray, always have the nostrils facing the floor and spray *up* the nose once or twice.) Wait about five minutes, have your youngster blow his nose, and then repeat the procedure. The first time will shrink the tissue near the opening of the nose, and the next time will shrink the membranes in the upper nose and clear the upper passageway. Repeat this procedure for the other nostril.

Caution should be advised in the use of various medicated, Vaseline-like preparations that parents frequently place inside their youngster's nose to help clear the nostrils. It is possible that these could irritate the inside of the nose in some children. If you are concerned, stop using them and see if your child breathes more easily. Then check with your physician about how or when to use various nose preparations.

Nose drops or sprays can help nose and ear allergies. Antihistamines can be used at the same time to see if they help relieve your child's symptoms. Both of these medications might help prevent earaches if used before airplane rides.

Steroids or Cortisone Drugs

Cortisone is a most powerful and helpful steroid medicine. It is used to treat allergies and many other diseases. It is sometimes the critical drug or key that helps to save lives. Like many strong drugs, it has great potential for helping, but it can also be very harmful. This drug should never be taken unless it is given *under a physician's close supervision*. Its major function is to diminish inflammation by decreasing swelling and redness, which can occur in almost any area of the body for multiple reasons. This drug relieves, but certainly does not cure, allergy.

Cortisone is prescribed mainly when a child cannot engage in normal activities related to everyday living in spite of the proper use of the usual medicines that relieve allergies. It is essential in the treatment of certain life-threatening or distressing allergic emergencies such as asthma.

A new method to diminish the amount of cortisone needed to control resistant asthma is to use a low dose of a cancer drug called methotrexate. Before this is tried, however, time should be spent trying to detect unsuspected food and chemical sensitivities. (See Megan, Chapter 25.)

In general, cortisone skin medications are not considered dangerous. They are most frequently used in low concentrations on relatively small areas of skin, so their effect is mainly local. Sometimes strong concentrations can cause atrophy scars on the skin, so they should be used with caution on the face. If strong concentrations of cortisone creams are applied over large portions of the body, an excessive amount of this drug can be absorbed. Because there is a great variation in the potency or strength of various cortisone salves or tablets, only your physician can decide which your child needs and how long it should be used. A list of some common cortisone preparations appear in Table 26.4.

A number of weaker cortisone preparations are available without a prescription. These include Cortaid and Hydrocortisone Cream.

Stronger cortisone skin preparations can be prescribed by your doctor. Be sure to ask your physician or druggist about the side effects of any skin preparation ordered for your child.

How Much Danger Is There If Cortisone Is Taken in Large Doses But for Only a Few Days?

Usually very little. In an emergency situation, the drug is often administered this way. As soon as a child is better, the dose is quickly tapered over a period of several days and then the drug is stopped. At times it is difficult to discontinue the use of this medicine, especially if the drug has been taken for weeks or months. Each time the dosage is lowered, the child's symptoms, such as asthma or eczema, become much worse. This is a real challenge for a physician and is a major reason why some physicians are most reluctant to start a child on this drug. *Never suddenly stop any cortisone drug*, except ointment, unless

Table 26.4

Common Cortisone Preparations

Betamethasone (Celestone)

Dexamethasone (Decadron, Hexadrol, Gammacorten)

Fludrocortisone (Florinef)

Methylprednisolone (Medrol)

Paramethasone (Haldrone)

Prednisolone (Delta-Cortef, Predne-Dome)

Prednisone (Deltasone, Delta-Dome)

Triamcinolone (Aristocort, Kenacort)

Cortisones combined with antihistamines are Aristomin, Dron-actin, and Metreton

Beclomethasone (Vanauceril) Aerosols

---

your physician has specifically advised you to do so. Under certain circumstances the drug *must* be tapered and stopped gradually. *Asthmatic deaths have occurred when this drug has been discontinued suddenly or the dose has been tapered too quickly.*

What Undesirable Minor Effects Can Cortisone Have?

It can cause acne, hairiness of the face or body, increased appetite, weight gain, a round face, abdominal pain, a rise in blood pressure, cataracts, dry mouth, bruising, fatigue, leg cramps, and increased perspiration. Sometimes the breasts or anus will itch. It causes bloating, the face becomes round, or a hump can develop on the back of the neck. Sometimes there will be sugar in the urine temporarily. These problems usually disappear if the dosage is lowered sufficiently or if the cortisone is stopped.

Newer forms of cortisone or steroids cause fewer symptoms. You can look in the *Physicians' Desk Reference* at the local library or bookstore to learn about the possible side effects of any steroid your child might be using.

What Is One of the Most Serious Problems Cortisone Causes?

It tends to allow infections that normally would be confined to a certain body area to spread to other parts of the body. While this happens, the patient usually has an associated feeling of well-being. This combination can be very dangerous. It means that infection can spread and the parents have little warning because their child feels fine. For this reason it must be stressed that children on cortisone should be closely and regularly supervised by their physician *regardless* of how well they feel. If a child is taking this drug and looks or feels unwell in any way or develops a fever, contact your physician immediately. Ask the doctor to check your child's blood pressure and urine, and to do a thorough physical examination.

Chicken pox, in particular, can be a major problem if it develops when a patient is on cortisone. If this happens, chicken pox, which usually appears on the skin, can spread inside the body and make a child very ill. For this reason it is always safer for a child to use this drug only after he has already had this childhood illness. Measles and tuberculosis can also be a challenge for this reason.

Can Cortisone Affect the Growth of a Child?

Yes. When taken in large doses for prolonged periods of time, the child's growth in height can be less than normal when certain cortisone drugs are used. When the drug is stopped, however, there will generally be a sudden, rather fast compensatory growth spurt in height. This only occurs, however, if children are still young enough that their bones are still growing. This tendency to interfere with growth can be diminished if the drug dosage is kept very low or if certain cortisone drugs are given every other day rather than daily. Some children are so ill that the physician has a difficult decision to make. In spite of the many possible problems related to the use of this drug, cortisone is sometimes essential so that a child can live a relatively normal life.

What About the Inhaled Cortisone Powder, Vanceril or Azmacort?

This drug can be breathed into the lungs to help control asthma. The absorption of the drug is less, and therefore the side effects are diminished. Some doctors suggest that routine asthma medications plus an inhaled cortisone be used at the first evidence of a wheezing attack to more effectively abort the attack. In other patients who have improved on cortisone tablets taken by mouth, some allergists taper the dosage by converting the patient to an inhaled form of cortisone. Again, if a patient feels unwell in any way during this conversion period, a physician should be contacted. The major side effect of inhaled cortisone is thrush, or white patches of yeast on the inside of the mouth. This can be diminished by rinsing the mouth with water after the drug is used.

How Long Can a Child Remain in Cortisone Therapy?

Some children are on cortisone for many years and into adulthood. This is certainly not desirable, but it may be absolutely essential for severely ill patients so that they can live a more normal life.

Is It Ever Necessary to Resume Cortisone After It Has Been Discontinued?

Yes. The most common reason is that a child develops another extremely severe allergic episode, such as asthma. This drug can be necessary repeatedly to help relieve and control some children's asthma. These episodes can sometimes be diminished if the *cause* of the asthma can be found, i.e., foods, molds, dust, chemicals, and so forth.

There are other occasions when this drug must be started again even though your child might not have a severe allergic problem. Let us suppose that your child was very ill with allergies or some other medical problem and had to use this drug. If large amounts have been received over a long period of time, this can cause the adrenal glands, which make cortisone, to shrink. Normally when the human body is under stress (such as when an operation is needed or there is a death in the family), the adrenal glands go into full production to make the extra cortisone needed to cope with the emergency. If these glands have shrunk, they are like a factory that has shut down. They may not be able to function adequately and produce emergency cortisone when it is needed. In this situation it must be supplied by your physician, who orders cortisone for your child. For this reason, if your child has received this drug within the past six to twelve months and a serious emotional or medical situation arises, you should discuss it with *all* physicians caring for your child. Depending upon which type of cortisone drug your child took and how long it was used, your physician will decide whether more is necessary and will advise you accordingly.

Is Cortisone the Best Treatment for Asthma?

Many allergists frequently believe that there have been dramatic improvements in the treatment of asthma during the past few years. Some consider the best treatment for asthma to be cortisone, preferably in tablet form, rather than by aerosol.

They suggest this be used if a child wheezes every day or even if the asthma is evident only on occasion, noted with exercise, or as an allergic cough at night. Good studies show that the cellular evidence of inflammation in the lung decreases with this form of treatment.

Many of these same doctors feel that traditional allergy extract therapy is helpful only for asthma attacks that occur a few hours after an allergic exposure. They doubt that most foods cause allergies unless they contain additives, such as sulfites or monosodium glutamate.

Recent studies, however, indicate that the death toll (now 1.9 deaths/100,000) from asthma has tripled since 1976.[2] The death rate in the United States for children aged five to nine years increased five-fold from 0.1 to 0.5 per 100,000 from 1979 to 1987, while in those aged fifteen to nineteen years, the rate doubled during that same time period. At about that time the use of theophylline and cortisone became preferred methods of treating asthma in the United States. Could there be a relationship? The cause of this mortality increase, however, is usually attributed to a delay in therapy or inappropriate treatment.

Maybe the use of powerful steroids or other drugs might be diminished if more emphasis was placed on *why* children are wheezing. Maybe changes in diet, home factors, and limiting exposures to the ubiquitous array of chemicals in today's world would be helpful.

One Last Caution

Cortisone or other strong drugs are often prescribed when a child is very ill. Sometimes they are helpful, *but only on a temporary basis*. If your child has a medical problem such as asthma, eczema, or colitis, notice how the child feels and acts when he or she does not eat or when your child is fed intravenously. Does the medical problem stop at these times? If the answer is yes, think about your child's favorite

2. Anne Walling, M.D., "Why Is Asthma Mortality Rising?" (editorial) *American Family Physician* 42 (2) 1990. pp. 358–359.

foods. Is it milk, cheese, bread, candy? What does your child repeatedly ask to eat? It might be possible that the asthma, eczema, or colitis would be relieved if a child's problem foods were taken from the diet for a week or two, and the use of drugs (or even surgery) might not be needed. *The aim of everyone must be detection of the cause of an illness, not treatment of the effect.*

Skin Preparations

For Insect Bites

Most people can relieve the itch associated with insect bites, either mosquito, fly, or bee stings, with a paste of meat tenderizer. An antihistamine also helps decrease the itch of hives, itchy eyes, and nose congestion. Calamine lotion can help stop itching. Try not to use any variation that contains phenol or menthol because that chemical, at times, can cause a sensitivity to develop to these chemicals. Also use an asthma preparation if any chest tightness or shortness of breath is noted after an insect bite.

For Atopic Dermatitis

For atopic dermatitis or eczema, a cream, such as Cortaid, or an ointment that contains cortisone is often helpful *temporarily*. Most children seem to tolerate creams better than ointments, but again notice which seems to be best for your child. If the cream or ointment burns or makes the skin feel worse, stop it until you check with your child's doctor.

The skin preparation should be applied sparingly over the involved skin areas several times a day. If the skin areas are open and oozing, soaks such as Domeboro are indicated, and you should consult your physician or a dermatologist. Regardless of what you use, if the cause of the eczema is not eliminated, the skin will break out repeatedly, shortly after the cortisone cream is discontinued.

If your child has eczema on the arms and/or legs, repeatedly check your child's armpits and groin area (where the legs meet the abdomen). If there are large, *tender* swollen nodes or lumps in those areas due to infection on the arms or legs, you need your child's doctor and skin specialist immediately. Children with eczema typically have swollen nodes, but tenderness in those areas normally indicates an infection that requires an antibiotic as soon as possible.

CHAPTER 27

Nutrition and Vitamins

Today many children and adults suffer from an unfortunate combination: They have an inadequate nutrient intake due to a relatively poor diet, combined with an increased need for nutrients because of our excessive exposure to chemicals and pollution. Some have inadequate digestion, which can lead to increased absorption of large food particles and a propensity to allergy. There is little doubt that our immune system can be impaired and damaged by pollutants. Trace metals such as copper, zinc, magnesium, selenium, and manganese, as well as B and C vitamins, are needed for the enzymatic breakdown or alteration of certain food substances into others needed by the body. Deficiencies of these nutrients are often unrecognized factors contributing to the ill health of some children and adults.

Recent studies by Gerald Ross, M.D., et al., in Dallas, Texas, confirm previous studies that persons of all ages who have environmental illness are often deficient in certain essential vitamins and trace metals.[1] In particular, patients who have environmental illness appear to be deficient in vitamins B_1 (thiamine), B_2 (riboflavin), B_3 (niacin), B_6 (pyridoxine), vitamin C, vitamin D, and folic acid. Females appear to have a B_6 deficiency twice as often as males. Vitamin B_6 is required for over sixty enzymatic cellular reactions. Common environmental

---

1. Gerald Ross, M.D., "Confirmation of Chemical Sensitivity by Double-Blind Inhalant Challenge," presented at the International Conference on Food and Environmental Factors in Human Disease, Buxton, Derbyshire, England, July 3–6, 1990.

pollutants such as benzene, carbon monoxide, and pesticides appear to increase our need for vitamin C.

Other contributing factors to nutrient deficiencies are the following:

- We lack nutrients because large amounts of vitamins are routinely removed from our bread and milk. They are replaced with minuscule amounts of nutrients, and ironically the bread is sold back to us as "nutritionally enriched."

- Allergic individuals are frequently intolerant of certain vitamins (see Table 27.1). Some children seem to be sensitive to yeast, which is a common source of vitamin B. Some children cannot tolerate corn, the usual source of vitamin C, so they must try varieties of vitamin C preparations made from sugar beets, sago palm, tapioca, potato, or carrots to see if one of these is well tolerated. Fish-sensitive individuals may not tolerate or be able to ingest essential fatty acids (see Table 27.2).

TABLE 27.1
Relatively Allergy-Free Multiple Vitamins

Name	Age	Dosage
Vital Life, Klaire Laboratories, Inc., P.O. Box 618, Carlsbad, Calif. 92008 (619-744-9680).		
Multi Vitamin with Chelated Minerals	3–10 years 10–adult	1 tablet/day 2 tablets/day
Multi Vitamin Complex	3–12 years Adult	1 capsule/day 2 capsules/day
Multi Mineral Complex	3 years– adult	2 capsules/day
Nutricology Inc., 400 Preda Street, San Leandro, Calif. 94577 (800-782-4274).		
Multi-Vi-Min	3–10 years 11–teens Adult	2–3 tablets/day 4–5 tablets/day 5–6 tablets/day
Vitaline Corporation, 722 Jefferson Avenue, Ashland, Ore. 97520 (800-648-4755).		

Vitaline's Maximum	3–10 years	2–3 tablets/day
	11–teens	4–5 tablets/day
	Adult	2 tablets 3×/day

Da Vinci (FoodScience label), 20 New England Drive, Essex Junction, Vt. 05452 (802-878-0072).

| Omni Jr. Chewable Vitamin/ Mineral | 3–10 years | 3 tablets/day (1 tablet with each meal) |

The Pain and Stress Therapy Center, 5282 Medical Drive, Suite 160, San Antonio, Tex. 78229–6043 (512-696-1674).

Kids' Companion Chewable Vitamin (natural fructose flavor)	Under 6 years	2 tablets/day
	Over 6 years	4 tablets/day
Floradix Liquid MultiVitamin (contains no fluoride)	Infant–1 year	1 teaspoon/day or 2×/day
	2–6 years	1 teaspoon 2×/day or 3×/day
	Over 6 years	2 teaspoons 2×/day or 3×/day

Freeda Vitamins, 36 East 41st Street, New York, N.Y. 10017 (212-685-4980).

| Vitalet Chewable Multi Vitamin | Under 4 years | 1 tablet/day |
| | Over 4 years | 2 tablets/day |

Other allergy-free vitamins are available through:

Carlson Lab, Carlson Division of J. R., Arlington Heights, Ill. 60004 (708-255-1600).

Nature's Place, 10 Daniel Street, Farmingdale, N.Y. 11735 (516-293-0030).

Wm. T. Thompson Co., 23529 S. Figueroa Street, Carson, Calif. 90749 (213-830-5550).

Bronson Pharmaceuticals, 4526 Rinetti Lane, La Canada, Calif. 91011 (818-790-2646).

- Some environmentally ill children are allergic or sensitive to particular nutritious foods, so they are therefore denied certain natural vitamins supplied in the diet. This contributes to vitamin deficiency (see Table 27.3).

- All humans are different and our needs for nutrients vary and should be individualized. Few parents or physicians request monitoring of children's vitamin levels to determine if too little or too much of a nutrient is a problem.

- Blood evaluation for individual nutrients is very expensive. For one reason, blood samples may not accurately reflect the level of specific essential nutrients needed at a cellular level in our body or in our brain tissues. These studies, however, sometimes provide very important clues. In time perhaps insurance companies will realize that children or adults who are well at a cellular level may be healthier in every respect. Over the long term people who have strengthened immune systems should actually save insurance companies money. If these companies would reimburse people for dietary analysis in an attempt to prevent potential nutrient deficiencies, it might also possibly prevent the onset of certain medical illnesses. Our concerted aim must be to prevent, as well as to treat disease.

- Improper utilization of ingested vitamins can be due to intestinal digestive or absorptive deficiencies and abnormalities. Some people take nutrients, but these merely pass through the bowels, so their deficiency persists.

- Our exposure to harmful chemicals increases our need for vitamins and trace metals in order to maintain normal function within our cells. Toxic chemicals increase our vitamin utilization because their presence creates an increased need for detoxification. Overworked detoxification systems can eventually lead to ill health because if they malfunction, our normal bodily processes cannot be kept in balance. We are also exposed to pollutants that can destroy digestive enzymes, and this in turn can contribute to deficiencies of essential nutrients. Pollutants not only increase our need for vitamins, but in addition, their toxicity can have a direct harmful effect on our immune system. The natural, organically grown crops of bygone years had more nutritive value than our present-day pesticided fruits and vegetables.[2]

2. Lawrie Mott and Karen Snyder, *Pesticide Alert: A Guide to Pesticides in Fruits and Vegetables,* 1987. Sierra Club Books, 730 Polk Street, San Francisco, Calif. 94109.

TABLE 27.2
Sources of Vitamin C

Name	Powder/Source	Tablets/Source
Vitaline C† 722 Jefferson Avenue Ashland, Ore. 97520	Sago Palm (noncorn) 2,270 mg/tsp.	Sago Palm (noncorn) 1,000 mg/tablet
The Pain and Stress Therapy Center 5282 Medical Drive Suite 160 San Antonio, Tex. 78229–6043	Ester C*† Super C*† Sugar Beet Sago Palm (noncorn) Tapioca 5,000 mg/tsp.	Ester C*† Super C*† Sugar Beet 275 mg/tablet Sago Palm (noncorn) 550 mg/tablet Tapioca 550 mg/tablet
Nutricology Allergy Research Group 400 Preda Street San Leandro, Calif. 94577	Buffered C Sago Palm (noncorn) 2,350 mg/tsp. Ascorbic C Sago Palm (noncorn) 4,000 mg/tsp.	Buffered C capsules Sago Palm (noncorn) 500 mg/capsule Ascorbic Acid capsules Sago Palm (noncorn) 1,000 mg/capsule

Doctors RX Dispensary (was Maxson Lab) 4426 Tilly Mill Road Atlanta, Ga. 30360	Vitamin C Ultra Fine Soluble Corn Base 2,400 mg/tsp. AllerBrand Vitamin C Carrot, Potato, or Sago Palm Base 2,400 mg/tsp.	Allerbrand Vitamin C Sago Palm (noncorn) 1,000 mg/tablet
FoodScience Lab 20 New England Drive Essex Junction, Vt. 05452		Potent C Corn Base 1,000 mg/tablet
Freeda Vitamins 36 East 41st Street New York, N.Y. 10017		Vitamin C† Vegetable Base 1,000 mg/tablet

* Short-acting
† Long-acting

Most of the above vitamins are also available through:

L & H Vitamins
37–10 Crescent Street
Long Island City, N.Y. 11101
(800-221-1152)

Table 27.3
Sources of Nutrients

Calcium

Green vegetables	Canned sardines and salmon
Mustard greens	Shellfish
Turnip greens	Broccoli
Egg yolk	Kale
Milk and dairy products	Soybeans

Iron

Dark molasses	Dried fruits
Enriched cereals	Green leafy vegetables
Dried apricots	Whole grain cereals
Wheat germ	Cocoa
All legumes	Peaches
Dried beans	Nuts
Soybeans	Shellfish
Lean meats	Seafoods
Egg yolk	

Copper

American cheese	Kale
Sweet potatoes	Lobster
Dried lima beans	Halibut
Dried prunes	Grapes
Citrus fruits	Flour
Beef liver	Oats
Pork chops	Pecans
Dried peas	Oysters
Mushrooms	Shrimp
White bread	Spinach
Mackerel	Turkey
Dried beans	Walnuts
Whole rye	Wheat
Chocolate	Cocoa

Asparagus
Almonds
Avocado
Cabbage
Chicken

Eggs
Apples
Bananas
Corn
Carrots

Magnesium

Raw tomatoes
Lima beans
Raw carrots
Roasted poultry
Roasted nuts
Whole wheat
Boiled spinach
Cashew nuts
Citrus fruits
Baked beans
Fresh peas
Codfish
Brazil nuts
Brown rice
Peas, beans, and lentils

Hazelnuts
Oatmeal
Peaches
Peanuts
Pecans
Potatoes
Soy flour
Walnuts
Almonds
Barley
Halibut
Beef
Corn
Cocoa

Manganese

Whole grain rye
Whole wheat flour
Wheat
Oatmeal
Whole corn
White flour
White rice
Dried peas
Dried prunes

Liver
Sweet potatoes
Snap beans
Spinach
Bananas
Beets
Lettuce
Kale
Dried beans

Potassium

All vegetables (especially potato skins and green leafy vegetables)
Bananas
Oranges
Whole grains
Sunflower seeds
Mint leaves

Sodium

Graham crackers
Cheddar cheese
Cottage cheese
Evaporated milk
French dressing
Popcorn
Pork sausage
Canned crab
Canned fish
Canned carrots
Canned asparagus
Canned sauerkraut
Canned spinach
Sweet pickles
Tomato catsup
Potato chips
Chipped beef
Frankfurters
Cream cheese
Boston brown bread
Cracked wheat bread
Canned baked beans
Canned lima beans
Canned mushrooms
Dried cod
Rye bread
Butter
Buttermilk
Blue cheese
Margarine
Olives
Saltines
Pretzels
Bacon
Bologna
Cured ham
Liverwurst
Rye wafers
Bran flakes
Cornflakes
Rice flakes
Wheat flakes
Wheat flour
White bread
Salted nuts
Corned beef
Canned green peas

Sulfur

Liver	Eggs
Meats	Cabbage
Fish	Dried beans
Legumes	Brussels sprouts
Nuts	

Zinc

Beef	Oat cereal (puffed)
Beans (common, mature, dried)	Peanuts (raw or roasted)
Brewer's yeast	Peanut butter
Chick-peas or garbanzos	Peas
Corn (sweet, yellow)	Popcorn
Cornmeal	Pumpkin seeds
Cowpeas (black-eyed)	Brown rice
Granola	Wheat (shredded)
Lentils	Wheat bran
Lima beans	Whole wheat bread
Rye bread	Wheat germ
Oatmeal (rolled oats)	

• Certain nutrients are utilized more completely if they are taken in a specific manner. For example, minerals, such as calcium and magnesium, are absorbed best if they are not combined with vitamins. The amino acid tryptophan needs B_6 to be properly utilized. Because nutrient utilization is complicated, many parents need the help of a nutrition specialist or a nutritionally oriented physician to decide how much of what to give when.

Hertha Hafer in Germany has suggested that phosphate additives in sausage, in particular, can cause some children to become hyperactive and hyperaggressive. One scientific German study confirmed her theory.

Dr. Stephen Schoenthaler of Stanislaus, California, has shown that the reading levels of children in 803 New York City schools representing over a million students improved after their diet was altered.[3] Before the two-year study, which decreased the sugar and food additives in their school diet, 21 percent read two years below school grade. After the study, that level had decreased to 6.5 percent. He showed that the academic ratings increased when children ate diets that excluded dyes, artificial flavors, additives, and sugar.

Dr. Schoenthaler has conducted a number of other studies on the diets of institutionalized adults and juvenile delinquents.[4] He has found that the combination of reduced sugar intake along with nutrient supplementation leads to decreased antisocial, uncooperative, and aggressive behavior. He is presently completing studies to evaluate the role of specific nutrients in relation to academic performance in normal children.

Conflicting scientific studies from England fail to give us clear-cut conclusions.[5] Some studies indicate that vitamins and nutrients increase academic performance, while others say exactly the opposite. Until we have more data, we simply can't be sure. It does not seem unreasonable to suppose that what children eat might affect not only how they feel and act but also their ability to learn. If a child's diet, for example, lacks zinc, there is no doubt that intelligence, as well as physical size and sexual development can be adversely affected. White specks on the fingernails or stretch marks on the skin suggest that an individual is zinc-deficient. Once again be cautious; more is not necessarily better. Check with your doctor.

Essential Fatty Acids

There are basically two types of essential fatty acids (EFA), called Omega-3 or Omega-6 oils. Many individuals appear to need both. Mature adults who have eaten deficient diets for prolonged periods of time may find these nutrients helpful. For further information I highly recommend *Superimmunity for Kids,* by Leo Galland, M.D. and

3. Stephen Schoenthaler, M.D., et al., "The Impact of a Low Food-Additive and Sucrose Diet on Academic Performance in 803 New York City Public Schools," *International Journal of Biosocial Research* 2 (1986), pp. 185–195.

4. Stephen Schoenthaler, M.D., "The Effect of Sugar on the Treatment and Control of Antisocial Behavior: A Double-Blind Study of an Incarcerated Juvenile Population," *International Journal of Biosocial Research* 3 (1982), pp. 1–19.

5. David Benton and Gwilym M. Roberts, "The Effect of Vitamin and Mineral Supplementation on Intelligence, the Sample of School Children," *Lancet* 664 (1988), pp. 140–143.

Diane Buchman.[6] In this book they explore how and why children can be healthier if they have an adequate supply of nutrients, especially essential fatty acids. He has kindly allowed us to provide the following revised and expanded information from his book.

Causes of an Essential Fatty Acids Deficiency

The usual cause is a diet poor in EFAs, that is, a diet that contains any of the following:

- Too much sugar, which increases the need for EFAs.
- White flour and other processed foods. Refined flour has had the dietary fiber, vitamins, and wheat germ removed, so the need for EFAs is increased.
- Margarine, crackers, or other snack foods that contain hydrogenated or partially hydrogenated vegetable oils, such as coconut or palm kernel oils. Hydrogenation extends the shelf life of oils but destroys the EFAs. It distorts the molecular shape of the oil. Hydrogenation allows a manufacturer to transform an inexpensive, low-quality source of oil into a product that competes with butter because of its taste and spreadability. The Dutch government has banned the sale of margarines with trans-fatty acids because of their potentially detrimental health effects.[7] Our vegetable-oil shortenings contain 14 percent to 40 percent trans-fatty oils.

Are You Confused About Hydrogenated Oils?

Many people are unsure about exactly what hydrogenated or partially hydrogenated oils are and how these are related to essential unsaturated or saturated fatty acids. We all need fatty acids to build or make body fat. Saturated fatty acids are solid at room temperature. These are not essential. Your body can make what you need. These are the fats that clog the vessels and interfere with our ability to use certain needed or essential fatty acids.

Unsaturated fatty acids are liquid at room temperature; some are needed or essential and others are not. This means that all essential fatty acids are liquid but some liquid oils are not essential. Again, the

6. Leo Galland, M.D., and Diane Buchman, *Superimmunity for Kids* (New York: E. P. Dutton, 1988).
7. Udo Erasmus, *Fats and Oils* (see Bibliography).

body can make all the nonessential fatty acids it needs. We need to know mainly which liquid oils contain the needed or essential fatty acids such as Omega-3 and -6.

Most vegetable oils in this country contain many nonessential fatty acids. These oils are hydrogenated to increase their shelf life. The hydrogen that is added to them converts the unsaturated or liquid fats into the undesirable saturated or solid fats. When an oil is partially hydrogenated, it means that the oil has been altered to create *artificial* essential fatty acids, which is undesirable, unnatural, and unnecessary. Margarine is a partially hydrogenated vegetable oil.

Clues That Suggest a Possible Essential Fatty Acids Deficiency

Although there are many causes for the complaints listed on Table 27.4, each symptom suggests a possible need for more EFAs. Prob-

TABLE 27.4
Symptoms Suggesting a Possible Need for Essential Fatty Acids

Excessive thirst

Insatiable appetite

Dry, flaking skin

"Chicken skin," or bumps on the outer upper arms, thighs, or cheeks

Calluses

Brittle, soft, or splitting fingernails

Nails with longitudinal lines

Dry hair

Dandruff

Excessive or hard ear wax

Dry scaling in the ear canal

Hyperactivity

Eczema

Asthma

lems other than a lack of EFAs, of course, can cause each of the listed symptoms as well, so other factors must be considered by your physician.

It is possible that those who are EFA-deficient may also:

- lack the enzymes needed to process EFAs;
- lack sufficient amounts of necessary cofactors, for example B vitamins, vitamin E, zinc, and magnesium that help convert one EFA to another;
- have a chronic yeast infection that further impedes normal body metabolism.

Tips for Supplementing Essential Fatty Acids

A child who has an EFA deficiency needs to take oils rich in Omega-3 and/or Omega-6. Check with your doctor if you want to try EFAs. Keep in mind that giving the wrong oil or not giving the amount your child needs (either too much or too little) may temporarily aggravate her or his symptoms. The following might provide some general basic background information:

- Evening primrose oil capsules are available at health food stores. The usual initial dose is one capsule per day. Another capsule is added at three-day intervals if all seems well. The maximum dose is two capsules, three times a day, for adults. Some hyperactive children respond favorably to one to three primrose oil capsules a day.

  Decreased thirst may occur within forty-eight hours after starting primrose oil. This is a good sign. Improvement in skin, food sensitivities, and behavior can occur within several weeks or months. If a child improves at a given dose, that dose should be maintained. Increased irritability, loss of appetite, acne, or diarrhea suggest that less primrose oil is needed. If in doubt, the dose should be stopped until you consult with your doctor.

- If a child's thirst increases, the skin becomes drier, or the behavior worsens on primrose oil or safflower oil, try medicinal linseed oil. Start with one teaspoon of linseed oil at breakfast. *If it is well tolerated,* raise the dose to two teaspoons after a few days. In a few more days, three teaspoons can often be tried. The dose is increased until the behavior, skin, and thirst improve. Check with a doctor if several tablespoons appear to be needed.

- Smell the oils you intend to use. If they smell rancid or have a bitter taste, throw them out. It helps prevent rancidity if you squeeze one 400 I.U. capsule of vitamin E into the oil. Don't shake it, however. Just refrigerate the oil. Vitamin E and refrigeration help delay spoiling.

- Some children won't swallow primrose oil capsules or take linseed oil. If that happens, prick and squeeze the oil from the capsule and rub it into the skin of the child's buttocks at bedtime. The underwear and bedding will be stained, but the oil will be absorbed through the skin.

- Avoid or limit hydrogenated oils, partially hydrogenated oils, margarine, refined flour, processed foods, and sugar.

Sources and Suggested Dosages of Omega-6

If your child's symptoms are caused by an EFA deficiency, these supplements sometimes help dramatically. A few children start to respond within hours; others may require several months before improvement is noted.

This type of essential fatty acid is found mainly in seeds grown in the temperate zone. Important sources include safflower seeds and their oil, sunflower seeds and their oil, corn oil, evening primrose oil, and sesame oil.

Evening primrose oil comes in 500-milligram capsules and is sold in health food stores. The suggested dosage per day is as follows:

Up to 1 year old	1 capsule
1–2 years old	2 capsules
3–5 years old	3 capsules
6–9 years old	4 capsules
10–12 years old	5 capsules
Teenager and older	6 capsules

Super GLA 240 (borage oil) is available through Nutricology,[8] L&H Vitamins,[9] and other nutrient suppliers. Each capsule is equivalent to six capsules of evening primrose oil, and one capsule supplies the entire daily supplement, but its use should be restricted to children thirteen years and older.

8. Contact: Nutricology, 400 Preda Street, San Leandro, Calif. 94577 (800-782-4274).

9. Contact: L&H Vitamins, 37-10 Crescent Street, Long Island City, N.Y. 11101 (800-221-1152).

GLA 40 (black-currant-seed oil) can be purchased through L&H Vitamins,[10] Doctors RX Dispensary,[11] and other nutrient suppliers. Each capsule is equivalent to one 500-milligram primrose oil capsule, and the same dosage can be used.

Sources and Suggested Dosages of Omega-3

The second type of EFA, known as Omega-3, is found in *fresh* oily cold-water fish, such as salmon, tuna, mackerel, herring, and sardines.

Another good source is flaxseed oil (also known as linseed oil). This must be obtained from a health food store, *not* hardware store. The suggested dosage of this oil per day is as follows:

Up to 2 years old	1 teaspoon
2–3 years old	2 teaspoons
3 years old and older	3 teaspoons

A third possible source is Fortified Flax, which comes in powder form and has a nice taste. The dosage for children over three years is 3 teaspoons/three times per day. It is available through Omega-Life, Inc.[12]

Another good source is cod liver oil, and it is available at health food stores. Because cod liver oil contains high amounts of vitamins A and D, the dosage must be limited to one-third that of flaxseed oil. In other words, children over three years should have 1 teaspoon per day.

The dose for walnut oil, another good source, is twice that of flaxseed oil. In other words, children over three years should have 3 teaspoons twice a day. Walnut oil is available at most health food stores.

Natural sources of Omega-3 and Omega-6 are found in kidney beans, navy beans, soybeans, and great northern beans.

Digestive Enzymes

Specialists in environmental medicine believe that food sensitivities can sometimes be decreased if the digestion or breakdown of foods

10. Ibid.
11. Contact: Doctors RX Dispensary, 4426 Tilly Mill Road, Atlanta, Ga. 30360 (404-451-4857).
12. Contact: Omega-Life, Inc., 15355 Woodbridge Road, Brookfield, Wis. 53005 (414-786-2070).

in the intestines and subsequent absorption can be improved. If large particles of undigested food are absorbed into the bloodstream, this can increase the tendency to develop allergies.

Clues That Suggest a Possible Digestive Enzyme Deficiency

Common signs of poor digestion can include bloating, belching, rectal gas, heartburn, nausea, constipation, diarrhea, undigested food particles in the bowel movements, and indentations from the teeth on the sides of the tongue. Sometimes these complaints subside if digestive enzymes are taken with each meal or hearty snack. If they do not, discuss with your physician the possibility of consulting a specialist in intestinal problems. There are only a limited number of ways that our intestines can complain or talk to us, and many different medical problems can cause the same symptoms.

Digestive enzymes are available by prescription or from health food stores and vitamin companies.

Sources and Suggested Dosages of Digestive Enzymes

Pancrease[13]

This is a prescription enzyme that is derived from pork. It is available in a capsule that contains granules that can be opened and sprinkled on food. The capsule is dye-free and delivers high levels of biologically active enzymes into the duodenum or small intestines.

The usual child's dose is one capsule taken with each meal or large snack.

Viokase Powder[14]

This is a prescription item similar to pancrease. This natural digestive enzyme hydrolyzes, or changes, fats into fatty acids and glycerol. It splits proteins into amino acids. It also converts carbohydrates such as baked goods and sweets to dextrins and short-chain sugars.

The usual dose for infants and young children is ⅓ teaspoon, and it can be mixed into foods. This has a pork base, so it could cause symptoms in pork-sensitive patients.

13. Contact: McNeil Laboratories, 7 Welsh and McNight Road, Spring House, Pa. 19477 (215-628-5000).
14. Contact: A. H. Robins Co., 1407 Cummings Drive, Richmond, Va. 23220 (804-257-2000).

Pancreatin[15]

These are nonenteric (uncoated) digestive-enzyme tablets that are available without a prescription. They are buffered to prevent destruction by the acids and gastric pepsin normally found in the intestines. This enzyme promotes more complete digestion of carbohydrates, proteins, and fats.

The usual dose is one tablet with each meal or large snack.

Tyme Zyme[16]

These enteric (coated) caplets can be purchased at many health food stores. This preparation has a vegetable base and is free of common allergens found in many commercial medications.

The usual dose is one caplet with each meal or large snack.

Digestive Aid[17]

This tablet is covered with a food dye. Wash off the colored coating with water and then dry and store the tablets for future use. They are derived from a plant source.

The usual dose is one tablet with each meal or large snack.

Vital-Zymes[18]

This preparation is free of common allergens and is derived from a plant source. The usual dose is one capsule immediately before each meal.

Lactase

Another digestive enzyme is lactase, which is used for a milk sugar (or lactose) intolerance. Some children and adults lack the enzyme lactase, which breaks down lactose. (See Linda, Appendix E.) If lactase is not present in the intestine, the abdomen bloats, and rectal gas, belching, and diarrhea are very common complaints. If these

15. Contact: Vitaline Corporation, 722 Jefferson Avenue, Ashland, Or. 97520 (800-648-4755).

16. Contact: Tyme Zyme, The Prozyme Co., Inc., 2567 Greenleaf Avenue, Elk Grove Village, Ill. 60007 (708-364-6366).

17. Contact: Neo Life, 20151 Haviland Avenue, Hayward, Calif. 94545 (415-278-5320).

18. Contact: Klaire Laboratories, Inc., P.O. Box 618, Carlsbad, Calif. 92008 (800-533-7255).

are not your child's symptoms, your child is probably not lactose intolerant. If milk appears to cause symptoms that are *not* associated with indigestion, the problem may be a milk allergy. This is one way to distinguish a lactose intolerance from a milk allergy.

Lactase can be purchased at any drugstore or health food store. Lactaid is one brand name. Add five to fifteen drops to one quart of milk and allow the milk to stand in the refrigerator for twenty-four hours. This will digest the lactose in the milk. If you prefer, you can purchase milk that has been pretreated with lactase. You can also purchase tablets that contain lactase. These are consumed before, during, or immediately after meals. Lactase-treated milk, cheese, and ice cream are available at some larger chain stores, but are more expensive than making it yourself.

If your child can drink lactase-treated milk but not regular milk, the problem is probably not an allergy to milk but a lactose intolerance or a deficiency of the enzyme lactase. Some children, however, appear to have a combined problem and are helped in part by lactase but also by appropriate milk allergy therapy. A milk allergy, as well as many other medical problems, can cause recurrent diarrhea. Constipation, however, is a more characteristic complaint, suggesting that a milk sensitivity needs to be seriously considered as a possible cause. A distended abdomen, excessive belching or rectal gas, nausea or vomiting, clucking throat sounds, bed-wetting, ear fluid, nose congestion, asthma, leg aches, or personality changes are all common complaints associated with a milk allergy. Some combination of these symptoms in a family that has allergies should suggest a possible milk sensitivity, especially if any family member loves or hates any form of dairy. Discuss your observations with your physician.

Amino Acids

Sometimes children are not feeling well and their bodies are not functioning normally because their metabolism is not normal. Amino acid analysis of the blood and/or urine can provide helpful information so that judicious individualized supplementation with amino acids is possible.

When we eat proteins and other foods, they are digested and broken down by various enzymes into peptide particles and eventually into amino acids. These are absorbed and transported in our blood, stored, and recombined in a number of complicated ways in the various areas of the body, such as the liver, muscles, and so forth.

Amino acids are used as building blocks to create new substances that supply energy, form antibodies, and/or produce other necessary substances, such as hormones, that our body needs.

Very simply, let us suppose that the body needs to convert an amino acid called X to a necessary substance called Y. To do this the body needs to supply certain B or C vitamins, and/or trace minerals such as zinc, magnesium, or manganese. If the blood examination shows too much X and too little Y, we have to determine the reason. One must ask if the body lacks the necessary vitamins or trace elements needed to convert X to Y. If an amino acid analysis suggests this, the answer is to supply the needed nutrients. If there is too little protein eaten or if it is not digested or absorbed properly, there may be an inadequate supply of X, so both X and Y will be too low. Sometimes the solution is simply to provide more X or use a digestive enzyme that will help to provide enough Y so that the cells function correctly. Sometimes there is some problem in the kidney so that X is lost in the urine before the body has a chance to make enough Y. This can also cause a low X and low Y. Sometimes the answer is to supply the body directly with more Y or to try to correct the cause of the "leaky" kidney.

By examining the amino acid levels in the blood and urine it is sometimes possible to pinpoint exactly where and why the body is not functioning correctly. Sometimes specific amino acid supplements or vitamin and trace-metal therapy can help the body to function more correctly at a cellular level.

Two laboratories that analyze and interpret the results of amino acids analysis are:

MetaMetrix, Inc.
Medical Research Laboratory
J. Alexander Bralley, Ph.D.
3000 Northwoods Parkway
Suite 150
Norcross, Georgia 30071
(404-446-5483)

Bionostics, Inc.
J. B. Pangborn, Ph.D.
P.O. Drawer 400
Lisle, Illinois 60532
(405-840-4968)

Amino acid studies (AA) are not required for all allergic children, but for some, they help us glean special information about possible specific metabolic errors related to our cellular function. If we can make each cell in our body feel well, the body as a whole will feel better. AA studies provide an inside glimpse at what our cells are doing, and from that we can sometimes learn what our bodies need to function at a higher level of performance so that we feel better.

Sometimes these types of studies, however, provide individualized help for children who have sleep, learning, or behavior problems in particular. The following patient illustrates how some children appear to be helped remarkably with amino acid therapy.

A FOOD-SENSITIVE ARTHRITIC CHILD WHO NEEDED THE AMINO ACID TRYPTOPHAN

Julie

Julie's mother came for an allergy evaluation because her child could not sleep. Julie was so sensitive to so many foods that it was difficult to find enough foods for her six-year-old to eat. They had many allergic relatives. Before Julie was born, she hiccupped much more than normal.

Early in infancy Julie would suddenly scream violently for about ten minutes as if she was in pain. This happened several times a day. In time her mother began to notice that as little as six sips of milk caused recurrent agitation and an upset about three hours later. She discontinued milk and instead gave her baby calcium and the baby seemed better. At about four months, however, as foods were added to her infant's diet, sleeplessness became a persistent problem. Then recurrent ear infections began. Her mother found that one formula after another seemed to bother Julie. When cow's milk was tried again she was rushed to the hospital. It caused extreme nose, eye, and throat congestion within fifteen minutes and she developed blisters on her tongue.

At about eight months Julie developed a tender right wrist. After extensive evaluations it was determined that she had rheumatoid arthritis. Later on, when the family moved to a damp area in the South, Julie intermittently developed red, swollen joints on very humid days. Routinely, the day before it rained, she would cry all day. A drug to treat arthritis helped, but the episodes still occurred.

Then her mother happened to read Dr. Collin Dong's arthritis book and she decided to try Julie on his diet when she was only two years old.[19]

One day after Dr. Dong's diet Julie did not cry as often as usual, had less joint pain, and was able to sleep better than she had since the age of three months. In time her mother found that whenever she made mistakes with this diet, Julie was worse. The diet was continued until she was about four years old.

This diet was tried in spite of the fact that most arthritis specialists strongly doubt that foods could cause arthritis. Some arthritics, however, appear to be helped by certain diets, and a few scientific studies tend to confirm this observation.[20] *Check with your doctor, however, before trying any diet on any infant or child.*

Because recurrent infections continued to be a major problem, Julie needed repeated antibiotics. Eventually this appeared to lead to a secondary yeast overgrowth.

Again, it was the *Donahue* show in 1988 that helped Julie. For the first time Julie's mother considered the possibility that her daughter's feeding and sleep problems could possibly be due to allergies. She found a specialist in environmental medicine to begin treatment.

At the age of four years Julie was treated for parasites and yeast, given allergy extract for common allergenic substances, and placed on amino acid therapy. Her amino acid analysis indicated a need for tryptophan, a natural sedative normally found in the brain. Within three weeks after this combined therapy was started, Julie was sleeping well again, and for the first time she could accidentally break her diet and not become ill. Once, Julie's mother forgot to reorder Julie's amino acids, and her sleep problems recurred. When they were restarted again, Julie was better in two weeks. With AA therapy, she could even tolerate damp, wet days without joint pain, so it appeared that the AA also helped her arthritis.

As the years have passed, milk continues to be a serious problem for Julie. If milk touches her skin, she develops blisters. Fortunately this degree of sensitivity is most extraordinary, but it suggests that dairy products will probably never be well tolerated by this child.

When Julie was five years old, her family doctor suggested that her AA be stopped. The sleep and joint problems recurred, and once again Julie awoke with terrible screaming episodes and nightmares.

This child appears to feel best if she maintains an allergy diet,

19. Collin Dong, M.D., and Jane Bank, *The Arthritic's Cookbook* (New York: Bantam Books, 1973).
20. See Bibliography at end of this book for details.

avoids certain foods, and rotates others. If she receives treatment with an updated food allergy extract, this should enable her to eat more foods without difficulty. Her ability to eat a varied diet without joint pain was best when she received both a food allergy extract and AA therapy, especially for tryptophan.

The Tryptophan Scare of 1989*

In 1989 there was a sudden appearance of an illness called eosinophilic myalgia in women using tryptophan. The FDA recalled and temporarily disallowed the sale of this amino acid. This meant that Julie and many other children could no longer receive this particular amino acid. There was no doubt that tryptophan relieved some sleep problems, but at that time, the safety of this drug was in question. When the drug was stopped, the child's symptoms reappeared.

After scientific evaluation it was ascertained that a large amount of tryptophan supplied by a single Japanese company had been accidentally contaminated with a toxic chemical. A medical article in July 1990 indicated that the contaminant, not the tryptophan, caused the illness.[21] Fortunately for Julie, this amino acid is available again and she has improved again.

21. Laurence Stutsker, et al., "Eosinophilia-Myalgia Syndrome Associated With Exposure to Tryptophan From a Single Manufacturer," *JAMA* 264 (1990), pp. 213–217.

* See Chapter 17.

CHAPTER 28

Counseling and
Psychotherapy

Many children who have brain allergies and have never felt well may not have responded effectively to psychotherapy and extensive counseling before we see them. After they have improved with comprehensive allergy care, however, many need and respond favorably to the same suggestions that were previously ineffective. Behavior-modification techniques simply cannot be applied at the time of a full-blown food-related outburst. These children often can't remember their actions during some of their extraordinary episodes. At times they truly do not seem to hear or understand when they are reacting to certain allergenic exposures. It is almost as if they were not in tune with reality.

After children have had their allergies recognized and treated, they and their parents need to continue counseling in order to cope with their children's present and future outbursts. In addition they need help modifying their previous learned responses to such reactions. Many children have had feelings of inadequacy, guilt, resentment, and anger for years and often are in desperate need of feeling better about themselves. Many have had a lifetime of rarely feeling well either physically or emotionally. Due to their social limitations, some have had few, if any, friends. Many never achieve in a manner commensurate with their ability. They believe they are "stupid" and "bad" and have low self-esteem. Without counseling they may never really realize their true worth. They need to appreciate that they, too, have special gifts, which often more than compensate for a few rough edges.

Many parents have expressed that their problem child is loved but not liked. Often the entire families of the children described in this book need some counseling. The siblings feel neglected because the "squeaky wheel" misbehaving child gets all the attention. The affected children and parents have developed habit patterns of response that need some modification. The stresses in families that have one child who has chronically vacillated between a delightful Dr. Jekyll and an impossible Mr. Hyde can be devastating. Some fathers work longer hours, have two jobs, become alcoholic, or find a new wife. The mothers typically are overwhelmed with feelings of being failures as both mothers and wives. Many husbands, relatives, friends, and even physicians repeatedly blame them for their child's behavior and they become victims of an impossible situation.

After both the child and the parents understand why reactions occur, it makes it much easier to tolerate sudden allergy-related changes in personality. For the first time parents realize they and their children are not at fault. The children often realize that they are really nice youngsters, and the older ones verbalize that they are so happy to learn they are not "crazy." After children have responded to allergy care, many need only a little behavior modification to create a state of peace and serenity in their home that was never possible previously.

A BATTERED ADOPTIVE MOTHER OF AN ABUSED CHILD WHO HAD PSYCHOLOGICAL PROBLEMS AND ALLERGIES

Wayne

Wayne was a very large, handsome, strong, healthy-appearing ten-year-old when we initially saw him. His mother was extremely distraught because he had beaten her on the head with a glass bottle while she was sleeping. She was constantly black and blue because of his aggressive behavior. She was the recipient of six black eyes, one broken rib, and countless arm and leg bruises, which began with his rages at about the age of four. She recalled one time when he was only five years old, he hit her so vigorously with an iron rod across her hip that she had a hard welt in that area for that entire summer. Although he also attacked his father if he interfered, as well as his small dog, it was his mother who was the major target for his aggression. Four weeks after he began his allergy treatment, his mother was in tears again in our office, but this time it was because she was pleased and relieved: Her son had not abused or hit her for about a month.

Wayne had been adopted at the age of about two years. His body had been seriously physically abused prior to that time. He had been deaf since birth, although this was not recognized until he was two years old. The last in the series of four foster mothers stated she could not "cope with his behavior." During an emergency call she said emphatically, "Get him out of my house immediately, now." His present mother went to retrieve him as quickly as possible from this foster home.

Wayne had classical hay fever, allergic coughing, asthma in the winter, and muscle aches. His bowel movements sometimes leaked onto his underwear, and he wet the bed if he was not awakened each night. He refused to sleep alone. He could not sit through a story, a meal, or a television show. In particular he bit, spit, hit, kicked, and beat his mother. He was hostile, aggressive, irritable, argumentative, unhappy, restless, uncooperative, and tended to have a glassy-eyed look when he became nasty. His mother said he had "two different children in the same body." At times he was extremely lovable. He would hug and kiss. Then suddenly for no apparent reason he would punch his mother in the stomach, kick her in the leg, jab her with a sharp object, bite her, or threaten her with a knife or both fists. He also drew aggressively at that time (see Figure 22.2).

During provocation allergy testing we precipitated some of his typical bouts of aggression, particularly when he was tested for his favorite foods. We could stop his attacks on his mother after he received the correct neutralization dose of allergy extract. After his mother recognized cause-and-effect relationships, she realized that apples, bananas, cola, or candy preceded many of his angry episodes. Behavior problems were typically evident after celebrations such as Halloween, after binging on junk food, and during the late summer months, suggesting that molds or weeds might also affect how he felt.

After allergy extract therapy he no longer wheezed unless he broke his diet. His schoolwork improved. One most unusual observation was that for the first time in his life he said he was able to hear something in his right ear. He could not identify the sound. When his mother discontinued his treatment, however, Wayne no longer heard anything in that ear. (On rare occasions ecologically oriented ear specialists have noted that some children who respond favorably to allergy therapy surprisingly begin to hear sound, even though they have nerve deafness.)

This child tended to be very manipulative. He desperately needed counseling, as well as his allergy extract treatment, a rotation diet, a more allergy-free bedroom, chemical avoidance, and better nutrition. In the past, repeated counseling alone was simply not very effective.

His mother tried to be as cooperative as possible in relation to his allergies. She stated that he had improved 50 percent in one month, 75 percent in four months, and one year later he continued to be 85 percent better. His Conner's Hyperactivity Score dropped from an abnormal high of 20 to a normal of 5 within three months of therapy. He could concentrate better in school, play more quietly, and his aggressive episodes were much less frequent and severe. His mother was no longer afraid to drive with him in the car or to be alone with him at home. For the first time his mother could go to work. In the past this was not possible because no one would baby-sit Wayne.

Even though Wayne was doing "so well," his mother discontinued his allergy treatment because he refused to take his sublingual allergy extract therapy and the treatment was too expensive. During the following late summer, when he was no longer treated for his mold and weed-pollen sensitivities, he began his violent attacks again. This type of seasonal flare-up had been noted in previous years. It was repeatedly obvious that not only did his hay fever seem worse each fall, but his attitude and behavior deteriorated at the same time. The police were called twice in less than two weeks, and finally he was hospitalized on a child's psychiatric ward for observation.

He remained in the hospital under the care of a well-trained psychiatric staff for about two weeks. They observed that Wayne seemed nonaggressive except when his adoptive mother came to see him. They eventually ascertained that he falsely believed that his present mother had caused the extensive physical injuries he had sustained as an infant and a toddler before he was adopted.

One year after his hospital psychiatric diagnosis and counseling he had stopped abusing and battering his mother. However, his mother continues to restrict his diet. She dares not allow a banana in their house and she sharply limits his ingestion of sugar because she knows that these two foods, in particular, continue to cause him to become angry, negative, and hyperactive. His room has remained somewhat allergy-free. Without his allergy treatment he has developed hay fever and recurrent ear infections, again during each mold and pollen season. However, he has not become aggressive and belligerent at these times, the way he had repeatedly in the past. Counseling, maturity, and avoidance of sugar and bananas are the most likely reasons for this improvement.

Obviously this youngster had many deep-rooted emotional problems related to his exceedingly traumatic early infancy, which caused him to direct his anger toward his adoptive mother. Once this was resolved, he was better able to manage many of the emotional aspects of his illness. Although certain foods continued to change his behavior or mood, he was better able to control his aggression after he was counseled. His physical symptoms, however, were not resolved without appropriate allergy extract therapy. The use of an air purifier in his bedroom during the late summer has helped to relieve some of his classical allergic symptoms.

In Chapter 22 some of the research correlating delinquency and aggression to foods, and additives in particular, was discussed. Our entire penal system needs to become aware of the role allergies can possibly play in the behavior and actions of some individuals. The challenge is to differentiate how much of a person's problems are social or emotional and how much are physical due to allergy or other medical problems that can alter normal brain function.[1] Wayne certainly desperately needed counseling. He responded best, however, when both the psychological and the allergic aspects of his illness were recognized and appropriately treated. By avoiding certain offending foods that cause his behavior to deteriorate and following the suggestions of his psychologist, he is certainly much less abusive and a more pleasant, even delightful child.

DOES THIS CHILD NEED A PSYCHIATRIC INSTITUTE OR ALLERGY TREATMENT?

Sidney

Sidney was only eight years old when we first saw him. He was truly an "impossibly angry" child. His mother described her son and herself as desperate. She said she didn't need a miracle, only a more normal child. He was irritable, wiggly, and argumentative. His parents were separated, in part because of the stress Sidney caused in their marriage. His mother knew that it was no longer safe for Sidney to remain

1. J. Satterfield, "Therapeutic Interventions to Prevent Delinquency in Hyperactive Boys," *Journal of American Academy of Child and Adult Psychology.* 26 (1987), pp. 56–64.

at home and that he might need placement in a psychiatric institute for violent children unless she could find out why he was so difficult. The doctors had told her that institutionalization might be the only plausible solution. Her family said it was needed and his teacher said Sidney was schizophrenic. There was no doubt that he acted strange at times. He had periods of extreme hostility. He frequently had sudden outbursts, during which he would hurt other children, as well as his parents and himself. He would climb on top of bookcases. He would routinely get on his bed, flip the mattress off onto the floor, and then proceed to tear the room apart. On one occasion he threw his tiny sister, complete with her walker, across the room. When she was three years old, he tried to shove her out of a moving car. At Christmas, he became upset and heaved an entire trimmed Christmas tree against a wall. Once he tossed a chair through a school window. His mother's arms were covered with his bite marks. At times, he feels so angry he even bites himself. His episodes often last over an hour.

He often states he is unhappy and for at least eighteen months has repeatedly said, "Let me die." He tried one time to hang himself with a shoelace, and grabbed knives and threatened to cut his wrists. He repeatedly ran into the street so the cars could run over him. The school officials do not want him to return. His mother was pushed beyond the limits of tolerance when the sheriff was called because Sidney had jumped from the first-story window and run away. Before he ran away he told his mother "to kill him or he would have to kill himself." When his behavior becomes intolerable, he has the characteristic allergic symptoms of brilliant red earlobes, wiggly legs, and a spacey look.

But there are many times when he is simply the nicest, cutest, calmest little child you could imagine. For example, once he took off his coat and gave it to a little boy who needed warmer clothes. But why does he have such violent, frightening episodes?

His parents both have allergies. One grandmother had hypoglycemia. His other grandmother was repeatedly suicidal, *usually, in September*. Could she have had seasonal mold or pollen brain allergies? (See Chapter 22.)

When his mother was pregnant with Sidney, he kicked so hard in the uterus that his father could not sleep. His mother was eating an excess of dairy at that time.

As an infant he cried constantly. He had prolonged colic until the milk formula was changed to a soy preparation. He walked at nine months. He could not be cuddled and still does not like to be held. As an infant, he had recurrent ear infections, as well as typical nose allergies. By the age of two, his intense, uncontrolled temper tantrums were clearly evident. Sleep was always a challenge and bedtime was known as "helltime." When he was at an early age, his mother realized sugar set him off, but no on believed her.

As time passed he developed typical hay fever, then headaches.

Once again, it was the *Donahue* show that gave his mother the insight she needed. His mother heard about the role diet played in relation to some children who had activity and behavior problems. A year before she saw us, she had tried the Multiple Food Elimination Diet, but he refused to cooperate. However, after the sheriff came to her home, she knew she had few choices. She had to find an answer. She tried the Multiple Food Elimination Diet again, but this time he was cooperative. Within four days his Conner's Hyperactivity score decreased from a highly abnormal 28 to a normal 8. His violence and irritability decreased markedly at home, but not at school. Sugar, wheat, milk, and preservatives were the major offenders during the second part of the Multiple Food Elimination Diet.

In time we found that he was definitely hypoglycemic late in the mornings and afternoons. He needed to eat at least every two hours.

We videotaped his responses to molds, sugar, orange juice, and plums during P/N allergy testing. He would scream, bite, hit, kick, race, crawl under furniture, refuse to be touched, and break anything within reach. Before and after testing he was truly adorable, once again the nicest youngster you could imagine, but during the provocation test, he could be truly impossible. With some provocation allergy tests, he showed little response, but when a major offender was found, he was suddenly totally uncontrollable. He reverted to the type of activity and behavior that made the school want him placed in an institution.

After only one day of allergy testing, his parents were delighted. He smiled for the first time in years and atually laughed and joked on the way home. He became more affectionate. His parents then began to note that chemicals such as auto fumes and correction fluid caused activity changes. In nine days his episodes were still evident, but less severe and less frequent, and his mother said he was 50 percent better.

Prior to the diagnosis of Sidney's allergies, his mother was repeatedly told she was not raising him correctly. She needed to be firmer and to discipline him better; others said he was just being a boy and was spoiled. Ritalin, Mellaril, Clonidine, and Desipramine were all tried. They all seemed to help at first, but after a short time his aggression, anger, and suicidal statements and actions would recut.

It is too soon to know the long-term effect of a comprehensive environmental treatment program in relation to Sidney's future, but we certainly know that food and mold allergies, chemical sensitivities, and hypoglycemia are major causes of at least some of his intolerable behavioral episodes. At present it appears hopeful that his mother no longer needs to fear that her son will be institutionalized because he cannot behave. The preliminary followup indicates he is definitely better.

What Is Needed to Help More
Children and Physicians

We desperately need a large, centrally located facility in a less polluted, relatively clean area of the United States to diagnose and treat infants and children who have environmental illness. Such a center could also be used to instruct young physicians about these newer concepts of treating allergies and chemical sensitivities. The facility should be staffed with both clinicians and scientists who will impartially research, evaluate, and further document or negate the efficacy of many aspects of this form of medicine. Educational material in pamphlet, book, audio, and video forms could be produced to help teach the public, educators, psychologists, counselors, and physicians. If anyone has any ideas in relation to how any of the above can be made a reality, please write to the Practical Allergy Research Foundation (PARF), P.O. Box 60, Buffalo, New York 14223–0060. This foundation has already produced the audio and video educational resources listed in Appendix C.

Food Sources of Some Allergenic Substances

Wheat and Eggs[1]

Wheat	Eggs
Baked goods	Albumen
Biscuits[c,d]	Baked goods[d]
Bread crumbs[b]	Bavarian cream
Breads (including rye, rice, etc.)[b]	Bread crumbs (at times)
	Candy[a]
Breakfast cereals[a]	Coffee[a]
Candy[a]	Creamed foods
Coffee substitutes[a]	Croquettes
Cracker meal	Crusts (if shiny bread, etc.)

Note: Read all food labels very carefully.

[a]Some, not all.

[b]Italian bread is often milk-free.

[c]Make unseasoned Ry-Krisp sandwiches; all bread contains wheat.

[d]When baking, substitute 1/2 teaspoon baking powder for each egg omitted from the recipe.

[1]We are grateful to the late Dr. Jerome Glaser, Rochester, N.Y., for a portion of this list.

Wheat	Eggs
Crackers	Custards
Dumplings	Egg white
Gravy	Powdered or dried egg
Macaroni, etc.	French ice cream
Malt (beer)	French toast
Noodles, spaghetti	Fritters
Salad dressing	Frostings
Sauces for vegetables or meats	Meringue
Soups (bisques or chowders)	Noodles
Stuffing	Pie filling
Swiss steak	Root beer[a]
Wieners or bologna	Salad dressing
	Sauces (hollandaise)
	Sausage
	Soups[a]

Corn[2]

Kernel corn	Confectioner's sugar
Corn cereal	Brown sugar
Cornstarch	Candy
Cornmeal	Carob (CaraCoa)
Corn sugar	Creamed pies
Corn syrup	Cookies
Sorbitol	Custards
Canned or bottled juice drinks	Frostings
Some frozen orange juice	Fritos
Coffee (instant)	Graham crackers
Tea (instant)	Jellies

[2]Sources of corn from Doris J. Rapp, M.D., *Allergies and the Hyperactive Child,* Practical Allergy Research Foundation (PARF), 1980, P.O. Box 60, Buffalo, N.Y. 14223–0060.

Coffee Rich

Some cranberry juice

Candied fruits

Canned fruits

Dried fruits

Frozen fruits (sweetened)

Fruit desserts

Cottage cheese

Ice cream

Milk in paper containers

Oleomargarine

Sherbet

Yogurt

Hominy

Succotash

Commercial baked goods

Biscuits

Bisquick

Cake, pancake, and pie mixes

Cookies

Donuts

All presweetened cereals

All commercial breads

Bacon

Cooked meats in gravies

Ham (cured)

Luncheon meats (bologna, etc.)

Sandwich spreads

Sausages

Wieners

Brown sugar

Gelatin mixes

Peanut butter

Popcorn

Puddings

All usual baking powders

All corn oils

Yeast

Aspirin

Capsules

Ointments

Suppositories

Most tablet medicine

Some vitamins

Bath or body powder

Paper cups and plates

Adhesives

Envelopes

Labels

Stickers

Tapes

Stamps

Liquids poured from paper cartons

Some plastic food wrappers

Toothpastes/powders

Foods fried in corn oil

Gravies

Monosodium glutamate

Zest soap

Beer, ale, gin, whiskey

Infant Formulas That Contain Corn

Infant Milk Formulas	Infant Soy Formulas	Other
Enfamil	Isomil	Pedialyte
Similac	Prosobee	
Advance	Nursoy Powder (not liquid)	
Portagen	Soyalac (not I-Soyalac)	
Lofenalac		

Hydrolyzed Casein

Nutramigen
Progestimil

Infant Formulas That Do Not Contain Corn

Infant Milk Formulas	Infant Soy Formulas	Other
Hydrolyzed Casein Alimentum	I-Soyalac (liquid and powder)	Ricelyte
	Nursoy (liquid only)	

Good Start contains soy, whey (milk), but no corn

Milk[3]

Milk Products

Whole, skim, 1 percent and 2 percent, lactase-treated, and acidophilus milk. Cream includes: half-and-half and heavy and light cream. Foods made from milk or cream include yogurt, sour cream, all types of cheese, butter, whipped cream, whipped topping, ice cream, ice milk, and milk sherbet.

[3]We are grateful to Judy Moyer for permission to use some of the material in her book, *Cooking for the Allergic Child*, Collegiate Pride, Inc., Publishing Division, State College, Pa. 16801.

Other Related Products Include

Casein or caseinate (a milk protein), whey or lactose (milk sugar)

Beverages

Malted milk, Ovaltine, powdered milk, condensed milk, evaporated milk, dried milk powder, buttermilk, most cocoa, all instant cocoa preparations. "Nondairy" substitutes such as Coffee-Mate, Prem and Cool Whip contain casein or caseinate, a milk protein.

Breads, Cereals, and Other Grain Products

All bread and rolls made with milk, such as muffins, popovers, baking powder biscuits; griddle cakes and waffles; donuts; zwieback; biscuit mixes; noodles, macaroni, and spaghetti; most commercially made breads, except Italian; dry cereals, if made with milk, and instant cream of wheat and rice, if made with milk; or the new high-calcium dry cereals such as Dairy Crisp

Fats and Salad Dressings

Butter and some margarines. Check salad dressing labels for cheese, buttermilk, or sour cream.

Meats, Fish, and Poultry

Breading, when milk is used as a coating, creamed meats, frankfurters, bologna or luncheon meats containing milk solids, some meat loaf

Vegetables

Creamed vegetables, mashed potatoes, au gratin and scalloped dishes

Desserts

Custards, puddings; cakes; cookies; ice cream, sherbets, frozen yogurt; cream pies; whipped cream and piecrusts made with butter; some candies or chocolate

Miscellaneous

Rarebits, curd; creamed or milk-based soups, bisques, cream sauces, milk gravies; fritters; soufflés and omelets; egg replacers; scrambled eggs, lactalbumen, and lactoglobulin; plus any combination dishes that might contain milk

Soy

Read all labels carefully. Soy is used as a protein filler (lecithin), emulsifier, or a "vegetable" oil in a wide variety of products, such as baked goods, soups, candies, cereals, roasted nuts, and so on.

Foods

Soybeans
Soy sauce (Worcestershire and Oriental)
Soy nuts
Soy noodles, spaghetti, macaroni
Soy sprouts (Chinese foods)
Tofu
Infant soy formulas
  Soyalac or I-Soyalac
  Nursoy
  Isomil
  Prosobee
Infant milk formulas
  Enfamil
  SMA
  Similac
  Advance
  Portagen
  Alimentum
  Good Start
Margarine
  Mrs. Filbert's soft margarine

Land O' Lakes
Imperial
Parkay
Promise
Farmdale
Blue Bonnet
Mazola
Crisco, Spry, Pam, Puritan oil
Ice cream, sherbet, and ice milk
Processed cheeses
Nondairy products (Coffee Rich, etc.)
Liquid protein foods

Contacts

Adhesives	Some dog and fish food
Blankets	Fertilizer
Candles	Soap
Celluloid	Automobile parts
Cloth	Oils, lubricating
Cosmetics	Paint
Glycerine	Enamel
Linoleum	Varnish
Fodder for animals	Massage creams
	Paper sizing and finishes

Sweets[4]

When purchasing alternative sweetening agents, be sure to choose ones that are not highly processed. Processing usually involves the use of chemicals that alter a food product. Look for labels that state "natural," "unprocessed," or "raw," and look for those products that are chemically less contaminated (organic).

[4] Sources of sweets from Ilene Buchholz, Karen Cook, and Theron Randolph, *An Alternative Measure* (see Bibliography for details). Used with permission.

Almond Syrup

A liquid syrup that is made from almond extract and 1 percent malt (barley). It is fairly mild in taste. It is light amber-beige in color and has the consistency of a thin maple syrup. Almonds are in the plum family. Do not use this if your child has an almond allergy.

Aquamiel

This is a naturally sweet, nutritious liquid derived from the maguey (century plant). It has approximately twenty calories per teaspoon versus sixteen calories in a teaspoon of table sugar. It is dark amber-brown in color, has the consistency of honey, and the taste of a blend of honey and molasses. Aquamiel is in the agave family.

Carob

This looks like chocolate but has a taste that is only similar to chocolate. It is available in a raw as well as a roasted form and is sold in both liquid and solid forms (carob chips). Carob is in the legume (peanut) family.

Date Sugar

This is made from pitted dates that are dried and then ground into a somewhat coarse dark-brown meal. It may be packaged in a dry, crystallized form or a moist, clumpy, coarse meal. It can be dissolved in boiled water to obtain a liquid sugar. It has a tendency to ferment and develop mold growth, so it is best to keep it refrigerated or frozen. Date sugar is in the palm family.

Dried Fruit

Dried apricot, pineapple, raisin, peach, papaya, and other fruits can be chopped or grated and added to cookies, quick breads, and pancake recipes, but additional baking powder and a slight amount of liquid may be needed. A concentrated syrup is derived from fresh, sun-ripened figs. Dried figs are in the mulberry family.

Fructose

This comes from a variety of natural fruits, such as apple, peach, plum. This is usually considered to be a corn derivative.

Honey

Although varieties are derived from sage, orange blossom, avocado, clover, and buckwheat, they are similar and must be rotated every four days. The darker the honey, the stronger the flavor. Honey should not be given to infants.

Licorice

This is much sweeter than sugar. Licorice is in the legume or pea family. Do not use if sensitive to peanuts.

Malt Syrup

Grain-sensitive patients need to be cautious if they use this because the starch added to the sprouted barley during fermentation is commonly derived from cornstarch. This could therefore be a problem for some corn-sensitive children. Malt syrup is in the grain/grass family.

Maple Sweeteners

This is available as liquid syrup, sugar granules, maple butter, and solid crystalline-sugar forms (candy). Buy only 100 percent pure maple. Common store varieties are made with a corn sweetener, artificial flavors, artificial colors, and preserving agents. Unless you know the American supplier, Canadian maple syrups are preferred because they do not use formaldehyde sanitizing pellets when the sap is obtained. You can check by using a kit to detect formaldehyde.[5] See Chapter 13.

---

[5] Northeast Center for Environmental Medicine, 2800 W. Genesee Street, Syracuse, N.Y. 13219 (315-488-2856).

Rice Syrup

Be cautious if you are grain-sensitive because some contain a small amount of barley malt. Mildly sweet commercial rice syrups contain 1 percent barley malt. Rice syrup is in the grass family.

Stevia Rebaudiana

This is a South American herb, with a slight licorice taste.[6] One serving equals the sweetness of two tablespoons of sugar and has less than one calorie. This may be used by adding the crushed leaves to recipes or as a liquid that is brewed.

Jaguary Sugar

This is derived from sugar cane. It looks like a block of honey-colored brownish sugar. It should not be kept refrigerated unless it is very hot because it cannot be sliced if it is too cold. If it becomes too hot, however, it can liquefy and ferment and thus become spoiled. It is sold in plastic bags. It can be used for baking, but the recipe must be altered because it is about 50 percent sweeter than regular sugar. When melted with sesame seeds and a form of clarified butter, it is sold as a candy.

It is available at the Indian Trade Center, Indian and Oriental Foods and Spices, 3359 Bailey Avenue, Buffalo, N.Y. (716-838-2149).

A Few Words About Artificial Sweeteners: How Safe Are They?

Aspartame is advertised as a safe, nutritive sweetener that has essentially no calories. It is made from two amino acids, aspartic acid and phenylalanine, and is not derived from natural sources but rather from hydrocarbons or from fermentation. It is said to be safe, but many people have raised questions about this. Dennis W. Remington, M.D., and Barbara W. Higa, in their book entitled *The Bitter Truth About Artificial Sweeteners*, will provide much upsetting food for thought.[7] MSG (monosodium glutamate) is so similar in molecular

---

[6] Allergy Resource, 62 Firewood Road, Port Washington, N.Y. 11050 (516-767-2000).
[7] Remington and Barbara Higa, *The Bitter Truth About Artificial Sweeteners*. 1986. (See Bibliography for details.)

structure to aspartic acid that a sensitivity to one could mean problems with the other. In particular, children who drink many low-cal soft drinks and whose diet is mainly fast foods (MSG) are at more risk than others.

Some investigations indicate that aspartame can damage the nervous system or brain, not only in rats but also in humans. It is said to cause mood and behavioral changes, epilepticlike seizures, insomnia, depression, headache, and even menstrual disorders. The use of this substance during pregnancy is questioned.

One must wonder why the FDA has allowed this drug to be marketed in view of the multiple serious negative reports regarding aspartame.

To Diminish Sugar Craving[8]

The following substances are said to diminish sugar cravings:

Gymnema Sylvestre

When taken before a meal, it is said to impede the absorption of a certain amount of the sugar or carbohydrates you eat and decrease the craving for sugar.

Glycine, 500 Milligrams

This amino acid has a sweet taste. It is used as a sugar substitute.

L-Glutamine, 500 Milligrams

This amino acid is used to prevent cravings for sweets.

Chromium

This is a trace metal that has also been said to decrease the desire for sugar. Check with your doctor about dosage.

[8] Available through the Pain and Stress Therapy Center, 5282 Medical Drive, San Antonio, Tex. 78229 (512-696-1674). (See also Appendix B.)

A P P E N D I X   B

Aids to Keep You
Ecologically Healthy[1]

Under each category, the organizations below are listed in order of years of experience.

General Information

Bruce Small, R.R. 1, Goodwood, Ontario, Canada L0C 1A0 (416-649-1356).
The Living Source, 3500 MacArthur Drive, Waco, Tex. 76708 (817-756-6341).
Allergy Product Directory, P.O. Box 640, Menlo Park, Calif. 94026-0640 (415-322-1663).
AFM Enterprises, 1140 Stacy Court, Riverside, Calif. 92507 (714-781-6861).
Baubiologie Hardware, 207 16th Street #B, Pacific Grove, Calif. 93950 (408-372-8626).

Vacuum Cleaners

Rainbow Vacuum Distributors: Aqua-Tex Enterprises, Raymond Ratliff, 4501 Ratliff Lane, P.O. Box 395, Addison, Tex. 75001 (214-250-0525).

---

1. These lists are not complete and include only a few of many possible providers.

Vita Vac Vacuum/Air Cleaning System: Vita Mix Corporation, Joseph A. Sulak, 8615 Usher Road, Cleveland, Oh. 44138 (216-235-4840 or 800-848-2649).
Amway Corporation, Ada, Mich. 49355-0001 (800-253-4463).
Impact Networking Services, 11 Robin Road, West Amherst, N.Y. 14228 (716-689-8034).

Small Electric Room Heaters

Micromar, The Heat Machine Plus, Model HMG–4000, 6680 Middlebert Road, Romulus, Mich. 48174.
Pelonis, Model P861-TC/VHC (electric heater): The Living Source, 3500 MacArthur Drive, Waco, Tex. 76708 (817-756-6341).
Duro Heat, Ceramic electronic heater. Available through Busy Beaver Building Centers, Corporate Offices, 701 Alpha Drive, Pittsburgh, Pa. 15238 (412-828-2323).
Electric Intertherm Heaters, Electric Stores, K-Mart, Corporate Offices, 3100 Big Beaver Road, Troy, Mich. 48084 (313-643-1000).
Value Home Centers, Corporate Offices, Clinton and Rossler Plaza, S. Cheektowaya, N.Y. 14206 (716-825-7377).

Air Purifiers

Sierra Group for Environmental Products, Inc., 433 Rivers Edge Court, Mishawaka, Ind. 46544 (800-234-9517).
AllerMed Air Purifier, 31 Steel Road, Wylie, Tex. 75098 (214-442-4898). Martinaire VH300 removes chemicals. Autoaire II is an air purifier for the car. This unit plugs into the lighter and removes chemicals, dust, pollen, and molds from the interior of the car.
Dust Free, Inc., 4824 Industrial Park Drive, P.O. Box 519, Royse City, Tex. 75089 (214-635-9565).
E. L. Foust Co., Inc., P.O. Box 105, Elmhurst, Ill. 60126 (708-834-4952 or 800-225-9549).
N.E.E.D.S. (National Ecological and Environmental Delivery System), 527 Charles Avenue 12-A, Syracuse, N.Y. 13209 (315-446-1122 or 800-634-1380). Aireox for cars removes chemicals, dust, pollen, and molds.

Ozone Generators

N.E.E.D.S. (National Ecological and Environmental Delivery System), 527 Charles Avenue 12-A, Syracuse, N.Y. 13209 (315-446-1122 or 800-634-1380). FMC 110 Odor Control Unit (available for rent or sale).
Ecology Box, Puretec Odor Control Unit, 425 East Washington #200, Ann Arbor, Mich. 48104 (313-662-9131 or 800-735-1371).

Water Purifiers

Herro Care International, 5121 North Central Avenue, Phoenix, Ariz. 85012 (602-274-6563). For specific details see end of Appendix B.

Diapers

Bio Bottoms, P.O. Box 6009, 3820 Bogeda Avenue, Petaluma, Calif. 94953 (707-778-7945).
Dimples, 35 Konrad Crescent, Suite 201, Markham, Ontario, Canada L3R 8T7 (800-387-4239).
The Ecology Box, 425 East Washington #202, Ann Arbor, Mich. 48104 (313-662-9131).

Nonodorous Crayons

Livos Plantchemistry, 1365 Rufina Circle, Santa Fe, N.M. 87501 (505-438-3448).
Childcraft Toys, Childcraft Education Corp., 20 Kilmer Road, Edison, N.J. 08818 (800-631-5657).
Toys "Я" Us (a national toy store chain; see your local listings).

Peak-Flow Meters

Keller Medical Specialists, 42609 Crawford Road, Antioch, Ill. 60002 (800-843-6226). Standard Mini Wright.
CDX Peak Flow Meter, CDX Corporation, 2 Charles Street, Providence, R.I. 02904 (800-525-3515). They provide one unit for small children, and another for older children and adults.

Ceramic Masks

The Living Source, 3500 MacArthur Drive, Waco, Tex. 76708 (817-756-6341).

Organic Vegetables, Fertilizer, Diatomaceous Earth

Oak Manor Farms, R.R. 1, Tavistock, Ontario, Canada N0B 2R0 (519-662-2385).

Organic Foods

Ener-G Foods, Inc., P.O. Box 84487, Seattle, Wash. 98124-5787 (800-331-5222).
Allergy Resources, P.O. Box 888, Palmer Lake, Col. 81033 (719-488-3630).
Americans for Safe Food, Center for Science in the Public Interest, 1501 Sixteenth Street N.W., Washington, D.C. 20036 (202-332-9110)
Arrowhead Mills, Inc., P.O. Box 866, Hereford, Tex. 79045 (806-364-0730).
Chico-San Inc., P.O. Box 810, Chico, Calif. 95927 (916-891-6271).
Clear Eyes Natural Foods, R.D. 1, Route 89, Savannah, N.Y. 13146-9790 (315-365-2816).
Deer Valley Farm, R.D. 1, Guilford, N.Y. 13780 (607-764-8556).
Elam's, 2625 Gardner Road, Broadview, Ill. 60153 (708-865-1612).
Good Food Guide, Natural Organic Farmers' Association, R.D. 1, Box 134 A, Port Crane, N.Y. 13833 (607-648-5557).
Shiloh Farms, P.O. Box 97, Sulphur Springs, Ark. 72768 (501-298-3297).
Special Foods, 9207 Shotgun Court, Springfield, Va. 22153 (703-644-0991).

Organic Baby Food

The Ecology Box, 425 East Washington #202, Ann Arbor, Mich. 48104 (313-662-9131).

Cellophane Bags

The Living Source, 3500 MacArthur Drive, Waco, Tex. 76708 (817-756-6431).
Erlanders, P.O. Box 106, Altadena, Calif. 19001 (213-797-7004).

Allergy-Free Cosmetics, Hair Color, Permanents

Most large chain drugstores or better department stores.
N.E.E.D.S. (National Ecological and Environmental Delivery System), 527 Charles Avenue 12-A, Syracuse, N.Y. 13209 (315-446-1122 or 800-634-1380).

Architecture

Dona Schrier (Designer), Dona Designs, 825 Northlake Drive, Richardson, Tex. 75080 (214-235-0485).
Good, Clint, and Debra Dadd. *Healthful Houses—How to Design and Build Your Own.* Guaranty Press, 4720 Montgomery Lane, Suite 1010, Bethesda, Md. 20814. (800-541-9185)

Cotton Bedding

Dona Designs, 825 Northlake Drive, Richardson, Tex. 75080 (214-235-0485).
Otis Bedding Co., 639 Exchange Street, Buffalo, N.Y. 14210 (716-842-1127).

Cotton Pillows

Dona Designs, 825 Northlake Drive, Richardson, Tex. 75080 (214-235-0485). (Her bedding is made with organically grown cotton. She also sells solid wood furniture and pure beeswax.)
KB Cotton Pillows, Inc., P.O. Box 57, DeSoto, Tex. 75115 (214-223-7193).
The Cotton Place, P.O. Box 75229, Dallas, Tex. 75229 (214-243-4149).

Mother Hart's, P.O. Box 4229, Boynton Beach, Fla. 33434-42229 (407-738-5866).

Cotton or Wool Carpets

Penny's, 3 Lincoln Center, 5430 LBJ Freeway, Dallas, Tex. 75240 (214-591-1000).
Sears, Roebuck & Co., Sears Towers, Chicago, Ill. 60684 (312-875-2500).
Speigel, P.O. Box 927, Oak Brook, Ill. 60522-0927 (800-345-4500).

Wool Mattresses, Futons, Comforters, Yarns

Pure Podunk, Inc., Podunk Ridge Farm, R.R. 1, Box 69, Thetford Center, Vt. 05075 (802-333-4256).

Sealants, Stains, Paint, Cleaning Products

The Living Source, 3500 MacArthur Drive, Waco, Tex. 76708 (817-756-6341).
Livos Plantchemistry, 1365 Rufina Circle, Santa Fe, N.M. 87501 (505-988-9111).
Pace Chemical Industries, 710 Woodlawn Drive, Dept. N.N., Thousand Oaks, Calif. 91360 (805-496-6224).
Miller Paint Company, 317 S.E. Grand Avenue, Dept. NNE, Portland, Ore. 97214 (503-233-4491).

Formaldehyde and Mold-Detection Kits

Formaldehyde Spot Test Kit and Mold Plates: Northeast Center for Environmental Medicine, 2800 West Genesee Street, Syracuse, N.Y. 13219 (315-488-2856).

Furnace–Air-Conditioning Units

Thurmond Air Quality Systems, P.O. Box 23037, Little Rock. Ark. 72221 (501-227-8888 or 800-AIR-PURE).

The Herro Care Water Purification System

First Stage

This first step makes the water more clear and less cloudy. This particular water purifier has an initially inexpensive, easily replaceable filter that removes dirt, scale, sediment, or other large particles from the water. It is located on the outside of a cartridge. You can therefore look at the cartridge and know when the filter needs to be replaced. The filter is effective for six to twelve months.

Second Stage

The water then passes through the second filter, which has a number of specialized functions. This cartridge contains electrically charged charcoal or carbon particles. The charge causes vegetable or animal debris in the water to stick to or adhere to the carbon.

The activated carbon is composed of a compressed block of powdered charcoal. In contrast to the usual granular forms of charcoal, the finer powder has the advantage of providing a greater surface area to remove objectionable tastes, odors, and colors, along with numerous organic materials and chemicals.

The activated charcoal also provides a medium to remove volatile organic chemicals such as chloroform, which cannot be removed by reverse osmosis or distillation. This system claims to help reduce some potentially health-threatening chemicals such as trichloroethylene (TCE), the carcinogenic trihalomethanes (THMs) such as chloroform, dichlorodiphenyl trichloroethane (DDT), polychlorinated biphenols (PCBs), as well as radioactive particles. This system will remove organic chemicals, such as pesticides, herbicides, solvents, phenol and so on, as well as specific chemicals such as chlorine. It will not, however, remove fluoride. A separate cartridge is now available that does this.

An optional ion exchange resin can be added to this cartridge to remove heavy metals such as lead, mercury, chromium, cadmium, silver, arsenic, and so on.

Third Stage

The third stage of this particular sequential filtration and purification system removes microorganisms that are larger than 0.3 microns in size. This would include certain bacteria, molds, fungi, and yeasts, as well as some organisms such as *Giardia lamblia* and other parasites. It probably will not remove viruses, which vary from 0.009 to 0.012 microns in size. Bacteria are about 0.2 to 30 microns, so some would be removed. (Red blood cells are 50 to 90 microns and the human hair about 25 to 200 microns).

This cartridge contains a biologically inert filter. These last two filter cartridges are more expensive to produce, so the cost-effectiveness of this unit is increased because the inexpensive first filter is designed to remove many impurities that could clog and diminish the life span of the more expensive two sequential filters.

The final result is water that is not cloudy or turbid. It has no objectionable taste or odor. No chemicals or sodium have been added, and essential minerals, such as calcium, have not been removed, as happens with distilled water.

Appendix C

Audiocassettes and Videotapes About Environmental Medicine

Audiocassettes[1]

Rapp, Doris J., M.D. *Allergy Diets.*
Focuses on food allergies, how to diagnose them, and the usefulness of common allergy diets. The advantages and disadvantages of a number of allergy diets and instructions for following them are discussed. Many helpful tips are provided.

———. *Environmental Aspects of Allergy.*
Focuses on the various environmental substances that can cause problems in susceptible individuals. It provides suggestions for creating a more allergy-free home environment and offers many alternatives to help relieve some of the illness due to today's "chemical world."

———. *General Aspects of Environmental Illness.*
Focuses on the recognition, manifestation, and treatment of allergy. Many useful hints are given. This easily understood tape contains general information. It was originally a lecture to the public.

———. *Infant Food Allergies.*
Focuses on some typical unrecognized symptoms of allergy that are often evident during the infant and toddler period. It discusses breast and formula feeding as well as suggestions about how and when to add specific foods to an allergic infant's diet. These suggestions can

1. All cassettes are available through: Practical Allergy Research Foundation (PARF), P.O. Box 60, Buffalo, N.Y. 14223-0060 (716-875-0398).

be discussed with your pediatrician. It provides practical information to hopefully prevent, delay, or relieve the onset of typical allergies and behavior and learning problems later in life.

Educational Videotapes for Parents, Educators, Psychologists, and Physicians[2]

Rapp, Doris J., M.D. and Dorothy Bamberg, Ed.D. *Allergies Do Alter Activities and Behavior.*
This is a three-tape series designed to simplify and clarify the relationship of unsuspected allergies to common physical and behavioral changes seen in children. *Guide for Libraries*, 1990, rated this series five-star, or "must have," for most libraries and called this series "extremely exceptional." Many of the children described in this book are vividly shown on these videotapes as they react to P/N testing.

Videotape I—*How You Can Recognize Unsuspected Allergies* (11 minutes). Shows how you can determine which children are affected and demonstrates sudden changes in how they look, act, behave, write, or draw. It vividly illustrates mood changes and Dr. Jekyll/Mr. Hyde behavior. It shows how allergic exposures can cause some children to act inappropriately.

Videotape II—*Make the Connection: What Causes Allergy and What You Can Do About It* (15 minutes). Instructs the viewer to suspect and detect cause-and-effect relationships. It explains how to recognize consistent patterns between exposures to pollen, mold, dust, food, or chemicals and the time when a child suddenly develops symptoms. This tape enables a parent or teacher to make the connection between the onset of inappropriate behavior and activity and the most probable cause of such a change.

Videotape III—*Clues to Predict Possible Allergies* (17 minutes). This tape is in six sections. Each section elucidates a different aspect of environmental illness. The first section demonstrates how one child's symptoms of Tourette's Syndrome decreased after proper allergy treatment with an extract made from his school's air. The second section illustrates how one retarded child's unrecognized allergies to molds interfered with her ability to learn and behave as well as she could. The third section vividly illustrates one child's fatigue at age four due to an allergy to cherry, and again at the age of twelve due to yeast. The fourth section shows a gifted child who appeared to be

2. All videotapes are available through: Practical Allergy Research Foundation (PARF), P.O. Box 60, Buffalo, N.Y. 14223-0060 (716-875-0398).

aggressive and slow until his need for allergy treatment was recognized. The fifth section clearly demonstrates how allergies can typically affect infants. Babies often have classical allergies and then develop the less frequently recognized physical and behavioral symptoms. In time these can lead to eventual learning and emotional problems, needless surgery, and chronic ill health if the basic problem is not recognized. The sixth section demonstrates a typical hyperactive toddler's reaction after eating sugar cubes.

Rapp, Doris J., M.D. *Impossible Child or Allergic Child?* (20 minutes). Designed to show how unsuspected allergies can alter the lives of affected children and their families. It will help the viewer gain a better understanding of how such sensitivities can cause severe behavioral, social, and educational problems.

————. *Why Some Children Can't Learn or Behave* (2 hours). This two-hour tape illustrates and explains the mild, moderate, or severe changes that can occur in some children who have unrecognized forms of allergy. Many movies, slides, and writing and drawing samples dramatically illustrate typical changes. The tape is a seminar presentation by Dr. Rapp. She vividly explains and demonstrates, in a systematic manner, how the viewer can develop competency in the recognition and management of a wide spectrum of unsuspected allergy related illnesses. This tape is only for educators, psychologists, or physicians who want practical, extremely comprehensive, and immensely detailed information. The quality of some of the movie and slide transfers, for technical reasons, is not always optimum. However, this tape is much more exhaustive and extensive than any other tapes presently available. It can be viewed either in small sections or in its entirety for personal instruction or for use in selected small or large conferences.

APPENDIX D

Specialists in
Environmental Medicine

Where Can Physicians Be Found Who Detect Food and Chemical Sensitivities, and Treat Environmental Illness?

Specialists who detect environmental and food sensitivities presently number about 2,600. These physicians include about 2,000 otolaryngologists, and the remaining 600 physicians include allergists, pediatricians, family practitioners, neurologists, gastroenterologists, surgeons, and psychiatrists. Of this entire group 51 percent are board-certified in one specialty, and 29 percent are board-certified in two specialties.

Most of the ear, nose, and throat allergy specialists use a method called End-Point Titration, another newer variation of allergy testing. Some combine this with provocation/neutralization to help in the detection and treatment of food sensitivities.

You can write the following to find the nearest well-trained ecologic physician. As with all medical specialists, each member practices in a somewhat individualized manner and some may be preferable to others because of your particular needs. They all, however, share one basic concept, namely they attempt to find the specific cause of each individual's particular illness and eliminate it if at all possible.

Environmental medicine or clinical ecology:
American Academy of Environmental Medicine
P.O. Box 16106
Denver, Colo. 80216

Ear Specialists (Otolaryngologists):
American Academy of Otolaryngic Allergy
Suite 302
1101 Vermont Avenue, N.W.
Washington, D.C. 20005

Various specialists who incorporate allergy in their practices:
Pan-American Allergy Society
P.O. Box 947
Fredericksburg, Tex. 78624

Additional Histories

Many parents of allergic children are truly saints in mortal form, because they have tried everything they can to make their youngsters content and happy. Their sacrifices have been above and beyond the call of parenthood in every sense of those words.

ADOPTED TODDLER
WITH MULTIPLE SENSITIVITIES,
TO ORANGE AND MILK IN PARTICULAR

Jay

Jay was only nineteen months old when his mother came to see us. He was a darling little youngster with a wide, friendly smile. He had been tried on several different milk and soy formulas prior to his adoption at the age of fourteen months. Although he seemed to feel better on a soy formula that did not contain corn, he still would never have been described as a quiet, contented toddler.

Within two weeks after adoption his mother realized he coughed and wheezed whenever he drank milk and whenever she took him shopping. Milk also caused him to have puffy eyes and dark eye circles. In time she determined that milk also caused constipation. Department stores, with their vast array of chemical odors, routinely caused him to become hyperactive and uncontrollable.

His mother tried to limit the amount of milk he drank and she avoided taking Jay shopping. By about fifteen months of age, however, he was irritable, hyperactive, and had frequent uncontrollable temper tantrums. At times he would throw himself violently onto the floor, into his sister, or against any piece of furniture that was nearby. Then he would kick and scream as hard as he could. When his mother tried to hold him, he would arch his head back and wiggle so vigorously that his mother could barely hold on to him. Later on his mother noted that milk and wheat seemed to cause his aggressive episodes.

Initially his new parents were also concerned because it was hard to rouse him from sleep. His mother even had difficulty rousing him enough so that he could be fed. Eventually his new mother noticed that this happened only after he ate turkey or drank pineapple juice. She also noticed that both soy and corn caused diarrhea. She found he developed a rash on his head and cheeks that became more severe whenever the family visited Puerto Rico. His mother said he had a "motor mouth," which is a typical complaint of allergic toddlers. He tended to rattle on and on and say very little.

When we used the newer provocation allergy testing, we clearly precipitated and reproduced his dramatic temper tantrums. These were particularly evident when we tested him for orange and dust. We documented on videotape his impressive response shortly after he drank one glass of orange juice. We vividly showed how easily we could eliminate this reaction with his neutralization dose of allergy extract for orange.

His blood RAST allergy tests for such items as dust and foods were *negative*, in spite of his remarkable reactions during single-blinded allergy testing. Except for orange juice, which routinely produced a reaction within a few minutes, most of the symptoms caused by eating allergenic foods occurred within one to two hours.

A few weeks after his treatment began, his father took Jay to the zoo. He absentmindedly gave Jay some orange juice. The child became totally uncontrollable, and his father had to rush to take his son home. Jay was promptly given his neutralization allergy extract treatment for orange, and in less than ten minutes he was back to normal.

Jay has shown slow, progressive improvement, and five years later his mother says he is 100 percent improved. When he has symptoms, his knowledgeable mother almost always knows exactly why. He presently does not have periods of unusual fatigue and rarely is overactive. If he eats an excess of either sugar or food coloring, however, he still becomes hyperactive. Orange juice is no longer a problem, but if he ingests too much milk or dairy, she knows he will wheeze. He rarely needs asthma medicines. Shopping in stores no longer creates a scene. His parents carefully monitor their home and their children's diets. The entire family feels much better because of their knowledge about how the environment and allergies can affect the activity and behavior of Jay and their other children.

AN EXTENSIVE EIGHT-YEAR HISTORY BEGINNING IN INFANCY WITH RECURRENT INFECTIONS, DROOLING, VOMITING MUCUS, AND NUMEROUS TYPICAL ALLERGIES

Laurie

Laurie came to see us when she was about three and a half years old. In spite of her tender age she had an exceedingly long medical history of illness. Other physicians had refused to see her because they found her mother was such a constant, chronic complainer. It seemed unlikely that all her previous doctors could have been wrong. I accepted Laurie as a new patient with trepidation. Was Laurie an impossibly sick child, or was her mother inordinately difficult to please?

Laurie had many allergic relatives. She was so active in the uterus that her mother complained of pain. She hiccupped and moved much more than normal. Her mother forced herself to drink two glasses of milk a day during her entire pregnancy because she was told to drink milk. She wanted to do everything she could to create a healthy baby.

After birth, when her mother tried to breast-feed Laurie and supplement that with Similac formula, Laurie seemed to be extremely cranky. Ironically she improved when she was no longer breast-fed, indicating that some food her mother had been eating, which passed into the breast milk, was probably bothering Laurie. By the time she was fifteen months old, she perspired in excess and was literally "soaked in drool." All her clothing had to be changed three times a day because she was so wet. She even needed a cloth diaper under her undershirt to help soak up the perspiration. Laurie needed a towel under her mouth when she napped to absorb the copious secretions of saliva. It was so extreme during her infant period that Laurie had a hospital evaluation to be certain she did not have a salivary gland problem. Her pediatricians said that Laurie was teething and was "too lazy to swallow." This problem continued to be extreme until she was about three and a half years old. At that time, milk was finally removed from her diet, and this eventually proved to be the major, but not the only, cause of this problem.

When we initially saw her, her mother said she had always had dark eye circles. By the time she was one and a half years old, she was wheezing and coughing whenever she laughed, played hard, or was exposed to moldy places. She had daily abdominal pain, vomiting, bloating, and routinely complained that she felt sick to her stomach. She frequently gagged and seemed to be able to vomit any time she liked. By two years of age she was wiggly, irritable, and hyperactive. At other times she was too tired to move. She had periods when she was so angry that she bit her younger brother and, one time, even the Sunday school teacher. She tended to be an unhappy child who cried easily and often.

Her dietitian mother was overwhelmed with feelings of inadequacy and depression. She had repeatedly been made to feel by the physicians and her critical relatives that her children's medical illnesses were entirely her fault. If only she were a better mother, her children would be well.

By the age of two and a half, Laurie had developed problems with her nose: She was always either stuffy or her nose ran. She sneezed often, rubbed her nose, and had one infection after another. By the time she was three and a half years old, she had headaches four to five times a week. She was a challenging behavior problem and always complained that she never felt well.

At about that time her mother called for an appointment in our office. While waiting for her first visit, Laurie was tried on the Multiple Food Elimination Diet. Within two days the child was more loving, attentive, and caring. Her behavior improved so dramatically that those closest to Laurie could not believe it. Her drooling stopped for the first time in her life; her cough diminished. Prior to the diet, Laurie had vomited across the room at least twice a day for years. By the third day on the diet this stopped. Now this happens maybe twice a year and is evident only when her allergy extract treatment needs adjustment.

When foods were added back during the second week of the Multiple Food Elimination Diet, her mother found that milk caused wheezing, fatigue, drooling, and headaches. Eggs and yellow-colored items such as Kool-Aid or yellow cough medicines or decongestants caused hyperactivity.

After P/N testing her parents treated her with an allergy extract for foods and other allergens under the tongue. Laurie was 95 percent improved within one to two weeks. Five years later, at the age of eight, she only drooled excessively when she was unavoidably exposed to certain substances to which she was sensitive. By the age of ten this was no longer evident.

She is now ten years old and remains 95 percent better. She needs selective retesting three to four times a year, mainly to prevent recurrences of her previous symptoms.

Her mother can now easily recognize and pinpoint offending foods or other substances. Often these can be removed from her diet or environment so that she remains well. For example, exposure to a Christmas tree caused immediate drooling and wheezing. Her mother removed the tree, the drooling stopped, and her asthma subsided without the need for drugs. If her sublingual mold allergy treatment needs adjustment, she will become nasal when she is in a damp place or on rainy days. After allergy retesting for molds, exposure to that same damp area will no longer cause symptoms. The secret for wellness in this child was, again, a combination of a caring and capable mother plus an ecologically sound, allergy-free home; selective food elimination; avoidance of chemicals; adequate nutrients; and P/N allergy testing and treatment. Laurie is now a beautiful, healthy child and has been well for the past seven years.

A Boy With Typical Allergies, Hyperactivity, Behavior Problems and Aggression, Who Was Repeatedly Told Not to See an Allergist

Charles

Charles had a number of allergic relatives. His entire history is typical of many children, and it shows how parents can recognize that something is wrong, suggest the right answer, and be misdirected by one well-meaning but skeptical and disbelieving physician after another.

When Charles was in the uterus, he was much more active than his sister during her fetal period. He hiccupped and he kicked so hard that he vibrated the bed when his mother tried to rest.

During the later part of his first year of life, he was much too active. He flitted from thing to thing and never seemed to be content. He was too wiggly and restless even to play with a toy.

By the age of two he was argumentative, biting, hitting, spitting, and refused to stay dressed. He had the classical red ear lobes and wiggly legs. Temper tantrums occurred whenever he was told no. By the time he was two and a half, his mother sought help because he was too difficult to control. He misbehaved so often that the family doctor suggested Ritalin. He was slightly more quiet after his initial morning dose of Ritalin, but as the day progressed, he became worse in spite of another dose at noon.

By the time Charles was four the Ritalin was stopped because a neurologist did not feel it was indicated and it really did not seem to be helping. He said the boy was not hyperactive and suggested it was a behavior problem. A pediatric psychologist counseled the parents for two months, at which time she told them that she had done all she could. Charles remained the same.

At about this time his mother saw our 1988 presentation on the *Donahue* show and recognized that her son was similar to the hyperactive children she saw. She asked her doctor again if her son could have allergies. She thought Charles seemed to have trouble handling food coloring. She was told once more there was no link between food dyes and his problems. Again, various doctors repeatedly discouraged her from evaluating the role of allergies in relation to her son's behavior in spite of his classical nose and respiratory allergies, which had begun when he was only four.

Within two weeks after Charles started kindergarten, the school behavior problems were evident. He was asked not to ride the school bus. The school had problems with his disruptive and distracting behavior in class. He was rejected by the other children because he bit them. He was still out of control, always fighting and misbehaving in school and at home.

His mother again contacted the doctor and was told to have him return to the neurologist. Once again she asked about the possibility of allergies affecting her son and the doctor shunned the idea, saying it had nothing to do with his problems. The neurologist felt that he had behavioral problems compounded with oppositional and conceptual difficulties. His parents found that discipline, punishment, rewards, and spankings were of no value. His father hated to pick him up at school because there was a daily stream of complaints about his behavior.

Then, when Charles was six years old, his mother met another mother whose child had been treated successfully for behavioral allergies. She tried our Multiple Food Elimination Diet and within eight days he was 85 percent better. His Conner's Hyperactivity Score decreased from a highly abnormal level of 28 at the beginning of the one-week Multiple Food Elimination Diet to a normal score of 8 after seven days. Cocoa, preservatives, and citrus all made him active or wild. Food coloring caused his behavior to become intolerable. After three pieces of cinnamon toast he changed from Dr. Jekyll to Mr. Hyde. This diet clearly indicated that, indeed, foods were probably a major part of her child's problems.

Three weeks after the diet she found that his activity and behavior became normal. Charles was calm, reasonable, much more responsive, and he "could sit and stand still for the first time in his entire life." His mother had tried unsuccessfully to teach him his ABCs for an entire year. After she eliminated the problem foods from his diet, he learned the alphabet within two weeks.

His mother expressed it very well when she said, "My heart breaks for my son." Everyone had always considered him to be a "bad" kid when he had simply had an unrecognized medical problem. She was tired of yelling at him. She realized he needed to be helped, for his sake as well as for hers.

His many allergic relatives and his own hay fever provided clues that Charles was an allergic child. His infant, toddler, and early-childhood history were classical for both typical and the less readily recognized forms of allergies. His rapid favorable response to an allergy diet indicated that his hyperactivity and behavior problems were to a large degree related to his food sensitivity. What a shame that so many well-trained specialists are reluctant to try a simple two-week allergy diet to help desperate mothers of hyperactive, unruly, obviously allergic youngsters.

His mother was perplexed, delighted, and angry because of her son's dramatic improvement after the first week of the diet. His improvement had been delayed for over one year because of the unreasonable discouragement of so many well-trained physicians. She repeatedly asked why they objected to a diet that might have helped when it was so simple and so effective?

ANOTHER *DONAHUE* SUCCESS: A FOOD- AND CHEMICAL-SENSITIVE FIVE-YEAR-OLD WITH EXTREME THIRST AND DROOLING

Bill

Bill was another patient whose life was changed dramatically by our *Donahue* show in 1988. His parents saw a hyperactive child who seemed similar to Bill on that show. Because the boy on that television program had been helped by the Multiple Food Elimination Diet, his parents tried their five-year-old son on the diet. His behavior was better in just one day, and by the end of the first week he had improved 80 to 90 percent. His Conner's Hyperactivity Score decreased from an abnormal high of 18 to a normal 9. His tantrums, which previously occurred at least ten times a day and lasted from fifteen to thirty minutes prior to the diet, now occurred only once every two to three weeks. He began to listen to stories and in addition he could suddenly write and draw better than ever before. His drooling decreased. When milk or dairy products were added back into his diet, he developed red cheeks, clung to his parents, and his typical temper tantrums returned.

After eight months of treatment his parents said he was 85 percent improved. He had a tantrum only once every week or two, and like the episode at the aquarium, which was due to the chlorine odor (see Chapter 18), his parents could usually determine exactly what caused each episode.

Bill's history was strikingly similar to that of many others. He was usually awake at least two to three times every night until he was treated for his allergies.

He seemed to have extreme thirst, drinking about a dozen eight-ounce bottles of soy milk a day when he was only five months old. (Excessive thirst can indicate many problems including infection, a kidney problem, diabetes, an essential fatty acid deficiency, or an allergy.) Some children who have ecologic illness seem to have an insatiable desire to drink or eat. These symptoms often subside after they respond to a comprehensive allergy treatment program if these problems are due to allergy or a chemical sensitivity.

After his adoption at five months of age Bill drank soy milk for about four months. Then he began to have periods of thrashing about and irritability. He cried easily and became a behavior problem. He would roll his head from side to side as he held his bottle in his stroller. Then he would arch his back and scream violently. By the time he was two years old, his parents noted glassy, glazed eyes, red cheeks, and red earlobes whenever he had his Dr. Jekyll/Mr. Hyde episodes. These episodes were characterized by clumsiness, irritability, high-pitched screaming, anger, whining, and saying the same phrase over and over and over. His tantrums were creating problems and concern for the entire family.

A sensitivity to cow's milk was considered when he refused to drink milk at one year of age, but he continued to crave cheese and ice cream. His provocation allergy skin test for milk caused him to drool and suddenly become very fussy and whiny. This precipitated one of his typical episodes, and we confirmed his parents' suspicion that milk was a problem.

A FOUR-YEAR-OLD TYPICALLY ALLERGIC BOY WHO "MOTHER-BATTERED" DUE TO FOOD AND CHEMICAL SENSITIVITIES

David

David was four years old when his mother brought him to see us. Her arms were covered with bruises from his repeated bites. David could be adorable and then suddenly, for no apparent reason, he would attack his mother. She had already tried the Multiple Food Elimination Diet, and he was remarkably better within one week. During the second week of the diet his mother determined that milk and wheat caused dramatic, at times unbelievable, personality changes.

Many relatives had typical allergies, and David was following his family pattern. He had hives as an infant from his soy formula. He had diarrhea from the age of one month until he was two years old. Typical nose allergies started during infancy. As he grew older, his mild year-round nose problems became much worse during the pollen seasons. He developed classical eye allergies by the age of two years. In time it was obvious that cats caused hay fever.

After milk was removed from his diet, his diarrhea decreased from four or five times a week to once every two or three weeks. The fact that it did not subside completely suggested that he was either still ingesting some form of dairy or that other foods or factors were related to this problem. Leg cramps were noted from the age of ten to sixteen months, which suggests a possible milk allergy.

By the time he was one year old, he tended to cough when he laughed, ran, or was exposed to cold air. This type of cough often precedes asthma by months or years. He had classical itchy eczema in the creases of his arm from the age of eighteen months to three years. He never slept all night until he was eighteen months old. His mother said that at one time he could not sleep for ten days.

In addition to all of this, David had bad breath, excessive drooling, temper tantrums, irritability, excessive crying, whining, and behavior and activity problems. He tended to throw or break his toys. He repeatedly hurt his mother. Many of these complaints are typical of children who have the allergic tension fatigue syndrome. Associated with his symptoms, he typically had puffy eyes, dark eye circles, and red earlobes.

Odors caused his behavior to change. David craved the smell of gasoline. His mother could not take him into one specific drugstore that had a characteristic odor because he became so "wound up."

He improved about 70 percent within a month and 100 percent after two months of our comprehensive allergy treatment program. He continued for years to be about 75 percent better except after weekend visits with his father. We suspected that the rotation diet was stopped at that time and that he was exposed to dust and molds.

After five years of treatment, his allergy extract was discontinued. Two years after his treatment was stopped, he developed asthma during the pollen season.

We wonder if this could have been avoided if his therapy had been continued. David is now thirteen years old, and his mother states that he is doing well. Bananas no longer cause symptoms. NutraSweet causes red ears and hyperactivity, so it must be avoided.[1]

When he was four year old, we attempted to document his changes in personality by taking movies of the changes that occurred when he ate specific foods. On one occasion we asked him to drink orange juice, which usually caused no difficulty, and nothing happened. Then we asked him to eat a hard-boiled egg. Within an hour he was whining, restless, hostile, aggressive, pulling, pinching, and biting. This is what his mother had noted in the past after he ate eggs. We told his mother we were giving him his allergy extract treatment for eggs, but instead gave him water. For twenty minutes he continued to bite, hit, and act inappropriately. Then we gave him his sublingual neutralization treatment for egg. Within fifteen minutes he was back to normal. Blood studies that were done before, during, and after the reaction revealed marked changes in the level of serotonin. This is a neurotransmitter that affects brain functions. Surprisingly his RAST blood test for egg was negative, so this allergy test missed his egg sensitivity. After his allergy extract treatment for egg, however, he could subsequently eat eggs without difficulty.

During the egg allergy test he whined and repeatedly stated over and over again that he wanted a banana. This made us think he was probably allergic to bananas because children often crave the foods to which they are allergic. The University of Buffalo Media Department agreed to videotape David before, during, and after he ate a banana. We hired a medical student to code two identical covered bottles. One contained his banana neutralization allergy treatment; the other contained water.

Within a half hour after he ate the banana his earlobes became bright red. Then he threw his toys around and bit his books, toys, clothing. He kicked and hit his mother. When his reaction peaked, he bit her so vigorously on the knee that she subsequently had to see a physician and receive antibiotics.

The medical student flipped a coin and David was given drops from one covered bottle labeled *H* (for heads). He continued to hit and throw his toys for the next twenty minutes. Then three drops from the *T* (for tails) bottle were placed under his tongue. He stopped whining five minutes later. In ten minutes he was able to sit on the floor and construct a toy. In eleven minutes he could write his name. When the code was broken on the videotape, the *T* drops continued his neutralization treatment for banana.

On one other occasion we taped what happened to David when he was allergy-tested for the type of preservatives found in many prepackaged foods. His response was typical. First his ears became red, then he whined, and finally he became very angry. He pinched and twisted the flesh of his mother's arm so hard that she had a three-inch black-and-blue mark. As she cried, she hugged her son. She knew he was reacting to the provocation allergy skin test. After

---

1. Dennis Remington and Barbara Higa, *The Bitter Truth About Artificial Sweeteners*. 1986. Vitality House International, 3707 N. Canyon Road, #8C, Provo, Utah 84604.

appropriate allergy treatment he said he was sorry and became his normal lovable self again.

This child was said not to have any allergies when he was evaluated by a highly respected traditional board-certified pediatric allergy professor. His blood showed evidence of ragweed allergy, but the RAST food blood tests did not reveal any sensitivities. In spite of this doctor's diagnosis he had a combination of both typical allergy and the less readily recognized types of allergy. These were also evident in his relatives. We could produce and eliminate his behavior changes during single- and double-blinded allergy testing. We showed that a few immunological blood changes did occur when we tested him for certain allergenic foods. When he adhered to the recommendations of our allergy treatment program, he was remarkably improved.

A Nine-Year-Old Child With Headaches and Extreme Fatigue Along With Typical Allergic Symptoms

Roger

Roger was nine years old when we initially saw him. His mother came to see us because he was chronically tired and complained about headaches. During infancy his mother was concerned because he drooled so much that he constantly had to wear a bib. He perspired much more than she thought was normal. One of her major concerns, even during infancy, was his extreme fatigue. He always seemed to be too tired. He slept more often than most infants and for longer periods of time. He was eight years old before his mother found out why. She did our Multiple Food Elimination Diet at that time and found out that milk caused his lethargy.

As a toddler he had had intensely puffy eyes and dark pink eye circles. When he was two years old, he would suddenly become so tired that his face would fall onto his dinner plate. At times, as he grew older, he would have trouble sitting still and he had perplexing periods of prolonged crying, irritability, and negativity.

When he was three years old, he began to have many abdominal complaints, and by the time he was six years old, the diagnosis of nonspecific colitis was made. A few months later his bowel problems subsided completely. His mother had ascertained that his terrible abdominal cramps and diarrhea occurred only when he ate sugar-free gum or candy that contained sorbitol, a form of corn. His abdomen was very distended and large until his mother determined which foods bothered him. By limiting the amount he ate of problem foods and treating him for his food allergies, his abdomen became flat.

By the age of about four he had recurrent ear and sinus infections. He developed an allergic cough and asthma by the time he was seven years old.

He was evaluated by a board-certified allergist when he was eight years old. His mother was told that his allergy tests were only slightly positive for dust and feathers. She was given a sheet of paper to explain how to make his bedroom and their home more allergy-free. She was told that he did not need to return unless he became worse. His cough, asthma, and ear problems subsided after his mother followed the recommended changes in their home to control his allergies. He definitely improved after his feather pillow was removed and he slept in a different bedroom.

At the age of nine his most serious complaint was excruciating headaches. At the time his brow was furrowed in pain, and he looked very uncomfortable and sickly. He had very pink eye circles. His headaches were so severe that his pediatrician ordered a brain scan. This showed no sign of a tumor. The headaches had been occurring every single day for months.

When his mother tried our Multiple Food Elimination Diet, he improved dramatically within one week. His daily headaches stopped for the first time in four months. His eye circles were less intense. During the second week of the diet his mother found that wheat, milk, and sugar seemed to cause him to become very tired. Corn and chocolate brought on his headache, and food coloring caused him to become stubborn and cranky.

Many of his dietary responses were confirmed during provocation/neutralization testing. Within six weeks after treatment he was 80 percent better, and during the past four years he has remained 90 to 100 percent better. Occasionally he has had a brief relapse, but after retesting he quickly improves again. His mother can usually detect the exact causes of any symptoms that arise.

This child had many classical symptoms of typical allergy plus the allergic tension fatigue syndrome for years. The evidence suggesting allergy dated back to his infancy. His dust- and feather-related symptoms improved quickly and dramatically after his mother merely changed his bedroom as suggested by the traditional allergist. His severe food allergies, however, were not detected for another year until he tried our simple two-week diet. His repeated psychiatric evaluations and counseling did not resolve his constant medical complaints or his behavior problems. Through the years he had been seen by many physicians. Their extensive repeated medical examinations, blood tests, and X rays did not reveal the cause of his illness. Much of his recurrent illness and heartache could have been prevented by a simple two-week diet and the suspicion and realization that food allergies might have been part of his problem.

AN UNHAPPY SUICIDAL CHILD HELPED BY A TWO-WEEK DIET

Bryan

We saw Bryan for the first time when he was six years old. He was a really nice little boy who had been adopted at nineteen months. Bryan had a truly infectious, lovely smile and some special quality that made all our office staff want to hug him.

Bryan could not drink milk as an infant, so he had been given Kool-Aid. We have noted that children who are given colored, dyed beverages to replace milk in infancy tend to have behavior and activity problems later on. They often develop a sensitivity, particularly to red dyes and sugar.

Bryan also had the usual history of stuffiness, nose rubbing, throat clearing, and hives. He coughed and wheezed when he ran. Frequently he had abdominal pain, nausea, belly gas, bowel problems, and bad breath. His temper tantrums often lasted two hours, and his extreme violence distressed everyone in his family. For example, if he was upset, he would urinate all over his bedroom. During these episodes he had very dark eye circles, puffiness below his eyes, red cheeks, and a spacey look.

His major problems, however, were that he was extremely unhappy. He simply never smiled. At the age of five and a half he had never slept through a night. He was so depressed that he showed me exactly where he wanted to put his friend's knife into his chest. His mother showed us a number of holiday photographs in which he appeared most unhappy, in contrast to her other children. His mother called him Bryan the Grouch because he was always so sad every morning when he arose. He had periods when he would not allow anyone to touch or hold him. Ritalin and other similar drugs did not make him feel better. When we tested him in our office for pineapple, he became untouchable. After we found his neutralization treatment dose for pineapple, he crawled onto his mother's lap and seemed to enjoy her loving hug.

When Bryan was five years old, he was seen by a well-trained traditional pediatric allergist, and the family was told that he was not allergic. The routine allergy blood (RAST) and skin tests failed to reveal that allergies might be the cause of his many medical and behavior problems.

In spite of this diagnosis his mother tried the Multiple Food Elimination Diet. Within one week she said he was 75 percent improved. His mother said that he had never smiled in his entire life until he had been placed on the diet. His bed-wetting stopped, as did his headaches. He slept all night for the first time and amazingly was happy when he arose in the morning. His temper tantrums and abdominal complaints were less frequent and severe. He no longer cried hour after hour. His headaches decreased from three times a week to once every few months.

During the second week she determined that milk caused hives, eggs caused nasal congestion, wheat caused irritability, and sugar caused him to become hyperactive and to wet the bed.

He responded so well to our allergy program that the psychologist who was seeing him called us to discuss his remarkable improvement.

On one occasion, shortly after we began his allergy extract treatment for foods, he acted extremely hostile, depressed, and suicidal at his own birthday party. His mother took a picture of how he was before and again a few minutes later after she gave him his food allergy extract treatment. The pictures clearly illustrated a change from a morose, despondent child to a happy, smiling boy within a few minutes.

The next year he continued to remain 75 to 95 percent improved, except if he ate the wrong food. For example, before treatment wheat caused extreme anger that lasted almost a day. After a year's treatment, if he forgot and ate a cookie, he would develop that funny look in his eyes and become angry, but it would only last about twenty minutes. On one occasion during the tree pollen season, he seemed worse when he was outside. At that time his mother found him taking knives into his bedroom. He needed to have his tree pollen extract adjusted.

Later on his mother noted that Bryan tended to be worse on rainy days. This is a frequent observation in mold-sensitive children. On one occasion the family stayed in a moldy cottage for two days. He reverted to his previous form of extreme anger and made suicidal statements again. His mold allergy treatment obviously needed adjustment, and after it was corrected, he improved again. At times he hid under his brother's bed and kept saying, "Nobody likes me." Similar to other allergic children, he had times when he tended to withdraw into dark corners and become untouchable, occasions when he was unbelievably aggressive and hostile, and periods when he was exceedingly sweet and lovable.

Bryan was certainly not perfect after treatment. However, because of his parents' increased knowledge about environmental illness, they could easily pinpoint the specific cause if his mood and behavior deteriorated. If his allergy extract did not relieve his symptoms, this indicated he needed to be retested so that his doses could be fine-tuned. After his treatment was rechecked for specific allergenic items, and appropriate changes were made in his allergy treatment, he quickly changed again into a lovely child. He routinely and repeatedly improved within a day or two after selective food, mold, or pollen allergy retests.

About fourteen months later Bryan stopped therapy. His parents had tried so very hard to help him, but they felt that everyone continued to blame them for Bryan's problems. They were even accused of being "overeducated" whenever they tried to explain why Bryan would change from an "angel" to a "devil" in minutes. The pressure, worry, and financial strain because the insurance company balked at payments simply became too much. Without emotional and financial support, few people could manage well under such pressure. The social workers urged that his parents stop all his allergy treatment. Within two months he regressed to the way he had been prior to his treatment. At one point he tried to set the living room carpet on fire. His parents were fearful for their other children and their home. They regretfully returned him to the adoption agency at the age of ten. In spite of all we could do, and movies that clearly demonstrated how Bryan's total personality could change during allergy testing, the agency decided not to continue his allergy treatment. They did not believe allergies were part of his problem. They stopped his diet and all his allergy treatment.

There is no doubt that this child's problems were more complicated than simple allergy and chemical sensitivities, but psychotherapy, counseling, and activity-altering drugs had been tried repeatedly and unsuccessfully prior to the time we initially saw him. Although he flared up with accidental or purposeful allergenic contacts and exposures, he was really much improved for long periods of time whenever he received comprehensive allergy and ecologic treatment. We must wonder how this exceptional child would be today if the powers who decided the course of his life had simply allowed his individualized allergy extract treatment to be updated every few months.

Was It a Lactase Problem or a Milk Allergy or Both?

Linda's Past Medical History

Some children can have an inability to digest milk sugar, or have a lactase deficiency, combined with a milk allergy or intolerance. Linda's initial milk-related symptoms were solely related to a lactose intolerance, but later on she developed additional symptoms that were typical of a milk allergy.

Linda's Early History

Linda had classical hay fever by the time she initially saw us when she was six years old. Her family had many allergic relatives. Her mother noted that Linda hiccupped excessively when she was in the womb. After she was born, she cried "constantly and intensely for up to sixteen hours per day." She had one formula change after another because of prolonged colic and diarrhea. She also seemed to have one infection after another. Typical of allergic infants, her buttocks appeared to be scalded, she drooled more than normal, and she had eczema. At eighteen months of age her concerned mother took her to see a pediatric gastrointestinal specialist who assured her that Linda did not have food allergies. The doctor did a biopsy of her bowel and definitely proved she was unable to digest milk sugar. Within six weeks after discontinuing all forms of milk sugar in milk or dairy products, her nausea, abdominal pain, bloating, excessive gas, rectal bleeding, and diarrhea all stopped. These complaints are typical of a lactase deficiency. (See Chapters 3 and 27.)

Total avoidance of all dairy products, however, would also have been effective if she had a lactose intolerance combined with a milk allergy. Why did her eczema also subside when milk and dairy products were no longer ingested? Her intestinal discomfort was obviously due to a lactase problem. Eczema, however, is not typically associated with an inability to digest milk sugar. Atopic dermatitis is usually considered to be due to an allergy. Skeptics, however, would say she "outgrew her eczema," and that is also a possibility.

At the age of three and a half years, dairy products were resumed in her diet again. Over the next few weeks her mother noted that Linda would suddenly change from pleasant to argumentative and negative. After the ingestion of milk or dairy products, Linda seemed to have leg aches, bad breath, diarrhea, head-aches, and nausea. This combination of symptoms strongly suggested that she had a milk allergy in addition to her former inability to digest milk sugar.

At the age of thirteen, after six years of milk allergy extract treatment, she still cannot tolerate a full cup of any form of dairy without developing intestinal complaints, such as cramps, bad breath, diarrhea, and a headache. As might be expected, she apparently continues to have an inability to digest milk sugar and although it's easier for her if she drinks lactase-treated milk, she still has to limit her intake of dairy products because of her associated milk allergy.

She did not sleep all night until she was placed on the Multiple Food Elimination Diet at the age of five and a half. During the second week of the diet, when foods were added back, her mother found that milk and sugar caused abdominal pain and within about twelve to twenty-four hours Linda would have a trace of rectal bleeding. Beef also caused abdominal cramps and made her crabby. (Once again, the milk and beef sensitivities seem to occur together.) Peanuts caused Linda to rush to the bathroom so that she would not wet her underpants. Later on her mother found out that rice caused Linda to become uncooperative, irritable, and nasty within ten minutes. When she had provocation allergy testing for rice, she retreated to a distant corner of our office hall. After her treatment dose for rice she was friendly and pleasant again.

Linda had always refused to eat eggs because she said they made her sick. After many months of allergy treatment for an egg allergy, she found she could eat them infrequently, in tiny amounts, in some cooked foods. This was helpful at times because eggs are often a hidden ingredient in many foods. Before treatment she was so sensitive to egg that she sometimes became ill from the mere odor of cooked eggs. This type of response always indicated a very strong allergy. Linda's great-grandmother had similar problems from the smell of a fried egg. It is common for the same foods to cause similar medical problems in more than one generation of some very allergic families.

Upon treatment it was found that Linda's entire family improved. Three months after they started the rotation diet, her father had fewer headaches and his dark eye circles disappeared, and her brother had less congestion and depression.

COLITIS SURGERY PREVENTED BY WHEAT-ALLERGY TREATMENT

Linda's Mother's History

Linda's mother's abdominal pain was diagnosed as colitis many years prior to the time her daughter came to see us. One day while she was in the office, she said the pain was so severe that she could stand it no longer. She had finally decided to have a colostomy. We asked what her favorite foods were, and she said bread, pasta, cake. I suggested she let us test her, and the nurse began to test her for wheat, without telling her what food she was injecting in her arm. In a few minutes I walked into the testing room, and Linda's mother was sobbing. I tried to console her and asked about her pain. She explained she was crying not because of the pain but because it was the first time in months she had no pain! The wheat neutralization dose had relieved her extreme distress. On a limited wheat diet, combined with wheat allergy extract, she avoided surgery. A few years later she ate too much wheat at Christmas and the pain recurred. She quickly decreased her wheat consumption. She no longer has colitis, and with wheat-extract treatment she can eat small amounts of wheat, every four days, without difficulty. One has to wonder how many other patients who have colitis might be helped with a simple one-week allergy-free diet.

BIBLIOGRAPHY

Books and Tapes for the Public

Many of these books are available in local bookstores or health food stores.

Pregnancy

Elkington, John. *The Poisoned Womb*. New York: Viking Penguin, Inc., 1987.

Maclennan, John. *Common Sense for the Sensitive*. 1981. Human Ecology Foundation of Canada, 465 Highway 8, Dundas, Ontario, Canada L9H 4V9.

McNicol, Jane. *Baby Beware!!* 1988. Alberta Children's Hospital, 1820 Richmond Rd. S.W., Calgary, Alberta, Canada T2T 5C7.

Rapp, Doris J., M.D. *Infant Food Allergies* (Audiocassette tape). 1989. Practical Allergy Research Foundation (PARF), P.O. Box 60, Buffalo, N.Y. 14223-0060.

Rapp, Doris J., M.D. *Screaming Infants, Desperate Mothers*. due 1991. Practical Allergy Research Foundation (PARF), P.O. Box 60, Buffalo, N.Y. 14223-0060.

Wunderlich, Ray C., Jr., M.D. *Help for New Parents and Parents-to-Be*. 1989. Published by Ray C. Wunderlich, Jr., M.D. 666 Sixth Street South, St. Petersburg, Fla. 33701-4845.

Household Information

Becker, Robert. *Cross Currents*. Los Angeles: Jeremy P. Tarcher, Inc., 1990.

Dadd, Debra L. *Earthwise Consumer Newsletter*. P.O. Box 279, Forest Knolls, Los Angeles, Calif. 94933.

———. *The Nontoxic Home*. 1986. P.O. Box 279, Forest Knolls, Los Angeles, Calif. 94933.

———. *Nontoxic, Natural and Earthwise*. 1990. P.O. Box 279, Forest Knolls, Los Angeles, Calif. 94933.

Golos, Natalie, and Frances Golbitz. *Coping With Your Allergies*. New York: Simon & Schuster, Inc., 1986.

Good, Clint, and Debra L. Dadd. *Healthful Houses—How to Design and Build Your Own*. 1980. Guaranty Press, 4720 Montgomery Lane, Suite 1010, Bethesda, Md. 20814.

Lewith, George, and Julian Kenyon. *Clinical Ecology: Therapeutic Approach to Understanding Food and Chemical Sensitivities*. 1985. Thorson Publishers Ltd., Wellingborough, Northamptonshire, England.

McGee, Charles T. *How to Survive Modern Technology*. 1979. Keats Publishing, Box 876, 27 Pine Street, New Canaan, Conn. 06840.

Mansfield, Peter, and Jean Munro. *Chemical Children*. 1987. Century Publishing, Brookmount House, 62-65 Chandos Place, Covent Garden, London, England.

Pfeiffer, Guy O., and Casimer M. Nikel. *The Household Environment and Chronic Illness*. 1980. Charles C. Thomas, 2600 South First Street, Springfield, Ill. 62794.

Rapp, Doris J., M.D. *Allergies and Your Family*. 1980. Practical Allergy Research Foundation (PARF), P.O. Box 60, Buffalo, N.Y. 14223–0060.

Rea, William, M.D. *Chemical Sensitivity*. 1991. Lewis Publishers, Inc., 121 S. Main, Chelsea, Mich. 48118.

Rogers, Sherry. *Tired or Toxic?* 1990. Box 3161, 3502 Brewerton Road, Syracuse, N.Y. 13220.

Rousseau, David, William J. Rea, and Jean Enwright. *Your Home Your Health and Well-Being*. 1989. Hartley & Marks, 3663 W. Broadway, Vancouver, B.C., Canada V6R 2B8.

Saifer, Phyllis and Merla Zellerbach. *Detox*. New York: Ballantine Books, 1986.

Small, Bruce. *The Susceptibility Report: Chemical Susceptibility and Urea Formaldehyde Foam Insulation*. 1982. Small and Associates Publishers, R.R. #1, Goodwood, Ontario, Canada LOC 1A0.

Travis, Nick and Ruth Hollady. *The Body Wrecker*. 1981. Don Quixote Publishing Co., P.O. Box 9442, Amarillo, Tex. 79105.

Zamm, Alfred V., and Robert Gannon. *Why Your House May Endanger Your Health*. New York: Simon & Schuster, 1980. Touchstone Books, 1982.

Diet

Buchholtz, Ilene, Karen Cook, and Theron Randolph. *An Alternative Measure*. 1984. Human Ecology Research Foundation, The Holmstad 1103-F, Fabyan Parkway, Rt. 31, Batavia, Ill. 60510.

Dong, Collin, and Jane Bank. 1988. *The Arthritic's Cookbook*. New York: Bantam Books, 1973.

Erasmus, Udo. *Fats and Oils*. 1989. Alive Books, P.O. Box 80055, Burnaby B.C., Canada V5H 3X5.

Galland, Leo, and Diane Buchman. *Superimmunity for Kids*. New York: E. P. Dutton, 1989.

Gerrard, John. *Food Allergy: New Perspectives*. 1980. Charles C. Thomas, 2600 First Street, Springfield, Ill. 62794-9265.

Golos, Natalie. *If This Is Tuesday, It Must Be Chicken*. 1983. Keats Publishing, 27 Pine Street, New Canaan, Conn. 06840.

Miller, Ann. *Who Needs Wheat?! A Guide for Successful Wheat-Free Baking*. 1990. *Organic Annie's Booklet Series*. Organic Annie's Wholefoods, P.O. Box 751, Baldwinsville, N.Y. 13027.

Mott, Lawrie, and Karen Snyder. *Pesticide Alert. A Guide to Pesticides in Fruits and Vegetables*. 1987. Sierra Club Books, 730 Polk Street, San Francisco, Calif. 94109.

Moyer, Judy. *Cooking for the Allergic Child*. Collegiate Pride Inc., 1987. Publishing Division, State College, Pa. 16801.

Oski, Frank A. *Don't Drink Your Milk*. 1983. Mollica Press, Ltd., 1914 Teall Avenue, Syracuse, N.Y. 13206.

Powell, Donna. *Why 5? A Complete Food Allergy Guidebook*. 1989. Donna Powell, Box 25, Waterdown, Ontario, Canada LOR 2HO.

Rapp, Doris J., M.D. *Rotary and Other Allergy Diets Made Easy for Children*. 1991. Practical Allergy Research Foundation (PARF), P.O. Box 60, Buffalo, N.Y. 14223-0060.

Remington, Dennis W., and Barbara W. Higa. *Back to Health*. 1986. Vitality House International, 3707 N. Canyon Road #8C, Provo, Utah 84604.

———. *The Bitter Truth About Artificial Sweeteners*. 1986. Vitality House International, 3707 N. Canyon Road #8C, Provo, Utah 84604.

Robertson, Laurel. *Laurel's Kitchen Bread Book*. New York: Random House, 1984.

Rockwell, Sally. *The Rotation Game*. 1981. S. J. Rockwell, P.O. Box 31065, Seattle, Wash. 98103.

Sahley, Billie J. *The Natural Way to Control Hyperactivity With Amino Acids and Nutrient Therapy*. 1989. The Watercress Press, 5282 Medical Drive, Suite 160, San Antonio, Tex. 78229-6043.

Sahley, Billie J., and K. M. Birkner. *Breaking Your Addiction Habit*. 1990. Pain & Stress Therapy Publication, 5282 Medical Drive, Suite 160, San Antonio, Tex. 78229-6043.

Schauss, Alexander, and Caroline Costin. *Zinc and Eating Disorders*. 1989. Keats Publishing, 27 Pine Street, New Canaan, Conn. 06840.

General

Ashford, Nicholas, Ph.D., and Claudia Miller, M.D. *Chemical Sensitivity: A Report to the New Jersey Department of Health*. 1989. New Jersey Department of Health, John Fitch Plaza, CN 360, Trenton, N.J. 08625.

Barkie, Karen. *Sweet and Sugarfree: An All-Natural Fruit-Sweetened Dessert Cookbook*. New York: St. Martin's Press, 1982.

Beasley, Joseph, M.D. *How to Defeat Alcoholism*. New York: Times Books, a division of Random House, Inc., 1989.

Beasley, Joseph, and Jerry Swift. *The Kellogg Report*. 1989. The Institute of Health Policy Practice, The Bard College Center, Annandale-on-Hudson, N.Y., 12504. For a copy of publication write, 221 Broadway, Suite 301, Amityville, N.Y. 11701.

Bell, Iris. *Clinical Ecology*. 1982. Commonwealth Research Institute, P.O. Box 3168, Bolinas, Calif. 94924.

Brostoff, Jonathan and Linda Gamlin. *Food Allergy and Intolerance*. 1989. Bloomsbury Publishing Limited, 2 Soho Square, London, England W1V 5DE.

Coca, Arthur. *The Pulse Test*. 1956. Lyle Stuart, 225 Lafayette Square, New York, N.Y. 10012.

Coles, Gerald. *The Learning Mystique*. New York: Pantheon Books, a division of Random House, 1987.

Condrell, K. *How to Raise a Brat*. 1985. Loiry/Bonner Press, 226 W. Pensacola St., Suite 301, Tallahassee, Fla. 32301.

Gaby, Alan, M.D. *B-Six: The Natural Healer*. 1987. Keats Publishing, 27 Pine Street, New Canaan, Conn., 06840.

Grant, Ellen. *The Bitter Pill*. 1985. Practical Allergy Research Foundation (PARF), P.O. Box 60, Buffalo, N.Y. 14223-0060.

Harkavy, Joseph. *Vascular Allergy and Its Systemic Manifestations*. 1963. Butterworth's, 7235 Wisconsin Avenue, Washington, D.C.

Higa, Barbara R. D. 1989. *Desserts to Lower Your Fat Thermostat*. Vitality House International, Inc., 3707 North Canyon Road, Provo, Utah 84604.

Hoffer, Abram, M.D., Ph.D. 1989. *Orthomolecular Medicine for Physicians*. Keats Publishing, 27 Pine Street, New Canaan, Conn. 06840.

Hubbard, L. Ron. *Clear Body, Clear Mind*. 1990. Bridge Publications, Inc., 4751 Fountain Avenue, Los Angeles, Calif. 90029.

Kingsley, Patrick. *Conquering Cystitis*. 1987. Ebury Press, Broadwick Street, London, England W1V 1FR, 27–37.

Mandell, Marshall. *Dr. Mandell's 5-Day Allergy Relief System*. New York: Pocket Books, 1981.

———. *Dr. Mandell's Lifetime Arthritis Relief System*. New York: Coward-McCann, 1983.

———. *It's Not Your Fault You're Fat Diet*. New York: Harper & Row, 1983.

Pauling, Linus. *How to Live Longer and Feel Better*. New York: Avon Books, 1986.

Randolph, Theron and Ralph Moss. *An Alternative Approach to Allergies*. New York: Harper & Row, 1989.

Rapp, Doris J., M.D. *Allergies and the Hyperactive Child*. 1980. Practical Allergy Research Foundation (PARF), P.O. Box 60, Buffalo, N.Y. 14223-0060.

———. *Allergies and Your Family*. 1980. Practical Allergy Research Foundation (PARF), P.O. Box 60, Buffalo, N.Y. 14223–0060.

———. *The Impossible Child*. 1989. (Available in English and Spanish.) Practical Allergy Research Foundation (PARF), P.O. Box 60, Buffalo, N.Y. 14223-0060.

———. *Recognize and Manage Your Allergies*. 1987. Practical Allergy Research Foundation (PARF), P.O. Box 60, Buffalo, N.Y. 14223-0060.

Wilkenfeld, Irene. *How Environmentally Safe Are Our Schools?* 1990. Heal of Michiana, 52145 Farmington Square Road, Granger, Ind. 46530.

Wright, Jonathan, M.D. *Dr. Wright's Guide to Healing with Nutrition*. Emmaus, Pa.: Rodale Press, 1984.

Legal Aspects of Environmental Medicine

Ecological Illness Law Report. P.O. Box 6099, Wilmette, Ill. 60091.

Delinquency

Reed, Barbara. *Food, Teens and Behavior*. 1983. Natural Press, P.O. Box 2107, Manitowoc, Wis. 54220.

Schauss, Alexander. *Diet, Crime and Deliquency*. Berkeley, Calif.: Parker House, 1981.

Candida

Connolly, Pat. *The Candida Albicans Yeast-Free Cookbook*. 1985. Keats Publishing, 27 Pine Street, New Canaan, Conn. 06840.

Crook, William. *The Yeast Connection*. 1989. Professional Books Inc., P.O. Box 3494, 681 Skyline Drive, Jackson, Tenn. 38301.

Lorenzani, Shirley. *Candida: a Twentieth Century Disease*. 1986. Keats Publishing, 27 Pine Street, P.O. Box 876, New Canaan, Conn. 06840.

Remington, Dennis and Barbara Higa. *Back to Health*. 1986. Vitality House International, 3707 N. Canyon Road #8C, Provo, Utah 84604.

Rockwell, Sally. *Coping With Candida Cookbook*. 1984. P.O. Box 15181, Seattle, Wash. 98115.

Trowbridge, John P., and Walker Morton, *The Yeast Syndrome*. New York: Bantam Books, 1986.

Truss, C. Orian, M.D. *The Missing Diagnosis*. 1985. The Missing Diagnosis. Inc., P.O. Box 26508, Birmingham, Ala. 35226.

Wunderlich, Ray, Jr., and Dwight Kalita. *Candida Albicans*. 1984. Keats Publishing, 27 Pine Street, New Canaan, Conn. 06840.

Hypoglycemia and Diabetes

Fredericks, Carlton, Ph.D. *New Low Blood Sugar and You*. New York: Putnam, 1985.

Philpott, William, and Dwight Kalita. *Brain Allergies: The Psychonutrient Connection*. 1980. Keats Publishing, 27 Pine Street, New Canaan, Conn. 06840.

———. *Victory Over Diabetes*. 1983. Keats Publishing, 27 Pine Street, New Canaan, Conn. 06840.

For Psychologists, Educators, and Physicians

Bahna, Sami, and Douglas Heiner. *Allergies to Milk*. 1980. Gene and Stratton, Inc., 111 Fifth Street, New York, N.Y. 10003.

Brostoff, Jonathan, and Stephen Challacombe. *Food Allergy and Intolerance*. 1987. Bailliere Tindall Publisher, 33 The Avenue Eastbourne, East Sussex, England BN21–3UN.

Department of Consumer Affairs. *Clean Your Room. A Compendium on Outdoor Pollution*. 1982. Department of Consumer Affairs, P.O. Box 310, 1020 North Street, Sacramento, Calif. 95802.

Department of Consumer Affairs. *Clean Your Room. A Compendium on Outdoor Pollution.* 1982. Department of Consumer Affairs, P.O. Box 310, 1020 North Street, Sacramento, Calif. 95802.

Freed, D. L. J., *Health Hazards of Milk.* Philadelphia, Pa.: W. B. Saunders, 1984.

Hoffer, Abram. *Orthomolecular Medicine for Physicians.* 1989. Keats Publishing, 27 Pine Street, New Canaan, Conn. 06840.

Lee, Carleton. *Allergy Neutralization.* 1987. Tri Sigma Press, Box 5098, St. Joseph, Mo. 64505.

Miller, Joseph. *Food Allergy: Provocative Testing and Injection Therapy.* Springfield, Ill.: Charles C. Thomas Publishing, 1972.

——. *Relief at Last.* Springfield, Ill.: Charles C. Thomas Publishing, 1987.

O'Banion, Daniel *The Ecologic and Nutritional Treatment of Health Disorders.* Springfield, Ill.: Charles C. Thomas Publishing, 1981.

——. *The Ecology and Nutritional Approach to Behavioral Medicine.* Springfield, Ill.: Charles C. Thomas Publishing, 1981.

Randolph, Theron. *Human Ecology and Susceptibility to the Chemical Environment.* Springfield, Ill.: Charles C. Thomas Publishing, 1962.

Rinkle, Herbert J., Theron G. Randolph, and M. Zeller. *Food Allergy.* Springfield, Ill.: Charles C. Thomas Publishing, 1951.

Rowe, Albert H., M.D. *Food Allergy, Its Manifestations, Diagnosis, and Treatment with a General Discussion of Bronchial Asthma.* Springfield, Ill.: Charles C. Thomas Publishing, 1972.

Articles for Physicians

Asthma

Soothill, J. F., and J. O. Warner. "Control Trial of Hyposensitization to Dermatophagoides Pteronyssinus in Children With Asthma." *Lancet* 9 (1978): 912–915.

Autism

O'Banion, Daniel B., B. Armstrong, et al. "Disruptive Behavior: A Dietary Approach." *Journal of Autism and Childhood Schizophrenia* 8 (1978): 325–337.

Arthritis

Darlington, L., and J. Mansfield. "Food Allergy and Rheumatoid Disease." *Annals of the Rheumatoid Diseases* 42 (1983):218.

Kroker, G. F. "Fasting and Rheumatoid Arthritis: A Multicenter Study." *Clinical Ecology* 2 (1984): 137–144.

Marshall, R. M., Robert M. Stroud, and G. F. Kroker. "Food Challenge Effects on Fasted Rheumatoid Arthritis Patients: A Multicenter Study." *Clinical Ecology* 2 (1984): 181–190.

Parke, A. L., and G. R. V. Hughes. "Rheumatoid Arthritis and Food: A Case Study." *British Medical Journal* 282 (1981): 2027–2029.

Ratner, D., E. Eshel, and K. Vigder. "Juvenile Rheumatoid Arthritis and Milk Allergy." *Journal of the Royal Society of Medicine* 78 (1985): 410–413.

Vaughan, William T., "Palindromic Rheumatism Among Allergic Persons." *Journal of Allergy* 14 (1943): 256–263.

Zeller, M., "Rheumatoid Arthritis: Food Allergy as a Factor." *Annals of Allergy* 7 (1949): 200–239.

Colitis

Soothill, J. F., et al. "Food Allergy: The Major Cause of Infantile Colitis." *Archives of Diseases in Children* 58 (1983):653.

Chemicals and Pollution

Dowty, Betty J., John L. Laseter, and James Storer. "The Transplacental Migration and Accumulation in Blood of Volatile Organic Constituents." *Pediatrics* 10 (1976): 696–701.

Lieberman, Allan, Patricia Hardman, and Patricia Preston. "Academic, Behavioral, and Perceptual Reactions in Dyslexic Children When Exposed to Environmental Factors—Malathion and Petrochemical Ethanol." 1981. Dyslexia Research Institute, Inc., 4745 Centerville Road, Tallahassee, Fla. 32308.

Rapp, Doris, J., M.D. "Double-blind Case Report of Chronic Headache Due to Foods and Air Pollution." Abstract 13. *Annals of Allergy* 40 (1978): 289.

Rea, William J. et al. "Food and Chemical Susceptibility After Environmental Chemical Overexposure: Case Histories." *Annals of Allergy* 41 (1978): 101–110.

———. "Pesticides and Brain Function Changes in a Controlled Environment." *Clinical Ecology* 2 (1984): 145–149.

———. "Toxic Volatile Organic Hydrocarbons in Chemically Sensitive Patients." *Clinical Ecology* 2 (1987): 70.

Rogers, Sherry. "Diagnosing the Tight Building Syndrome or Diagnosing Chemical Hypersensitivity." *Environmental International* 15 (1989): 75–79.

Root, David, M.D., et al. "Excretion of a Lipophilic Toxicant Through the Sebaceous Gland: A Case Report." *Journal of Toxicology* 6(1) (1987): 13–17.

Depression

Randolph, Theron. "Allergic Factors in the Etiology of Certain Mental Symptoms." *Journal of Laboratory & Clinical Medicine* 36: (1950): 977.

———. "Depression Caused by Home Exposures to Gas and Combustion Products of Gas, Oil, and Coal." *Journal of Laboratory & Clinical Medicine* 46 (1955): 942.

———. "Ecologic Mental Illness—Psychiatry Exteriorized." *Journal of Laboratory & Clinical Medicine* 54 (1959): 936.

———. "An experimentally induced acute psychotic episode following the intubation of an allergic food." 7th Annual Congress, American College of Allergists, Chicago, Ill. February 1951.

Diet

Atherton, D., et al. "A Double-Blind Controlled Trial of an Antigen Avoidance Diet in Atopic Eczema." *Lancet* 1(1978): 401–403.

Goldman, J., et al. "Behavioral Effects of Sucrose on Preschool Children." *Journal of Abnormal Psychology* 14 (4) (1986): 565–577.

Levy, F., et al. "Hyperkinesis and Diet: A Double-Blind Crossover Trial With a Tartrazene Chellenge." *The Medical Journal of Australia* 1 (1978): 61–64.

Prinz, R., et al. "Dietary Correlates of Hyperactive Behavior in Children." *Journal of Consulting and Clinical Psychology* 48 (1980): 760–769.

Rapp, Doris J., M.D. "A Prototype for Food Sensitivity Studies in Children." (abstract) *Annals of Allergy* 47 (1981): 123–124.

Radcliffe, M., et al. "Food Allergy in Polysymptomatic Patients." *The Practitioner* 225 (1981): 1651–1654.

Rowe, K. "Synthetic Food Coloring and Hyperactivity: A Double-Blind Crossover Study." *Australian Pediatrics* 24 (1988): 143–147.

Shaywitz, B., et al. "Effects of Chronic Administration of Food Coloring on Activity Levels and Cognitive Performance in Normal and Hyperactive Developing Rat Pups." *Annals of Neurology* 4 (1978): 196.

Swanson, J. "Food Dyes Impair Performance of Hyperactive Children on a Laboratory Learning Test." *Science* 207 (1980): 1485–1487.

Tryphonas, H., et al. "Food Allergy in Children with Hyperactivity, Learning Disabilities and/or Minimal Brain Dysfunction." *Annals of Allergy* 42 (1979): 22–27.

Weiss, B., "Behavior Responses to Artificial Food Colors." *Science* 207 (1980): 1487–1489.

Williams., J., et al. "Relative Effects of Drugs and Diet on Hyperactive Behaviors: An Experimental Study." *Pediatrics* 61 (1978): 811–817.

Epilepsy

Crayton, John W. "Epilepsy Precipitated by Food Sensitivity: Report of a Case With Double-Blind Placebo-Controlled Assessment." *Clinical Electroencephalography* 12 (1981): 192.

Davidson, Hal. "Allergy and the Nervous System." *Quarterly Review of Allergy and Applied Immunology* 6 (1952): 157.

Egger, Joseph, M.D. et al. "Oligoantigenic Diet Treatment of Children With Epilepsy and Migraine." *Journal of Pediatrics* 114 (1) (1989): 51–58.

General

Boris, Marvin, M.D., et al. 1985. "Antigen-Induced Asthma Attenuated by Neutralization Therapy." *Clinical Ecology* 3 (1985):59–62.

Brostoff, John, M.D., et al., "Low-Dose Sublingual Therapy in Patients with Allergic Rhinitis Due to House Dust Mite." *Clinical Ecology* 16 (1986): 483–491.

Campbell, M. Brent. "Neurologic Manifestations of Allergic Disease." *Annals of Allergy* 31 (1973):485–498.

Crayton, John. "Anti-Candida Antibody Levels in Polysymptomatic Patients." Presented at The Candida Update Conference, Memphis, Tenn., September 16–18, 1988.

Gerrard, John W. et al. "Double-blind Study on the Value of Low-Dose Immunotherapy in the Treatment of Asthma and Allergic Rhinitis." *Clinical Ecology* 6 (1989): 43–46.

Jewett, Don, et al. "A Double-Blind Study of Symptom Provocation to Determine Food Sensitivity." *JAMA* 323 (7) (1990): 429–433.

King, D. "Can Allergic Exposure Provoke Psychological Symptoms? A Double-Blind Test." *Biological Psychiatry* 16 (1981): 3–19.

King, D., "The Reliability and Validity of Provocative Food Testing: A Critical Review." *Medical Hypotheses* 25 (1988): 7–16.

King, William, M.D., et al. "Provocation/Neutralization: A Two-Part Study." Part I. The Intracutaneous Provocative Food Test: A Multi-

Center Comparison Study. *Otolaryngology Head Neck Surgery* 99 (1988): 263–277.

———. "Provocation/Neutralization: A Two-Part Study." Part 2. Subcutaneous Neutralization Therapy: A Multi-Center Comparison Study. *Otolaryngology Head Neck Surgery* 99 (1988): 272–277.

Lagrue, G., et al. "Food Sensitivity and Ideopathic Nephrotic Syndrome." *Lancet* 2 (1987), p. 277.

Laseter, John, Ph.D. "Monitoring of Aromatic and Chlorinated Solvents in Blood Following Inhalant Abuse in Juveniles." Presented at the National Inhalant Abuse Prevention Conference, San Antonio Tex., March 13–16, 1990.

Mandell, Marshall. "Unsuspected Allergies Play a Major Role in Tourette's Syndrome." Presented to Society for Clinical Ecology, November 1984.

Mandell, Marshall, M.D., et al. "The Role of Allergy in Arthritis, Rheumatism, and Polysymptomatic Cerebral, Visceral, and Somatic Disorders: Double-Blind Study." *Journal of International Academy of Preventative Medicine* 1982.

Moore, Patricia. "Clinical Ecology: Medicine for the Chemical-Sensitive." *Coming Clean at Home—Garbage—The Practical Journal for the Environment* (1990): pp. 30–35.

O'Shea, J., et al. "Double-Blind Study of Children With Hyperkinetic Syndrome Treated With Multi-Allergen Extract Sublingually." *Journal of Learning Disabilities* 14 (1981): 189.

Rapp, Doris J., M.D. "Double-Blind Confirmation and Treatment of Milk Sensitivity." *Medical Journal of Australia* 1 (1978): 571–572.

Rapp, Doris J., M.D. "Environmental Medicine: An Expanded Approach to Allergy." *Buffalo Physician* 2 (1986): 15–24.

Rapp, Doris J., M.D. "Food Allergy Treatment For Hyperkinesis." *Journal of Learning Disabilities* 12 (1979): 42–50.

Rapp, Doris J., M.D. "Water as a Cause of Angio-Edema and Urticaria." *JAMA* 221 (1972): 305.

Rapp, Doris J., M.D. "Weeping Eyes in Wheat Allergy." *Trans American Society of Ophthalmology and Otolaryngology* 18 (1978): 149.

Rea, William, M.D. et al. "Elimination of Oral Food Challenge Reaction by Injection of Food Extracts: A Double-Blind Evaluation." *Archives of Otolaryngology* 110 (1984): 248–252.

———. "The Environmental Aspects of the Post-Polio Syndrome." World Conference on Post-Polio, 1986.

Ross, G. "Confirmation of Chemical Sensitivity by Double-Blind Inhalant Challenge." Presented at International Conference on Food and Environmental Factors in Human Disease. Buxton, Derbyshire, England, July 3–6, 1990.

Russell, Michael, et al. "Learned Histamine Release." *Science* 23 (1984): 733–734.

Satterfield, J. "Therapeutic Interventions to Prevent Delinquency in Hyperactive Boys." *Journal of American Academy of Child and Adult Psychology* 26 (1987), pp. 56–64.

Scarnati, Richard, D. O. "An Outline of Hazardous Side Effects of Ritalin (Methylphenidate)." *The International Journal of the Addictions* 21 (7) (1986): 837–841.

Schmidt, Kenneth, Wendy Weir, and Michael Asch. "Clinical Ecology Treatment Approach for Juvenile Offenders." For copy of article, write to: Kenneth Schmidt, Box 693, Atascadero, Calif. 93422.

Shaw, H. Batty, M.D. "Hypersensitiveness: The Parallelism in the Phenomena of Hypersensitiveness and Certain Clinical Manifestations of Obscure Nature." *Lancet* 1 (1912): 713–719.

Shirakawa, S., William J. Rea, M.D., Satoshi Ishikawa, and A. Johnson. "Evaluation of the Autonomic Nervous System Response by Pupillographical Study in the Chemically Sensitive Patient." *Clinical Ecology* 7 (2) (1990).

Slutsker, Laurence, et al., "Eosinophilia-myalgia Syndrome Associated With Exposure to Tryptophan From a Single Manufacturer." *JAMA* 264 (1990): 213–217.

Walling, Anne, M.D. "Why Is Asthma Mortality Rising?" Editorial. *American Family Physician* 42 (2) (1990): 358–359.

Headaches

Egger, Joseph, M.D. et al. "Is Migraine Food Allergy? A Double-Blind Controlled Trial of Oligoantigenic Diet Treatment." *Lancet* 11 (1983): 865–869.

Hyperactivity

Coleman, Mary. "Physiology and the Neurosciences." Editorial. *Biological Psychiatry* 14 (1979): 1–2.

Egger, Joseph, M.D., et al. "Controlled Trial of Oligoantigenic Treatment in the Hyperkinetic Syndrome." *Lancet* 1 (1985): 540–545.

Hagerman, R. J., and A. R. Falkenstein. "An Association Between Recurrent Otitis Media in Infancy and Later Hyperactivity." *Clinical Pediatrics* 26 (1987): 253–257.

Kaplan, B. J., et al. "Dietary Replacement in Preschool-Aged Hyperactive Boys." *Pediatrics* 83 (1989): 7–17.

Ott, John. "Influence of Fluorescent Lights on Hyperactivity and

Learning Disabilities." *Journal of Learning Disabilities* 9 (1976): 417–422.

Rapp, Doris J., M.D. "Does Diet Affect Hyperactivity?" *Journal of Learning Disabilities* 11 (1978): 56–62.

————. Rapp, Doris J., M.D. "Hyperactivity and Food Allergy: Are They Related?" Abstract 46. *Annals of Allergy* 40 (1978): 297–298.

Nutrition and Learning

Benton, David. "Vitamin/Mineral Supplementation and Intelligence." *Lancet* 335 (1990): 1158–1160.

Benton, David, and Gwilym M. Roberts. "The Effect of Vitamin and Mineral Supplementation on Intelligence, the Sample of School Children." *Lancet* 664 (1988): 140–143.

Schoenthaler, Stephen J. "The Effect of Sugar on the Treatment and Control of Antisocial Behavior: A Double-Blind Study of an Incarcerated Juvenile Population." *International Journal of Biosocial Research* 3 (1982): 1–19.

Schoenthaler, Stephen J., et al. "The Impact of a Low Food Additive and Sucrose Diet on Academic Performance in 803 New York City Public Schools." *International Journal of Biosocial Research* 2 (1986): 185–195.

Otitis

Shambaugh, G. "Serous Otitis: Are Ear Tubes the Answer?" *American Journal of Otology* 5: (1983): 63–65.

Vascular Disease

Rea, William J. "Environmentally Triggered Small Vessels Vasculitis." *Annals of Allergy* 38 (1976): 245.

————. "Recurrent Environmentally Triggered Thrombophlebitis." *Annals of Allergy* 47 (1981): 338–344.

Rea, William J., and O. D. Brown, "Mechanisms of Environmentally Vascular Triggering." *Clinical Ecology* 3 (1985): 122–127.

Rea, William J., and C. W. Suits. "Cardiovascular Disease Triggered by Foods and Chemicals." Chapter 5 from *Food Allergy: New Perspectives,* (Gerrard, John, ed.) Springfield, Ill.: Charles C. Thomas Publishing, 1980.

Rea, William J., et al. "Environmentally Triggered Large-vessel Vasculitis." *Annals of Allergy* 38 (1977): 245–251.

Ross, Gerald, and William J. Rea. "Environmentally Triggered Hypertension. Part II. Environmental Health Center—Dallas Treatment Experience. Presented at the 8th Annual International Symposium on Man and His Environment in Health and Disease. Dallas, Tex., Feb 22–25, 1990.

Index

Accu-Chem Laboratories, 268, 277, 288, 317
acne, 106, 153, 441, 447
adaptation, 63–64, 289
ADD (attention deficit disorder), 23, 327–329, 349, 351, 352, 426
addictions, 23, 91, 136–137, 161, 166, 192, 256, 403
  to chocolate, 77–78, 256, 267
  to grains, in alcoholism, 94
  masking and, 63–64, 162, 174, 265–267, 289
  premenstrual, 152, 256
  to Ritalin, 354, 356, 497–498
  withdrawal and, 166, 174, 265, 354, 356
additives, food, 164, 226, 242, 329–330, 528, 539, 540, 557
ADHD (attention deficit hyperactivity disorder), 23, 327, 329, 344, 351, 352, 353, 372, 387
adolescent allergies, 8, 139, 142–153, 349
  adulthood and, 148–149
  allergy testing of, 147–148
  behavior problems in, 143, 145, 146, 149–152
  depression in, 142, 143, 145, 146
  emotional problems in, 143, 146, 149
  family history in, 144, 151
  fatigue in, 395–396, 397–398
  gender differences in, 152
  independent behavior and, 148, 149–152, 170, 350, 420, 422, 434–435, 496
  motherhood after, 149
  peer pressure in, 150, 170, 496
  physical complaints in, 145, 147
  premenstrual tension (PMS) and, 145, 152
  recurrent ear infections in, 144
  school problems and, 143, 145–146, 148, 151–152
  sleep problems in, 133
  sound sensitivity in, 146–147

  suicidal episodes in, 142, 146
  symptom change at puberty in, 145, 152–153
  worries about craziness in, 147, 554
  yeast infections in, 443
  see also child allergies; delinquency; infant allergies; toddler allergies
adopted children, 34
  case example of, 554–557
adrenaline, 76, 185, 460, 492
  indications for use of, 516
aerosol drugs, 513
aerosol-mist therapy, 76, 517–520
aggression, 8, 146, 327, 331–332, 363, 367–379, 381, 540
  case examples of, 367–378, 554–560
  contact sports and, 378–379
  counseling for, 124, 371–372, 375–376, 554–560
  drawing changes in, 376–378
  father battering in, 376
  mother battering in, 367–376, 384, 414–415, 416, 554–557
  self-battering in, 123
  in toddlers, 123, 125, 130–131, 134, 413
  see also delinquency
air purifiers, 236, 237, 252, 298, 497, 575
albuterol, 520
alcoholism, 68, 94
Alimentum, 107, 566
aliphatic hydrocarbons, 279, 281
alkali preparations, 23, 79, 169–172, 184
  Alka-Aid, 23, 168, 373
  Alka-Seltzer Antacid Formula, 23–24, 168, 417
  baking soda, 167, 168–170, 435
  cautions about use of, 169–170
  dosage of, 168–169
  preventive use of, 170